Rapid R

Physiology

Rapid Review Series

Series Editor
Edward F. Goljan, MD

Behavioral Science, Second Edition
Vivian M. Stevens, PhD; Susan K. Redwood, PhD; Jackie L. Neel, DO;
Richard H. Bost, PhD; Nancy W. Van Winkle, PhD; Michael H. Pollak, PhD

Biochemistry, Second Edition
John W. Pelley, PhD; Edward F. Goljan, MD

Gross and Developmental Anatomy, Second Edition
N. Anthony Moore, PhD; William A. Roy, PhD, PT

Histology and Cell Biology, Second Edition
E. Robert Burns, PhD; M. Donald Cave, PhD

Microbiology and Immunology, Second Edition
Ken S. Rosenthal, PhD; James S. Tan, MD

Neuroscience
James A. Weyhenmeyer, PhD; Eve A. Gallman, PhD

Pathology, Second Edition
Edward F. Goljan, MD

Pharmacology, Second Edition
Thomas L. Pazdernik, PhD; Laszlo Kerecsen, MD

Physiology
Thomas A. Brown, MD

USMLE Step 2
Michael W. Lawlor, MD, PhD

USMLE Step 3
David Rolston, MD; Craig Nielsen, MD

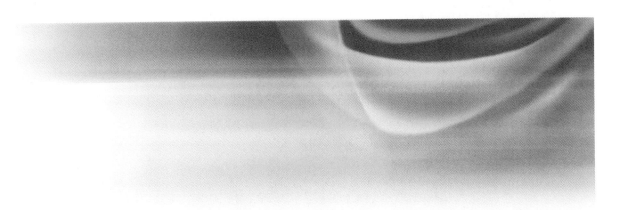

Rapid Review
Physiology

Thomas A. Brown, MD
Senior Resident, Internal Medicine
Dartmouth-Hitchcock Medical Center
Lebanon, New Hampshire

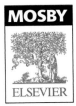

MOSBY

ELSEVIER

1600 John F. Kennedy Blvd.
Suite 1800
Philadelphia, PA 19103-2899

RAPID REVIEW PHYSIOLOGY

ISBN-10: 0-323-01991-9
ISBN-13: 978-0-323-01991-0

Copyright © 2007 by Mosby, Inc., an affiliate of Elsevier Inc.

Notice

Knowledge and best practice in this field are constantly changing. As new research and experience broaden our knowledge, changes in practice, treatment and drug therapy may become necessary or appropriate. Readers are advised to check the most current information provided (i) on procedures featured or (ii) by the manufacturer of each product to be administered, to verify the recommended dose or formula, the method and duration of administration, and contraindications. It is the responsibility of the practitioner, relying on their own experience and knowledge of the patient, to make diagnoses, to determine dosages and the best treatment for each individual patient, and to take all appropriate safety precautions. To the fullest extent of the law, neither the Publisher nor the Authors assume any liability for any injury and/or damage to persons or property arising out or related to any use of the material contained in this book.

Library of Congress Cataloging-in-Publication Data

Brown, Thomas A.
  Physiology / Thomas A. Brown.—1st ed.
    p. ; cm.—(Rapid review series)
  Includes index.
  ISBN 978-0-323-01991-0
  1. Physiology—Outlines, syllabi, etc. 2. Physiology—Examinations, questions, etc. I. Title. II. Series.
  [DNLM: 1. Physiology—Examination Questions. QT 18.2 B881p 2007]
  QP41.B86 2007
  612—dc22

                                                                    2006037539

Publishing Director: Linda Belfus
Acquisitions Editor: James Merritt
Developmental Editor: Katie DeFrancesco
Design Direction: Steven Stave

Printed in the United States of America.

Last digit is the print number: 9 8 7 6 5 4 3 2 1

Working together to grow
libraries in developing countries

www.elsevier.com | www.bookaid.org | www.sabre.org

ELSEVIER | BOOK AID International | Sabre Foundation

To Vidya and Maya, my best friends.

TAB

Contributors

TEXT

David D. Brown, DO
Resident, Department of Neurology
University of Califormia, Irvine
Irvine, California

Thomas A. Brown, MD
Resident, Internal Medicine
Dartmouth-Hitchcock Medical Center
Lebanon, New Hampshire

Courtney Cuppett, MD
Resident, Obstetrics and Gynecology
West Virginia University School of Medicine,
    Ruby Memorial Hospital
Morgantown, West Virginia

Jason B. Harris, MD, MPH
Instructor in Pediatrics, Harvard Medical School
Assistant in Pediatrics, Massachusetts General Hospital
Boston, Massachusetts

Jennie J. Hauschka, MD
Resident, Obstetrics and Gynecology
Carolinas Medical Center
Charlotte, North Carolina

Karen MacKay, MD
Associate Professor of Medicine and Nephrology
West Virginia University School of Medicine,
    Ruby Memorial Hospital
Morgantown, West Virginia

Ronald Mudry, MD
Fellow, Pulmonary and Critical Care Medicine
West Virginia University School of Medicine,
    Ruby Memorial Hospital
Morgantown, West Virginia

John Parker, MD
Chief, Section of Pulmonary and Critical Care
    Medicine
West Virginia University School of Medicine,
    Ruby Memorial Hospital
Morgantown, West Virginia

QUESTIONS

David D. Brown, DO
Resident, Department of Neurology
University of Califormia, Irvine
Irvine, California

Thomas A. Brown, MD
Resident, Internal Medicine
Dartmouth-Hitchcock Medical Center
Lebanon, New Hampshire

Courtney Cuppett, MD
Resident, Obstetrics and Gynecology
West Virginia University School of Medicine,
    Ruby Memorial Hospital
Morgantown, West Virginia

John Haughey, MD
Resident, Emergency Medicine
Albert Einstein College of Medicine
Beth Israel Medical Center
New York, New York

Ched Lohr, MD
Resident, Department of Radiology
Mercy Hospital
Pittsburgh, Pennsylvania

Quincy Samora, MD
Resident, Orthopedic Medicine
West Virginia University School of Medicine,
    Ruby Memorial Hospital
Morgantown, West Virginia

Alex Wade, MD
Resident, Internal Medicine
West Virginia University School of Medicine,
    Ruby Memorial Hospital
Morgantown, West Virginia

Melanie Watkins, MD
Resident, Department of Gynecology and Obstetrics
Emory University School of Medicine
Atlanta, Georgia

Series Preface

The *Rapid Review Series* has received high critical acclaim from students studying for the United States Medical Licensing Examination (USMLE) Step 1 and high ratings in *First Aid for the USMLE Step 1*. We have created a learning system, including a print and electronic package, that is easier to use and more concise than other review products on the market.

SPECIAL FEATURES

Book

- **Outline format:** Concise, high-yield subject matter is presented in a study-friendly format. In addition, key words and phrases appear in bold throughout.
- **High-quality visual elements:** Abundant two-color schematics, black and white images, and summary tables enhance your study experience.
- **Two-color design:** The two-color design helps highlight important elements, making studying more efficient and pleasing.
- **Two practice examinations:** Two sets of 50 USMLE Step 1–type clinically oriented, multiple-choice questions (including images where necessary) and complete discussions (rationales) for all options are included.

New! Online Study and Testing Tool

- **350 USMLE Step 1–type MCQs:** Clinically oriented, multiple-choice questions that mimic the current board format are presented. These include images where necessary and complete rationales for all answer options. All the questions from the book are included so you can study them in the most effective mode for you!

- **Test mode:** Select from randomized 50-question sets or by subject topics for an exam-like review session. This mode features a 60-minute timer to simulate the actual exam, a detailed assessment report that can be printed or saved to your hard drive, and direct links to all or only incorrect questions. The links include your answer, the correct answer, and full rationales for all answer options, so you can fully analyze your test session and learn from your mistakes.
- **Study mode:** Like the test mode, in the study mode you can select from randomized 50-question sets or by subject topics to create a dynamic study session. This mode features unlimited attempts at each question, instant feedback (either on selection of the correct answer or when using the "Show Answer" feature), complete rationales for all answer options, and a detailed progress report that can be printed or saved to your hard drive.
- **Online access:** Online access allows you to study from an Internet-enabled computer wherever and whenever it is convenient. This access is activated through registration on www.studentconsult.com with the pincode printed inside the front cover.

Student Consult

- **Full online access:** You can access the complete text and illustrations of this book on www.studentconsult.com.
- **Save content to your PDA:** Through our unique Pocket Consult platform, you can clip selected text and illustrations and save them to your PDA for study on the fly!
- **Free content:** An interactive community center with a wealth of additional valuable resources is available.

Preface

This book focuses on human physiology: how the human organism functions. A basic understanding of this field is crucial to the informed and competent practice of medicine. The book is intended for medical students preparing for Step 1 of the United States Medical Licensing Examination. Although the core material is physiology, great efforts have been taken to present it in a clinical context and in an integrated fashion with respect to anatomy, pathology, and pharmacology.

As medical students progress through their clinical training they will encounter numerous scenarios in which an understanding of basic physiology will substantially improve the care they are able to provide. This book is designed with this in mind.

- **Clinical notes** stress the clinical significance of the underlying physiology, which facilitates comprehension and makes the material more enjoyable.
- **Basic science notes** act as a bridge between physiology and closely related concepts in anatomy, pathology, and pharmacology—essential for a deeper understanding of the underlying physiology of a condition, and invaluable preparation for the boards.
- **Tables** facilitate understanding and act as quick summaries of concepts.
- **Illustrations** in simple and elegant format summarize essential concepts.
- **Practice tests** emulate the USMLE Step 1 format and include detailed explanations of the answers.
- **Access to additional tests via the Internet (with the password provided)** allows online practice in a realistic USMLE format. Questions can be accessed in a subject-specific manner to review a given system or in a random manner to review all areas of physiology.

I hope you find this clinically oriented approach enjoyable. Good luck on the boards!

Thomas A. Brown, MD

Acknowledgment of Reviewers

The publisher expresses sincere thanks to the medical students and physicians who provided many useful comments and suggestions for improving both the text and the questions. Our publishing program will continue to benefit from the combined insight and experience provided by your reviews. For always encouraging us to focus on our target, the USMLE Step 1, we thank the following:

Jacob Babu, Sophie Davis School of Biomedical Education, City University of New York

Jay Bhatt, Philadelphia College of Osteopathic Medicine

Stephen Dolter, University of Iowa College of Medicine

Timothy Fagen, University of Missouri–Kansas City

Katherine Faricy, Jefferson Medical College

Veronica L. Hackethal, Columbia College of Physicians and Surgeons

Caron Hong, University of Hawaii at Manoa

Michael Hoffman, Robert Wood Johnson Medical School, University of Medicine and Dentistry New Jersey

Justin Indyk, State University of New York Stony Brook

David A. Kasper DO, MBA, Philadelphia College of Osteopathic Medicine

Tyler J. Kenning, MD, Albany Medical Center

Maria Kirzhner, Kresge Eye Institute

Caroline Koo, State University of New York Downstate Medical Center

Michelle Koski, MD, Vanderbilt University Medical Center

Barrett Levesque, New York Medical College

James Massullo, Northeastern Ohio Universities College of Medicine

Todd J. Miller, University of Utah School of Medicine

Tiffany Newman, New York University School of Medicine

Adaobi Nwaneshiudu, Temple University School of Medicine

Josalyn Olsen, University of Iowa College of Medicine

Daniel Osei, University of Pennsylvania School of Medicine

Sachin S. Parikh, Robert Wood Johnson Medical School, University of Medicine and Dentistry New Jersey

Neil Patel, David Geffen School of Medicine, University of California, Los Angeles

Brad Picha, Case Western Reserve University School of Medicine

Stephan G. Pill, MD, MSPT, Hospital of the University of Pennsylvania

Keith R. Ridel, University of Cincinnati College of Medicine

Arjun Saxena, Jefferson Medical College

Sarah Schlegel, MD, Stony Brook University Hospital

Tana Shah, School of Osteopathic Medicine, University of Medicine and Dentistry of New Jersey

Yevgeniy Shildkrot, Kresge Eye Institute

Julia C. Swanson, Oregon Health & Science University

Ian Wong, MD, St. Vincent Hospital, Indiana University

Michael Yee, Sophie Davis School of Biomedical Education, City University of New York

Acknowledgments

Writing a physiology text has been a privilege as well as an amazing educational experience, and I have many people to thank for this opportunity. Jason Malley, the previous acquisitions editor at Elsevier, had confidence in me from the very beginning. For this I am eternally grateful. Susan Kelly, the managing editor for many of the texts in the *Rapid Review Series*, played an enormous role in the early stages. Her professionalism, work ethic, and attention to detail substantially improved the quality of this book and numerous others and have earned her the respect of her colleagues. Then there are the contributing authors. Dave Brown—my partner and confidant in the early stages of this project, as well as my partner in crime for *USMLE Step 1 Secrets*—deserves special recognition. His contributions were enormous. In addition to coauthoring several chapters, Dave helped me design a textual style—a merging of traditional outline and textbook format—that I believe works best for teaching physiology.

Special thanks to Dr. John Parker and Dr. Ronald Mudry for putting the finishing clinical touches on the respiratory chapter. My sincerest thanks as well to Dr. Karen MacKay for revamping the renal chapter from a nephrologist's perspective. Because of their contributions, I believe these chapters have a clinical feel that medical students will greatly appreciate. Additionally, I would like to thank Dr. Tim Gardner and Dr. Jeff Olsen for their reviews of the gastrointestinal and cardiovascular chapters, respectively. Their feedback was immensely helpful, and I am grateful for their time.

The talented Matt Chansky deserves enormous credit for the wonderful diagrams that appear throughout the book. The transformation from the rough sketches I provided him to the finished products is truly amazing, and the book is substantially improved as a result of his efforts. An enormous debt of gratitude is owed to Alison Whitehouse, developmental editor. Her impressive editorial and organizational skills contributed enormously to the book, and for this I am grateful. I would also like to thank James Merritt, acquisitions editor, and Kathryn DeFrancesco, developmental editor, for ensuring this project went through the production process in a smooth and timely manner. Finally, I would like to thank the many student physician reviewers; their input was invaluable.

Thomas A. Brown, MD

Contents

1

Cell Physiology

I. **Cell Structure and Function** (Fig. 1-1)
- Cells are the basic structural and functional unit of the body.
- Most cells contain a **nucleus,** surrounded by cytoplasm.
- The **cytoplasm** contains **cytosol,** within which sit various types of **organelles.**
- The cytoplasm is enveloped by a **cell membrane (plasma membrane).**
- An understanding of physiology at the cellular level is necessary for comprehending physiology and pathophysiology alike.
  A. **The cell membrane**
  1. **Structure** (Fig. 1-2)
     - The cell membrane is a **lipid bilayer** that separates the internal cellular environment from the extracellular fluid.
     - The lipid bilayer is composed of **phospholipids,** arranged as a hydrophilic glycerol backbone and two hydrophobic fatty acid tails.
       (1) **Fat-soluble (hydrophobic) substances** such as steroid hormones can dissolve in the hydrophobic bilayer and therefore can freely cross the membrane.
       (2) In contrast, **water-soluble (hydrophilic) substances** such as Na^+ and glucose cannot dissolve in this bilayer and must pass through pores or use carrier proteins.
     - Embedded in the lipid bilayer are proteins (Table 1-1), carbohydrates, and cholesterol.
     - The cell membrane is commonly described as a **fluid mosaic** because proteins can freely move within the phospholipid bilayer.
  2. **Morphology**
     - The cellular surface may be **smooth** or **folded.**
     - **Folding** of the membrane increases the **surface area** available for transport of substances in and out of the cell.
     - For example, the cells of the brush border of the small intestine have microvilli along their luminal surface. This provides the markedly increased surface area necessary for adequate absorption of ingested nutrients.
  B. **The nucleus** (Fig. 1-3)
     - The **nucleus** is centrally located within the cell and is surrounded by a two-layer **nuclear envelope,** which separates the cytoplasm from the **nucleoplasm.** Each layer of the envelope is a lipid bilayer.
     - It contains almost all the DNA of the cell, complexed with proteins (histones) in a form called **chromatin.**
     - It has several functions, including **messenger RNA synthesis (transcription)** and the regulation of cell division.

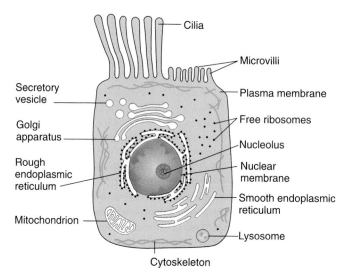

1-1: *Structure of the generalized cell. Cells have specialized structures depending on their origin and function; the components common to most human cells are shown here.*

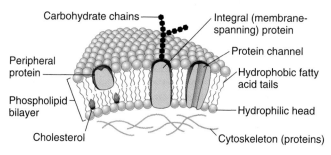

1-2: *The cell membrane.*

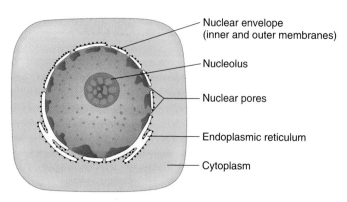

1-3: *The nucleus. The outer layer of the nuclear envelope and the space between the two layers are continuous with rough endoplasmic reticulum (rER). Both the rER and the outer layer are studded with ribosomes. Chromatin is seen as heterochromatin, a highly compacted form that appears dark in micrographs, and euchromatin, a less compact form containing DNA sequences that are transcriptionally active.*

TABLE 1-1:
Types of Membrane Proteins

Type	Function	Example	Pathophysiology
Channel proteins	Transport of substances into the cell	Nicotinic receptor on muscle cells (ligand-gated Na⁺ channel)	Myasthenia gravis
Enzymes	Catalyze reactions	Luminal carbonic anhydrase in the proximal convoluted tubule of the nephron	Proximal renal tubular acidosis
Receptor proteins	Mediate an intracellular response to extracellular ligands (e.g., hormones)	Insulin receptor	Insulin insensitivity in type II diabetes mellitus
Anchor proteins	Cell stabilization	Spectrin Dystrophin	Hereditary spherocytosis Duchenne muscular dystrophy
Carrier proteins	Required for facilitated transport	GLUT4 (glucose-sodium symporter)	Diabetes mellitus
Identifier proteins	Identify a cell as "self" or "foreign" to the immune system	Major histocompatibility complex I	Expression down-regulated in virally infected cells

TABLE 1-2:
Comparison of Intracellular and Extracellular Fluid Composition

Component	Intracellular Fluid	Extracellular Fluid
Sodium (mmol/L)	5–15	145
Potassium (mmol/L)	140	5
Calcium (mmol/L)	10^{-4}	1–2
Mg^{+2} (mmol/L)	0.5	1–2
Cl^- (mmol/L)	5–15	110
pH	7.2	7.4

- It also contains the **nucleolus,** a prominent, RNA-containing dense body that synthesizes **ribosomal RNA (rRNA).**
C. **The cytoplasm**
  1. **The cytosol**
     - The cytosol consists of the **intracellular fluid,** which contains many soluble proteins, ions, and metabolites, and **cytoskeletal elements.**
     - It contains non-membranous organelles, such as microvilli and centrioles.
     - Membranous organelles sit within the cytosol, but their membranes separate them from the cytosolic compartment, so the term "cytosol" does not encompass them.
     - Cytosol composition differs greatly from that of the extracellular fluid, as shown in Table 1-2.

2. **Membrane-enclosed organelles**
   a. **Endoplasmic reticulum (ER)**
      - This vesicular network is continuous with the nuclear envelope.
      - It is classified according to whether ribosomes are present (rough ER) or absent (smooth ER) on the membrane.
      - **Rough ER (rER)** is responsible for the **synthesis of proteins**, both secreted and intracellular.
      - **Smooth ER (sER)** functions in the **detoxification of drugs** and in the **synthesis of lipids** and **carbohydrates.**
      - Transport vesicles deliver the synthetic products of the ER to the Golgi apparatus.
   b. **Golgi apparatus**
      - This vesicular network has the appearance of flattened membranous discs and is located between the nucleus and the cell membrane.
      - Functions of the Golgi apparatus include the following:
        (1) **Post-translational modification of proteins,** such as addition of **mannose-6-phosphate (M6P) "tags"** to lysosomal enzyme precursors, which targets them for lysosomes
        (2) **Packaging of substances** destined for secretion and/or intracellular organelles (e.g., lysosomes)
        (3) **Maintenance of the plasma membrane** by the fusion of vesicles consisting of a phospholipid bilayer to the cell surface

        > **Clinical note:** In **I-cell disease,** there is impaired post-translational modification. The Golgi apparatus is unable to tag proteins with M6P due to a deficiency of the phosphorylating enzyme. Lysosomal enzyme precursors are therefore secreted from the cell instead of being taken up by lysosomes, resulting in impaired lysosomal function. The characteristic pathologic finding is the presence of inclusions within the cytoplasm. Death commonly results from cardiopulmonary complications (due to inclusions in heart valves) during childhood.

   c. **Lysosomes** (see Fig. 1-7)
      - Cytoplasmic, membrane-bound vesicles that contain hydrolytic digestive enzymes
      - Functions include the digestion of extracellular substances (**endocytosis** and **phagocytosis**) and intracellular substances (**autophagy**).
      - The interior of the lysosome is maintained at a pH of approximately 4.8 by a hydrogen ion pump.
      - This low pH removes the M6P tags attached to lysosomal enzyme precursors in the Golgi apparatus.

        > **Clinical note:** There are more than 45 **lysosomal storage diseases,** caused by impairment of lysosomal function, usually secondary to an inherited deficiency in a hydrolytic enzyme (Table 1-3). The resulting **lipid accumulation** within lysosomes

TABLE 1-3:
Lysosomal Storage Diseases

Disease	Defect	Pathophysiology	Inheritance
Niemann-Pick disease	Deficiency of sphingomyelinase	Accumulation of sphingomyelin and cholesterol	Autosomal recessive; death by age 3 yr
Tay-Sachs disease	Absence of hexaminidase	Accumulation of GM2 ganglioside	Autosomal recessive; death by age 3 yr; cherry-red spot on macula
Krabbe's disease	Absence of galactosylceramide β-galactosidase	Accumulation of galactocerebroside	Autosomal recessive; optic atrophy, spasticity, early death
Gaucher's disease	Deficiency of β-glucocerebrosidase	Glucocerebroside accumulation in liver, brain, spleen, and bone marrow	Autosomal recessive; "crinkled paper" appearance of cells
Fabry's disease	Deficiency of α-galactosidase A	Accumulation of ceramide trihexosidase	X-linked recessive
Hurler's syndrome	Deficiency of α-L-iduronidase	Clouding of cornea, mental retardation	Autosomal recessive
Hunter's syndrome	Deficiency of iduronate sulfatase	Mild form of Hurler's; no corneal clouding, mild mental retardation	X-linked recessive

eventually hinders the activity of cells in many organs, including liver, heart, and brain. As with I-cell disease, clinical symptoms are severe, and average life expectancy across the entire group of diseases is approximately 15 years, reflecting the importance of normal lysosomal function.

d. **Mitochondria**
 • These membranous organelles are composed of outer and inner membranes, intermembranous space, and inner matrix; they contain their own genetic material, mitochondrial DNA, which codes for mitochondrial proteins and transfer RNAs.
 • Responsible for energy production via aerobic metabolism and ketogenesis
 • Mitochondria and their DNA are inherited **maternally** (i.e., mitochondria are received only from the egg, not from sperm).

Clinical note: When **mitochondrial dysfunction** is inherited maternally via mitochondrial DNA, all offspring are equally affected but only female offspring pass on the disorder. However, other types of mitochondrial dysfunction result from defects in specific proteins that are coded by nuclear DNA but function in the mitochondria, such as **Leber's hereditary optic neuropathy (LHON)**, which is characterized by loss of vision in the center of the visual field. LHON is believed to be a result of decreased mitochondrial function and resulting lack of energy in the optic nerve and retina.

TABLE 1-4:
Overview of Cytoskeletal Proteins

Structure	Protein	Structure	Cell Location	Functions	Pathophysiology
Microfilaments	G actin	Small (5–9 nm), thin and flexible	Form cortex layer just under the plasma membrane	Mechanical support of cell membrane, cell flexibility, cell motility, polarity of the plasma membrane	*Listeria monocytogenes* spreads from cell to cell by inducing actin polymerization.
Intermediate filaments	Heterogeneous group of proteins	Intermediate (~10 nm)	Widely distributed	Mechanical stability of cells	Epidermolysis bullosa: blister formation in response to mechanical stress
Microtubules	Tubulin	Large (~25 nm), wide and stiff	One end attached to a centrosome	Cell division, intracellular movement of organelles; Components of cilia and flagella	Antimitotic drugs (e.g., colchicine, vincristine, vinblastine) inhibit microtubule function. Dysfunction can lead to disorders such as immotile cilia syndrome and male infertility.

3. **Cytoskeleton** (Table 1-4)
   - This network of filaments provides mechanical support, cell flexibility, and cell motility and aids in cell division.
   a. **Microfilaments**
      - Small-diameter, flexible, helical polymers composed of **G actin** and located just beneath the plasma membrane
      - Function in cell motility, organelle transport, cytokinesis, and muscle contraction
   b. **Microtubules**
      - Large-diameter, rigid cylinders composed of polymers of the protein **tubulin**
      - One end of the microtubule is attached to the **centrosome,** a densely filamentous region of cytoplasm at the center of the cell and the major microtubule-organizing center of the cell; the other end is free in the cytoplasm.
      - Serve as **scaffolding** for the movement of particles and structures within the cell (e.g., chromosomes during mitosis)
      - Are components of **cilia** and **flagella**
   c. **Intermediate filaments**
      - Comprise a large, heterogeneous family of proteins and are the most abundant of the cytoskeletal elements
      - Important in the **stability** of cells, especially epithelial cells

- Form **desmosomes,** structures that attach one epithelial cell to another, and hemidesmosomes, structures that anchor the cells to the extracellular matrix
- An example of a constituent of a membrane-bound intermediate filament is the protein **spectrin.**

> **Clinical note:** In **hereditary spherocytosis,** a form of **hemolytic anemia,** most patients have mutations in the **spectrin gene,** which causes impaired function of the membrane protein spectrin in red blood cells (RBCs). The characteristically spherical, mechanically unstable, and relatively inflexible RBCs tend to rupture within blood vessels and, because of their inflexibility, become lodged and subsequently scavenged within the splenic cords, resulting in a decrease in the number of circulating RBCs. The classic presentation is jaundice, splenomegaly, and anemia that typically resolves after surgical removal of the spleen (splenectomy).

4. **Non–membrane-enclosed organelles**
   a. **Microvilli**
      - Small, finger-like projections of the plasma membrane
      - Function to increase the **surface area** for absorption of extracellular substances
      - Examples of cell types with microvilli are the brush borders of the intestinal epithelium and the proximal convoluted tubule (PCT) of the nephron.
   b. **Centrioles**
      - Bundles of **microtubules** linked by other proteins
      - At least two are present in the **centrosome** of each cell that is capable of cell division.
      - Function in **cell division** by forming spindle fibers that separate homologous chromosomes.
   c. **Cilia**
      - Long, finger-like projections of plasma membrane, differing from microvilli in that they are supported by **microtubules**
      - Function to **move fluid and/or secretions** along the cell surface

   > **Clinical note:** In **Kartagener's syndrome (immotile cilia syndrome),** ciliary dysmotility results in the clinical triad of bronchiectasis, chronic sinusitis, and situs inversus. Respiratory tract infections occur as a result of impaired mucociliary clearance. The reason for situs inversus is unknown, although normal ciliary function is postulated to be a requirement for visceral rotation during embryogenesis. Deafness and male infertility may also result from the impaired ciliary function.

   d. **Flagella**
      - Similar in shape to cilia, but longer
      - Like cilia, they are supported by **microtubules.**

- Function in the **movement of cells** through a medium
- The **sperm cell** is the only human cell with a flagellum.
  e. **Ribosomes**
  - Consist of **ribosomal RNA** and **protein**
  - Function in protein synthesis (translation)
  - Fixed ribosomes are bound to the ER, whereas free ribosomes are scattered throughout the cytoplasm.

D. **Junctions between cells**
- **Tight junctions:** They seal adjacent epithelial membranes to prevent movement of most dissolved molecules from one side of an epithelial layer to the other. They also function to prevent membrane proteins from diffusing to other sections of membrane (i.e., they maintain membrane polarity between the apical and basolateral membranes).
- **Gap junctions:** Two lipid bilayers are joined by transmembrane channels (**connexons**) that permit passage of small molecules such as Na^+, Ca^{2+}, and K^-; various second messenger molecules; and a number of metabolites. Cells interconnected via gap junctions are electrically coupled and generally act in a coordinated fashion (i.e., as a syncytium).
- **Desmosomes:** They are plaquelike areas of intermediate filaments that create very strong contacts between cells (e.g., the junctions between epithelial cells).
- **Hemidesmosomes:** Resembling desmosomes, they anchor cells to the extracellular matrix.

E. **Transport across membranes**
1. **Simple diffusion**
   - The process whereby a **substance moves down its concentration gradient** across a semipermeable membrane
   - This tends to equalize the concentration of the substance on both sides of the membrane.
   - No metabolic energy or carrier protein is required.
   a. **Diffusion of uncharged substances**
   - The **rate of diffusion (J)** is dependent on the **concentration gradient** (ΔC), the **surface area** available for diffusion (A), and the **membrane permeability** (P):

$$J = PA(\Delta C)$$

   - **Permeability** (P) is directly proportional to lipid solubility of the substance and inversely proportional to the size of the molecule and the thickness of the membrane.
   - **Small hydrophobic** molecules have the **highest permeability** in the lipid bilayer.
   b. **Diffusion of charged substances**
   - If the diffusing substance is charged (e.g., ions), the net rate of diffusion (J) depends on the electrical potential difference across the membrane as well as ΔC (i.e., charged molecules will not necessarily flow down their concentration gradient).

- Positively charged ions (**cations**) tend to diffuse into the cell, whereas negatively charged ions (**anions**) tend to diffuse out of the cell, because the inside of the cell (at rest) is negatively charged.
  c. **Diffusion of nonpolar and polar substances**
  - Diffusion of **nonpolar substances** such as oxygen and carbon dioxide gases across a membrane is **more rapid** than the diffusion of polar substances such as water.
  - This is due to their relative solubility in lipids: nonpolar gases easily dissolve into the lipid bilayer, but water is insoluble because of its polarity.
  d. **Diffusion of gases**
  - Gases have a greater surface area available for diffusion: gases can diffuse across the entire surface area of the cell, whereas water must enter the cell through pores.
  - The **diffusion rate of a gas (V_g)** depends on the **pressure difference** across the membrane (ΔP), the **surface area** of the cell (A), the **diffusivity coefficient** (d), and the **thickness** of the membrane (T):

$$V_g = \frac{\Delta P \times A \times d}{T}$$

> **Clinical note:** Gas exchange in the lungs normally occurs very efficiently across the thin, lipid-rich pulmonary capillary and alveolar walls. However, in pathologic states such as **pneumonia,** gas exchange becomes less efficient because the accumulation of fluid increases the distance over which oxygen must diffuse.

2. **Osmosis**
   - Osmosis is the **movement of water,** not dissolved solutes, across a semipermeable membrane.
   - A **difference in solute concentration** across the membrane generates **osmotic pressure,** which causes the movement of water from the area of low solute concentration (**hypotonic solution**) to that of high solute concentration (**hypertonic solution**) (Fig. 1-4).

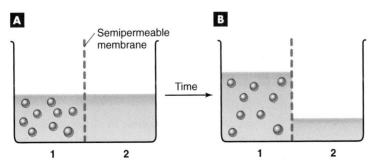

1-4: *Osmosis.* **A,** *Solution 1 has higher osmotic pressure (hypertonic) than solution 2 (hypotonic).* **B,** *Water has flowed from the hypotonic solution into hypertonic solution due to the driving force of osmotic pressure.*

- Osmotic pressure depends on the following:
    (1) the concentration of osmotically active particles: Osmotic pressure increases with increased solute concentration.
    (2) the ability of these particles to cross the membrane, which depends on particle size and charge.
- If the solutions on either side of the membrane have equal osmotic pressure, they are said to be **isotonic.**

a. **van't Hoff's Law**
   - Osmotic force (pressure) of a solution (π) depends on the number of particles per mole in solution (g), the concentration of the dissolved substance (C), the reflection coefficient of the solute across the membrane (σ; varies from 0 to 1), the gas constant (R), and the absolute temperature (T).
   - van't Hoff's law estimates osmotic force as

$$\pi = gC\sigma RT$$

   - If $\sigma = 0$, the solute is freely permeable across the membrane.
   - If $\sigma = 1$, the solute is impermeable, so osmotic pressure is indirectly proportional to solute permeability.

3. **Carrier-mediated transport** (Table 1-5)
   a. **Characteristics of carrier-mediated transport**
      - **Stereospecificity of carrier proteins:** Only one isomer of a substance is recognized by the carrier protein; for example, D-glucose but not L-glucose is transported by the GLUT4 transporters in muscle and liver.
      - **Competition for carrier binding sites:** Substances with similar structure can compete for binding to the carrier protein; for example, D-galactose binds to and is transported by the same GLUT4 transporter as D-glucose, thereby inhibiting the transport of glucose.
      - **Saturation of carrier proteins:** Once all of the transport molecules for a particular substance are occupied, the **transport maximum (T_m)** has been reached; the substance can no longer bind to its carrier and therefore cannot pass through the membrane (Fig. 1-5).
   b. **Facilitated transport (diffusion)**
      - Occurs **down an electrochemical gradient** and therefore **does not require metabolic energy**
      - Stops if the concentration of the substance inside the cell reaches the extracellular concentration or if carrier molecules become saturated.
      - For example, the GLUT4 transporter carries glucose into skeletal muscle and the liver; this proceeds for as long as a concentration gradient for glucose is present.
   c. **Active transport**
      - "**Uphill**" transport of a substance **against its electrochemical gradient**
      - **Energy** from hydrolysis of adenosine triphosphate (**ATP**) is required.
      - **Primary active transport:**
         (1) The transport of a substance across the plasma membrane **directly coupled to ATP hydrolysis**

TABLE 1-5:
Examples of Transmembrane Transport Molecules

Mechanism and Energy Source	Transporter	Function	Clinical and Therapeutic Relevance
Facilitated diffusion: No additional energy required	Glucose-facilitated transporter 4 (GLUT4)	Transports glucose into cells	Deficient expression in diabetes results in impaired glucose metabolism
	Voltage-gated Na^+ channel	Generates and propagates action potentials	Inhibited by tetrodotoxin (puffer-fish) and saxitoxin (contaminated shellfish)
Primary active transport: ATP hydrolysis	Na^+, K^+-ATPase pump	Electrogenic pump that contributes to maintenance of resting membrane potential	Inhibited by digitalis (naturally occurring toxin); a derivative, digoxin, is used in treatment of congestive heart failure.
	Ca^{2+}-ATPase	Maintains low cytoplasmic concentration of calcium	Inhibited by dantrolene (used in treatment of malignant hyperthermia)
	H^+, K^+-ATPase pump	Contributes to low pH of gastric secretions and acid secretion of distal convoluted tubule of the nephron	Inhibited by omeprazole (used to treat GERD and peptic ulcer disease)
Secondary active transport (cotransport): Energy derived from transport of Na^+ down its concentration gradient	Na^+-glucose cotransporter	Actively transports glucose into cells against concentration gradient, along with 2 Na^+. Located in gastrointestinal mucosa and PCTs of the nephron	Oral rehydration therapy exploits ideal Na : glucose ratio → uptake of salts, fluids, and glucose into intestinal epithelium. High-glucose, low-Na^+ solutions do not provide optimal rehydration, because cotransporter does not function without Na^+
	Na^+-K^+-2Cl^- cotransporter	Pumps 1 Na^+, 1 K^+, and 2 Cl^- into cells. Important role in thick ascending limb of loop of Henle	Inhibited by loop diuretics (e.g., furosemide). The nephron becomes unable to concentrate urine, resulting in loss of NaCl, K^+, and fluid

ATP, adenosine triphosphate; GERD, gastroesophageal reflux disease; PCT, proximal convoluted tubule.

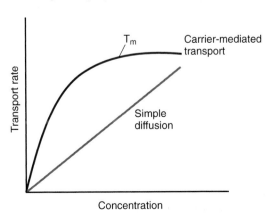

1-5: *A comparison of simple diffusion and carrier-mediated transport. T_m, transport maximum.*

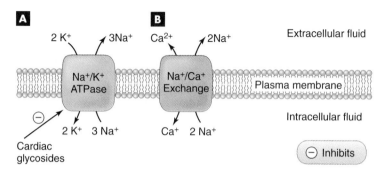

1-6: Examples of active transport in the myocardium. **A,** Primary active transport: the Na⁺-K⁺ transporter can be inhibited by cardiac glycosides. **B,** Secondary active transport: the Na⁺-Ca²⁺ countertransporter.

(2) Examples include the **Na⁺,K⁺-ATPase (sodium) pump** in the plasma membrane of all cells, the **H⁺,K⁺-ATPase (proton) pump** of gastric parietal cells, and the **Ca²⁺-ATPase pump** in muscle cells.

> **Pharmacology note: Proton pump inhibitors** such as **omeprazole** are used to treat peptic ulcer disease. These drugs directly inhibit the H⁺,K⁺-ATPase in gastric parietal cells. This reduces the acidic content of the stomach and allows for healing of the damaged mucosa.

- **Secondary active transport:**
  (1) The **simultaneous movement** of two substances across the cell membrane **indirectly coupled to ATP hydrolysis:** One substance moves **down** its concentration gradient, and this drives the "**uphill**" transport of the other substance against its concentration gradient.
  (2) In **cotransport (symport),** both substances move in the same direction (e.g., **Na⁺-glucose cotransport** in the epithelial cells of the brush border of the small intestine).
  (3) In **countertransport (antiport),** the substances move in opposite directions (e.g., the **Na⁺-Ca²⁺ countertransporter** of heart muscle cells moves Ca²⁺ against its concentration gradient as Na⁺ moves down its concentration gradient) (Fig. 1-6).

> **Pharmacology note: Cardiac glycosides** such as **ouabain** and **digitalis** inhibit the Na⁺,K⁺-ATPase in the myocardium (see Fig. 1-6). This increases the amount of sodium inside the cell, triggering the Ca²⁺-Na⁺ countertransporter. More calcium is brought into the cell, which increases the contraction of atrial and ventricular myocardium and increases cardiac output.

4. **Vesicular transport** (Fig. 1-7)
   a. **Endocytosis (membrane invagination)**
      - The cell membrane forms a new membrane-bound vesicle, enclosing extracellular material, which is then internalized.

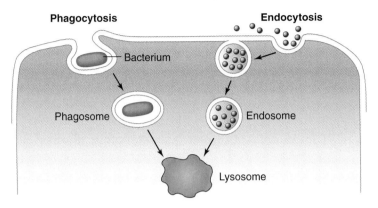

Phagocytosis

Endocytosis

Bacterium

Phagosome

Endosome

Lysosome

1-7: *Vesicular transport.*

- Most eukaryotic cells utilize this type of transport.
- In **pinocytosis,** the cell randomly samples the external environment by nonspecifically taking up droplets of extracellular fluid and transporting them into the cell in endocytotic vesicles.
- In **receptor-mediated endocytosis,** specific receptor-ligand interactions trigger endocytosis.
  (1) The receptors sit on a pitlike area of the membrane that is lined on its inner surface with the protein **clathrin.**
  (2) When a ligand binds to its receptor, this clathrin-coated pit invaginates and forms an endocytotic vesicle in which the entire receptor-ligand complex is included. As the vesicle buds from the membrane, it is stabilized by clathrin.
  (3) After the vesicle has been internalized, it fuses with an **early endosome,** which lowers the pH of the vesicle. This causes clathrin and the receptor molecule to be released and recycled to the cell surface.
  (4) Two medically important particles transported into the cell by receptor-mediated endocytosis are low-density lipoprotein (LDL; the "good" cholesterol) and transferrin (which delivers plasma iron to cells).

> **Clinical note: Familial hypercholesterolemia** is caused by a variety of mutations in the LDL receptor protein. The result is that plasma LDL particles cannot be effectively taken up by cells and therefore accumulate in the blood at high levels. Patients who are homozygous for these mutations typically die at an early age from atherosclerosis-induced myocardial infarction.

b. **Phagocytosis (engulfing)**
  - Actin-mediated process in which cytoplasmic finger-like extensions (**pseudopodia**) are extended into the extracellular fluid and surround solid particles, which are then internalized

- The internalized vesicle (**phagosome**) fuses with a **lysosome** that contains digestive enzymes. The phagosome contents are degraded (**"oxidative burst"**), and the waste products are released from the cell by **exocytosis.**
- Phagocytosis is carried out by a select group of cells, including **neutrophils and macrophages,** and is an important component of innate immunity.

> **Clinical note:** In **chronic granulomatous disease**, mutations in proteins of the NADPH oxidase system result in a reduced ability of phagocytic cells to produce the superoxide radical (O_2^-) and its products, the hydroxide radical and hydrogen peroxide. The enzyme catalase breaks down the hydrogen peroxide produced by the phagocytic cell and further decreases the cell's ability to destroy the offending microbe. Microbial killing is severely impaired in these patients, and phagocytic cells accumulate (forming granulomas) in areas of infection, commonly in skin, lungs, gastrointestinal tract, liver, spleen, and lymph nodes. The immune system often attempts to contain and wall off the clusters of phagocytic cells by creating a fibrous capsule around the affected area, forming abscesses.

c. **Exocytosis**
- **Intracellular vesicles fuse with the plasma membrane,** and vesicle contents are released into the extracellular space.
- This process is often triggered by an increase in intracellular **calcium.**
- For example, in the neuron, action potentials cause a calcium influx that triggers the fusion of neurotransmitter-laden vesicles with the cell membrane. The neurotransmitters are then exocytosed into the synaptic cleft.

5. **Other types of transport**
   a. **Paracellular** (Fig. 1-8)
   - The transport of substances **between cells**
   - For example, substances transported through **tight junctions** (such as those in the PCTs of the nephron) are transported via paracellular transport.
   b. **Transcellular (transcytosis)** (see Fig. 1-8)
   - The transport of substances **across cells**
   - Occurs because of differences in composition of the membrane on either side of the cell; the presence of different proteins on the apical versus the basal side of the cell is responsible for this polarity.
   - For example, the polarized nature of the membrane surfaces of epithelial and endothelial cells enables the transcytotic transport of substances from the lumen of the intestine to the bloodstream.
   c. **Convection**
   - The transport of substances via the **movement of a medium**
   - For example, the circulatory system uses the blood as a medium for transport of numerous substances, providing long-distance communication between organs.

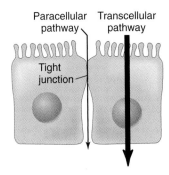

1-8: *Transcellular and paracellular transport.*

II. **Membrane Potentials, Action Potentials, and Nerve Transmission**
   A. **Resting membrane potential (RMP)**
   - RMP is determined by the concentration difference of **permeant ions** (ions able to pass through a particular semipermeable membrane) across the cell membrane, which depends on **membrane permeability** to the ions and the **equilibrium potential** of the ions.
   - It is a **negative value,** approximately −60 to −90 mV in most cells.
   - This polarized RMP is important for numerous cellular functions, including **cotransport** processes and **generation of action potentials.**
   1. **Selective membrane permeability and equilibrium potential**
      - The term "**selective permeability**" expresses the different permeability of membranes for different ions in different circumstances; this is a **dynamic** property of membranes.
      - Each ion tends to drive the membrane potential toward that ion's **equilibrium potential.**
      - The **equilibrium potential** for an ion is the membrane potential that would counter the tendency of the ion to move down its concentration gradient (i.e., the membrane potential at which there will no longer be *net* diffusion of the ion across the membrane).
      - The equilibrium potential for ion X (E_x) can be calculated from its concentration in extracellular fluid ($[X_{out}]$) and in the cytoplasm ($[X_{in}]$) using the **Nernst equation:**

$$E_x = \frac{-61\log[X_{in}]}{[X_{out}]}$$

   - For example, given the intracellular concentration of K^+ of approximately 150 mmol/L and the extracellular concentration of approximately 5 mmol/L, the equilibrium potential for K^+ is:

$$E_{K^+} = \frac{-61\log 150}{5}$$

$$= -90\,mV$$

- Thus, it is the concentration gradient of K^+, coupled with the relatively high membrane permeability to K^+, which determines the negative RMP of most cells. When the membrane potential is at $-90\,mV$, there will be no net potassium flux.

2. **Calculating RMP: the Gibbs-Donnan equation**
   - RMP (Em) is determined by the **permeability** (P) and **equilibrium potential** (E) for each of the **major permeant ions** (Na^+, K^+, and Cl^-):

$$Em = P_{Na}(E_{Na}) + P_K(E_K) + P_{Cl}(E_{Cl})$$

   - Thus, RMP reflects the equilibrium potential of the ions with the highest permeability and equilibrium potential (and concentration gradient across the membrane).
   - For example, in the **resting state of the neuron,** the membrane is **primarily permeable to potassium,** so K^+ makes the largest contribution to RMP. This explains why the RMP (roughly $-70\,mV$) of a cell approximates the equilibrium potential for K^+ ($-90\,mV$).

3. **Intracellular fixed anions**
   - Cytoplasm of the cell contains negatively charged organic ions **(anions)** that cannot leave the cell (i.e., they are "fixed").
   - These anions attract extracellular positively charged ions **(cations)**, particularly K^+ because of the high membrane permeability to K^+ in the resting state of excitable cells.
   - This results in a higher concentration of intracellular K^+ than extracellular K^+ and contributes to the negative RMP of cells (because there are more fixed anions than intracellular K^+ at the equilibrium potential for K^+).

4. **Na^+,K^+-ATPase pump**
   - This pump maintains the concentration gradient for Na^+ and K^+. Without it, Na^+ and K^+ have a tendency to leak through channels in the membrane, resulting in a net influx of extracellular sodium and efflux of intracellular potassium down their respective concentration gradients.
   - The constantly active electrogenic Na^+,K^+-ATPase pump removes 3 Na^+ ions for every 2 K^+ ions pumped into the cell to counteract leakages, thereby maintaining the concentration gradients across the membrane and preserving the RMP.

B. **Action potential** (Fig. 1-9)
   - A **rapid change in membrane potential** in response to a variety of stimuli
   - Occurs in excitable tissue (e.g., **neurons, muscle cells**) and is the **"language" of the nervous system** (the electrical signals that encode all information in the nervous system)

1. **Generation of an action potential**
   - The membrane potential reaches a threshold value (approximately $-55\,mV$) which is required for **activation** of **fast, voltage-gated sodium channels.**
   - Rapid influx of sodium occurs, causing **depolarization** of the cell. This corresponds to the sharp **upstroke** of the action potential.
   - The membrane potential becomes increasingly less negative as it depolarizes and approaches the equilibrium potential for Na^+. The **overshoot potential** is at the apex of the action potential spike and corresponds to the period during which the membrane potential becomes positive (+).

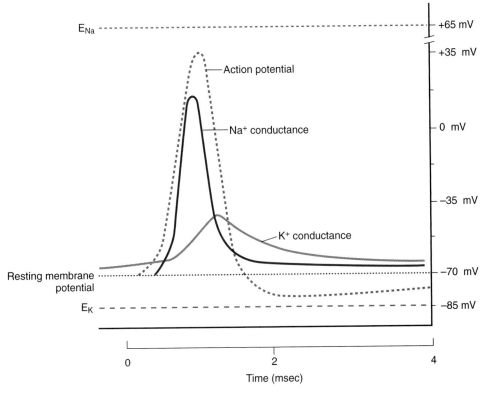

1-9: *Changes during generation of an action potential. E_K, equilibrium potential for K^+; E_{Na}, equilibrium potential for Na^+.*

- Next, the membrane becomes more permeable to K^+, causing efflux of potassium down its concentration gradient. This causes **repolarization** of the membrane potential.
- The final phase of the action potential is characterized by a slight **hyperpolarization** phase, during which the Na^+,K^+-ATPase reestablishes the original sodium and potassium electrochemical gradients across the plasma membrane.

2. **Properties of action potentials**
  a. **"All or none"**
     - Generation of an action potential is determined solely by the ability of the stimulus to cause the cell to reach **threshold** (i.e., it is "all or none"). If the threshold potential is reached, an action potential is generated; if it is not reached, no action potential is generated.
     - Regardless of **stimulus intensity** or **energy content,** the action potential will have the **same amplitude.**
  b. **Frequency**
     - Increasing **stimulus intensity** increases the **frequency** of action potential generation.
     - For example, in a mechanoreceptor of the skin, the more the receptor is deformed (i.e., the greater the mechanical energy applied), the higher the

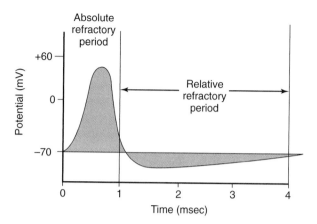

1-10: Refractory periods.

frequency of action potential generation (action potential amplitude remains unchanged).

c. **Refractory periods** (Fig. 1-10)
  • During refractory periods, **the cell is unable to generate an action potential.**
  • This is an important property of excitable tissue because it prevents overly rapid generation of action potentials.
    (1) **Absolute refractory period:** An action potential cannot be generated, regardless of stimulus intensity. This occurs during the **depolarization phase** of the action potential and is due to closure of the sodium channel inactivation gates.
    (2) **Relative refractory period:** Only a stimulus with intensity much greater than threshold can stimulate another action potential. This occurs during the **repolarization phase** and is due to the inactivated conformation of the voltage-gated sodium channels. The conductance of K^+ is higher than in the resting state, so the membrane potential becomes more negative.
    (3) **Accommodation:** When cells are held in the **depolarization phase** or are **depolarized very slowly,** the inactivation gates on sodium channels automatically close, and there is no sodium current. Even if the cell has reached its normal threshold potential, it is impossible for the cell to generate another action potential because too few sodium channels are open.

> **Clinical note:** In **hyperkalemia**, the extracellular potassium concentration is higher than normal, so there is less of a driving force for K^+ to leave the cell and keep the membrane potential at $-70\,mV$. The cell depolarizes enough to trigger the closure of sodium inactivation gates. This depolarization brings the membrane closer to threshold, but no action potential is generated.

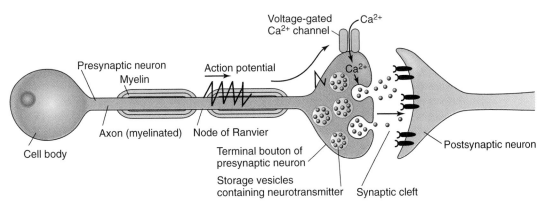

1-11: *Chemical transmission at a synapse. The basic structure of a myelinated neuron synapsing with another neuron is shown. Neurotransmitter is released from vesicles in the terminal bouton of the presynaptic neuron and taken up by receptors in the postsynaptic neuron.*

    d. **Conductance without decrement**
- Action potentials travel along a neuron with no decrease in signal strength because of the presence of the protein **myelin,** which acts as an electrical insulator (Fig. 1-11).
- At sites along the axon where myelin is absent, the **nodes of Ranvier,** the action potential must "jump" from one node to another, a process referred to as **saltatory conduction.**

> **Clinical note: Multiple sclerosis** is an autoimmune disease characterized by **inflammation** and **demyelination of nerves** in the central nervous system. It manifests in many different forms; some patients have cognitive changes, whereas others have paresis, optic neuritis, or depression.

C. **Transmission of action potentials between cells**
- Action potentials can be transmitted between cells by either electrical or chemical transmission.
1. **Electrical transmission**
   - This is a relatively **rare form of action potential transmission** in which current travels through openings between the cells, termed **"gap junctions."**
   - Occurs mainly in cardiac and smooth muscle, tissues in which there is cytoplasmic continuity between constituent cells (i.e., the cells function as a **syncytium**).
2. **Chemical transmission** (see Fig. 1-11)
   - Primary form by which action potentials are transmitted
   - Binding of the neurotransmitter (secreted from the presynaptic cell) to a **ligand-gated receptor** on the postsynaptic membrane results in localized depolarization and generation of an action potential in the postsynaptic cell.

(1) An action potential travels down the axon to **the terminal bouton** of the **presynaptic neuron,** causing opening of **voltage-gated calcium channels.**

(2) The resulting **Ca^{2+} influx** into the presynaptic nerve terminal causes **fusion** of neurotransmitter-containing vesicles with the presynaptic membrane and subsequent **release** of neurotransmitter into the synaptic cleft.

(3) The neurotransmitter **diffuses across the synaptic cleft.**

(4) The neurotransmitter binds to **ligand-gated receptors** located on the postsynaptic cell. This causes either an **excitatory postsynaptic potential (EPSP)** or an **inhibitory postsynaptic potential (IPSP).** EPSPs are a result of localized depolarization caused by increased conductance to (and influx of) Na^+, whereas IPSPs are a result of localized hyperpolarization caused by increased conductance to Cl^- or K^+.

(5) If **summation** of EPSPs and IPSPs at the **axon hillock** brings the membrane potential to **threshold,** generation of an action potential occurs via opening of voltage-gated sodium channels.

(6) The action potential travels toward the terminal bouton (**anterograde transport**).

(7) The action potential arrives at the terminal bouton, and the process repeats.

• To prevent repetitive stimulation, chemical neurotransmitters are either degraded in the extracellular environment or taken up by endocytosis into the presynaptic cell.

> **Clinical note:** In **Lambert-Eaton syndrome**, antibodies are made against the voltage-gated calcium channels on the terminal bouton of the presynaptic motor neuron. Binding of these antibodies to the calcium channels impairs neurotransmitter (acetylcholine) release by inhibiting calcium influx, resulting in generalized muscle weakness. Proximal muscles are affected more than distal muscles.

D. **Conduction velocity**
  • Conduction velocity is primarily dependent on the presence or absence of **myelin** and the **diameter of the axon.**
  • Large-diameter, **myelinated** axons conduct impulses much more **rapidly** (1–100 m/second) than small diameter, unmyelinated axons (<1 m/second).
  • Not having nodes of Ranvier, **unmyelinated** axons have to continually regenerate action potentials along the entire length of the axon, resulting in a much **slower** conduction velocity.
  • If the **distance between the nodes of Ranvier** is decreased along the length of an axon (i.e., there are more nodes of Ranvier), the conduction velocity will be reduced, because more action potentials need to be produced.

> **Clinical note:** In **Guillain-Barré syndrome**, segmental demyelination of peripheral nerves, nerve roots, and their associated ganglia occurs. It typically manifests as ascending weakness and paralysis, starting in the

distal extremities and rapidly traveling proximally. Paralysis may occur because of immunologic destruction of the myelin sheath, effectively **decreasing nerve conduction velocity.** The disease can cause fatal respiratory paralysis, so prompt respiratory care and support are crucial; once the inflammation has subsided, the nerves can remyelinate and normal function can be recovered.

E. **Types of neurotransmitters**
  1. **Acetylcholine: cholinergic transmission**
     - Acetylcholine (ACh) is used by all motor axons, autonomic preganglionic neurons, and postganglionic parasympathetic nerves and by some cells of the motor cortex and basal ganglia.
     - Depending on the postsynaptic receptor, ACh can be either **stimulatory** (e.g., at the neuromuscular junction via motor neurons) or **inhibitory** (e.g., in parasympathetic postganglionic fibers to cardiac muscle).

       > **Clinical note:** In the autoimmune disease **myasthenia gravis,** antibodies are made against ACh receptors of the neuromuscular junction in skeletal muscle. These antibodies bind to the ACh receptor on the postsynaptic membrane and block ACh binding, resulting in **muscle weakness** and **easy fatigability**. Treatment includes administration of **acetylcholinesterase inhibitors** such as **neostigmine** to increase the amount of ACh in the synaptic cleft.

     - Enzymes (synaptic cholinesterase and plasma cholinesterase) rapidly degrade ACh.
     - ACh also functions extensively in the brain to maintain **cognitive function.**

       > **Clinical note**: In **Alzheimer's disease,** there is degeneration of the basal forebrain nuclei that normally have extensive cholinergic projections throughout the brain. There is also evidence of a cortical deficiency of choline acetyltransferase, the enzyme that combines choline and acetyl coenzyme A to produce ACh. The resulting **lack of acetylcholine** appears to play a primary pathologic role in the learning and memory deficits.

  2. **Amino acids**
     a. **Glutamate: glutamatergic transmission**
        - Glutamate is the **primary stimulatory neurotransmitter** of the brain.
        - It binds to both **inotropic** (stimulatory) and **metabotropic** (modulator) receptors.
        - Excess glutamatergic activity is associated with **excitotoxicity** and **seizures.**
     b. **Gamma aminobutyric acid (GABA)**
        - GABA is the **primary inhibitory neurotransmitter** in the brain. It is abundant within the basal ganglia and cerebellum.
        - It is derived from the amino acid glutamate by action of the enzyme **glutamate decarboxylase.**

- Deficient GABA activity may result in movement abnormalities, anxiety disorders, seizures, and muscle spasms.

> **Pharmacology note:** Because GABA is an inhibitory neurotransmitter, GABA agonists such as **benzodiazepines, alcohol,** and **barbiturates** are frequently used (prescribed or not) as antianxiety agents (**anxiolytics**), suppressing cortical function.

> **Clinical note:** In **Huntington's disease,** there is progressive deterioration of the caudate nucleus, putamen, and frontal cortex, but clinical symptoms do not appear until the fourth or fifth decade, by which time many patients have already passed on the autosomal dominant gene to their children. Deterioration starts with hyperkinetic (choreiform) movements, progressing to hypertonicity, incontinence, anorexia, dementia, and death. **Loss of GABA-secreting neurons** between the striatum and globus pallidus is one of the factors responsible for the **abnormal movements.**

c. **Glycine**
   - Glycine is the **primary inhibitory neurotransmitter** of the **spinal cord.**
   - It **increases chloride conductance** in the postsynaptic membrane. This results in hyperpolarization of the postsynaptic membrane and inhibition of action potential generation.

> **Clinical note:** Glycine secretion in the spinal cord is inhibited by the **tetanus toxin**, exposure to which results in excessive stimulation (*disinhibition*) of the lower motor neurons, producing spasmic muscle contraction (i.e., **spastic paralysis**). The nerves must sprout new terminals before the patient can regain normal function.

3. **Monoamines**
   - These neurotransmitters contain a **single amine group** in their chemical structure and include norepinephrine, serotonin, and dopamine.
   - Monoamines are degraded by intracellular (presynaptic) **monoamine oxidase** (MAO) and postsynaptic **catechol-O-methyl transferase** (COMT).

> **Clinical note:** The **monoamine deficiency theory of depression** links depression to a deficiency in at least one of the three monoamine neurotransmitters: norepinephrine, serotonin, and dopamine. Extensive pharmacologic support for this theory has been obtained over the years, as evidenced by the efficacy of **monoamine oxidase inhibitors** and **tricyclic antidepressants,** which increase levels of monoamine neurotransmitters in the brain. However, these drugs affect levels of other neurotransmitters and have numerous side effects. More recently, **serotonin-specific reuptake inhibitors (SSRIs)** have been shown to be extremely effective in the treatment of depression with minimal side effects.

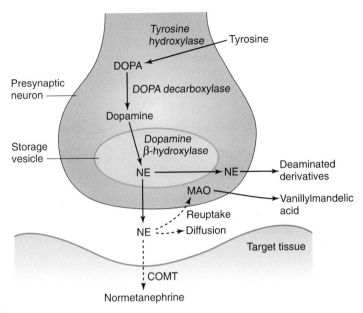

1-12: Adrenergic transmission: the norepinephrine pathway. COMT, catechol-O-methyl transferase; DOPA, L-dihydroxyphenylalanine; MAO, monoamine oxidase; NE, norepinephrine.

a. **Norepinephrine: adrenergic transmission** (Fig. 1-12)
   - Derived from the amino acid **tyrosine**
   - Synthesized and released by the **sympathetic nervous system, adrenal medulla,** and **locus ceruleus** of the central nervous system

   > **Clinical note:** Cocaine is a centrally acting norepinephrine reuptake inhibitor.

b. **Serotonin (5-HT)**
   - Serotonin is derived from the amino acid **tryptophan** (Fig. 1-13). The vast majority of the body's serotonin is found in the **enteric nervous system** of the gut.
   - The serotonin in the brain plays an important role in **control of mood.**

c. **Dopamine: dopaminergic transmission**
   - Dopamine is derived from the amino acid **tyrosine** (Fig. 1-14).
   - Dopamine is an important neurotransmitter in the brain.
   - There are three primary dopaminergic pathways.
     (1) The **nigrostriatal** pathway: transmits dopamine from the substantia nigra of the midbrain to the striatum and is important in the control of **voluntary movement**
     (2) The **mesolimbic** pathway: dopaminergic transmission between the midbrain and the limbic system. This is important in the **control of emotions** and also in **voluntary control of movements associated with emotion** (e.g., smiling, frowning).

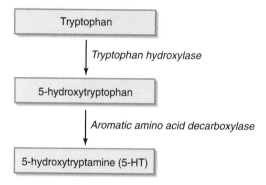

1-13: Synthesis of serotonin (5-hydroxytryptamine).

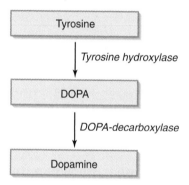

1-14: Synthesis of dopamine. DOPA, L-dihydroxyphenylalanine.

(3) The **tuberoinfundibular** pathway: dopaminergic transmission from the hypothalamus to the pituitary
- Dopamine is now known to be the **prolactin inhibitory factor** that inhibits prolactin secretion by the anterior pituitary.

> **Pharmacology note: Dopamine agonists** such as bromocriptine are used clinically to treat **prolactinomas,** the most common type of pituitary tumor; they are also the mainstay of treatment of **Parkinson's disease**. Conversely, the dopamine system may become overly active, as in **schizophrenia; dopamine antagonists** such as risperidone (Resperidol) and clozapine are widely used to reduce symptoms of schizophrenia such as hallucinations and delusions.

4. **Neuropeptides**
   - These have a **longer duration of action** than the smaller molecular neurotransmitters mentioned earlier, partly because neuropeptides act by **altering gene expression,** so their effects may continue after they are degraded.

- Neuropeptides may be secreted at the same time as a small molecule neurotransmitter such as norepinephrine (**cotransmission**). This results in an immediate, rapid response (due to the smaller neurotransmitter) and a delayed but prolonged response caused by the neuropeptide.
- For example, glutamate and the neuropeptide **substance P** are cotransmitted in the pain pathway; glutamate causes immediate inhibition of neurotransmission of pain, whereas substance P causes changes in gene expression to produce a lasting effect.
- Other examples of neuropeptides include **neuropeptide Y, enkephalins, endorphins,** and **nitric oxide**.

III. **Neuromuscular Junction**
  A. **Structure of the neuromuscular junction (NMJ)**
   - The NMJ is composed of a presynaptic motor neuron, the synaptic cleft, and the postsynaptic membrane (i.e., the plasma membrane of the muscle cell, termed the **sarcolemma**).
   - The NMJ is also called the **motor end plate**.
  B. **Mechanism of neuromuscular transmission** (Table 1-6)
   - An action potential triggers the fusion of ACh storage vesicles and corresponding **release of acetylcholine from the presynaptic neuron**.
   - ACh then diffuses across the **synaptic cleft** and binds to **nicotinic receptors** on the sarcolemma; the time required for this diffusion is responsible for **synaptic delay**.
   - Nicotinic receptors are slow, **ligand-gated sodium channels;** opening them produces a local depolarization along the sarcolemma, termed the **"end plate potential."**

TABLE 1-6:
Comparison of the Steps Involved in Synaptic Transmission at Neuron-to-Neuron Junctions and at the Neuromuscular Junction

Neuron to Neuron	Neuromuscular Junction
An action potential in the presynaptic neuron causes release of neurotransmitter from vesicles stored in terminal bouton	An action potential in the presynaptic neuron causes release of acetylcholine (ACh) from vesicles stored in terminal bouton
Diffusion of neurotransmitter across synaptic cleft	Diffusion of ACh across synaptic cleft
Neurotransmitter binds to postsynaptic ligand gated receptor, resulting in EPSP or IPSP. If summation of EPSPs and IPSPs exceeds threshold potential at the axon hillock, an axon potential is generated	ACh binds to postsynaptic nicotinic receptor, a ligand-gated receptor that, when activated, allows facilitated diffusion of Na^+ and K^+ ions, having a net depolarizing effect referred to as end plate potential (EPP)
To prevent repetitive stimulation, neurotransmitters are either degraded in the extracellular environment or taken up by endocytosis in the presynaptic cell	Acetylcholinesterase breaks down ACh into acetyl coenzyme A and choline, which are taken up into the presynaptic cell

EPSP, excitatory postsynaptic potential; IPSP, inhibitory postsynaptic potential.

TABLE 1-7:
Drugs and Toxins Acting at the Neuromuscular Junction

Toxin/Drug	Action	Clinical Effect
Botulinum toxin	Blocks release of acetylcholine (ACh) from presynaptic nerve terminal	Weakness and paralysis until new nerve terminals have sprouted
Organophosphates	Inhibit ACh, leading to persistently elevated ACh and tonic activation of ACh receptors	Diarrhea, urination, miosis, bronchoconstriction, excitation (muscle paralysis), lacrimation, and salivation
Curare (toxin)	Competitively antagonizes binding of ACh to the postsynaptic nicotinic receptor	Skeletal muscle paralysis
Nondepolarizing neuromuscular blocking drugs (similar to curare), such as atracurium	Competitively antagonize binding of ACh to the postsynaptic nicotinic receptor	Skeletal muscle paralysis. Used to cause paralysis in preparation for intubation
Depolarizing neuromuscular blocking drugs (e.g., succinylcholine)	Competitive agonist of the postsynaptic nicotinic receptor	Binds so strongly to nicotinic receptor that prolonged depolarization occurs, initially causing generalized skeletal muscle contraction that is short-lived; flaccid paralysis follows

- If the end plate potential reaches threshold, it triggers the opening of **voltage-gated sodium channels,** and an action potential is produced.
- A number of drugs and toxins block transmission at the NMJ (Table 1-7).

IV. **Skeletal Muscle**
  A. **Structure** (Fig. 1-15)
  - Skeletal muscle joins bone to bone.
  - The cells are large in diameter and multinucleated.
  - Cells contain a network of membrane invaginations called the **transverse tubules (T tubules);** these tubules interconnect the plasma membrane (**sarcolemma**) and ER (**sarcoplasmic reticulum**), which is filled with calcium at rest.
  - Actin-myosin myofilaments are arranged into **sarcomeres** (see Fig. 1-15):
    (1) Sarcomeres are the functional unit of skeletal muscle.
    (2) They are composed of overlapping **thick filaments (myosin)** and **thin filaments (actin),** which gives skeletal muscle its striated appearance under the light microscope.
  B. **Contraction**
    1. **Mechanism of contraction: the sliding-filament theory**
    - Conduction of an action potential along the sarcolemma and throughout the T tubules results in **release of calcium by the sarcoplasmic reticulum.**

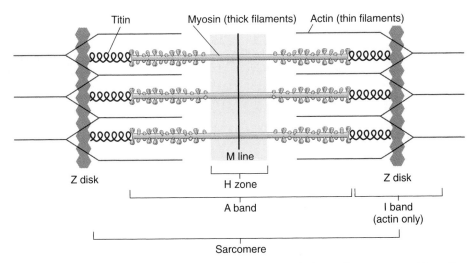

Titin   Myosin (thick filaments)   Actin (thin filaments)

M line

Z disk

H zone

Z disk

A band

I band
(actin only)

Sarcomere

1-15: *Sarcomere structure. Z disks are platelike protein structures into which actin filaments are inserted; two Z disks form the outer boundaries of one sarcomere. A bands, located in the center of the sarcomere, contain myosin filaments and appear dark under the light microscope. I bands are composed entirely of actin; they lie between A bands and are transected by the Z disks. Actin and myosin filaments overlap to form cross-bridges. However, the H zone (or bare zone), located in the center of the sarcomere, is composed entirely of myosin filaments; there is no overlap of actin and myosin filaments in this region. The M line lies in the center of the H zone and therefore consists only of myosin filaments. "Titin" is a protein important in striated muscle contraction that connects the Z disk to the M line in the sarcomere.*

- **Ca^{2+} binds to troponin,** causing a conformational change of troponin, which in turn causes **tropomyosin** to be displaced. The displacement of tropomyosin exposes myosin-binding sites on the actin, which allows temporary covalent bonds to form between actin and myosin (**cross-bridging**).
- Repetitive **cycles of cross-bridging,** pivoting, and detachment of actin and myosin result in the sliding of the filaments with respect to each other.
  (1) **ATP** is required for the detachment phase of the cycle. It causes a conformational change in myosin that decreases its affinity for actin.
  (2) Cross-bridge cycling occurs for as long as Ca^{2+} is bound to troponin.
  (3) When filaments slide over each other during cross-bridge cycling, the **Z disks are pulled toward one another,** the **sarcomere shortens,** and the **muscle contracts.**
  (4) Each sliding cycle shortens the sarcomere, and thus the entire muscle fiber, by ~1%; many cycles are required to produce significant muscle contraction.
- **Relaxation** occurs when Ca^{2+} has been pumped back into the sarcoplasmic reticulum via a **Ca^{2+}-ATPase** pump in its membrane. Ca^{2+} no longer binds to troponin, and tropomyosin goes back to its original conformation, blocking the interaction between actin and myosin.

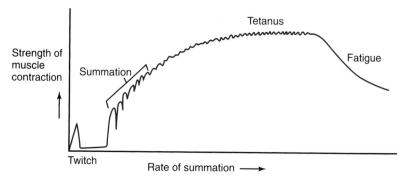

1-16: Types of muscle contraction.

> **Clinical note:** The importance of ATP in skeletal muscle relaxation, or the detachment phase of contraction, is evidenced by **rigor mortis,** which occurs as a result of the absence of ATP after death has occurred. The actin-myosin **myofilaments remain locked together** because ATP had been depleted.

2. **Types of contraction**
   - **Graded:** The **strength** of contraction depends primarily on the number of muscle fibers recruited rather than the strength of the muscle fibers.
   - **Twitch:** Electrical stimulation of myocytes above the threshold potential results in a limited efflux of Ca^{2+} from the sarcoplasmic reticulum into the cytoplasm, stimulating a **single contraction.**
   - **Summation and tetanus** (Fig. 1-16): If muscle is stimulated at a high enough frequency, individual muscle twitches combine (summate) to produce **sustained** contraction (tetanus).
   - **Isotonic muscle contraction:** A constant force is produced while the **muscle length is changing.** As muscle tension increases, the muscle shortens and lifts the load (e.g., biceps curls in weight lifting).
   - **Isometric muscle contraction:** A constant force is produced while the muscle is held so that it **does not change in length** and can only exert tension. Active tension is produced by cross-bridge cycling, but muscle length does not change (e.g., pushing against an immovable object such as a wall).
3. **Regulation of contraction**
   - Muscle contraction is regulated by the **somatic nervous system** (i.e., it is under voluntary control). The motor neuron (with cell body in the spinal cord or brainstem nuclei) and the muscle fiber or fibers it innervates are called the **motor unit,** the **functional unit of skeletal muscle.**
   - The fewer muscle fibers innervated by a given motor neuron, the greater the **precision** of the control of contraction. For example, motor neurons that innervate laryngeal muscles supply only a few muscle fibers, whereas motor units that innervate the gluteus maximus supply thousands of muscle fibers.

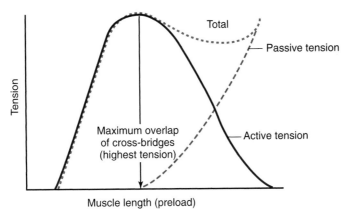

1-17: *Length-tension relationship in skeletal muscle.*

TABLE 1-8:
Types of Skeletal Muscle Fiber

Characteristic	Slow-Twitch	Fast-Twitch
Appearance	"Red" muscle	"White muscle"
Example	Soleus	Stapedius
Metabolism	Primarily aerobic	Primarily anaerobic
Diameter of fiber	Small	Large
Mitochondria	More	Fewer
Capillary supply	Higher	Lower
Myoglobin	Higher	Lower
Sensitivity to hypoxia	Higher	Lower
Resistance to fatigue	Higher	Lower

- The **strength** of skeletal muscle contraction is determined by four factors: metabolic condition (e.g., fatigue), amount of load, recruitment of motor units, and initial length of muscle fibers.
- The amount of **tension** that can be generated is determined by the extent of actin-myosin myofilament overlap. This is termed the **"length-tension relationship"** (Fig. 1-17). If the sarcomere is shortened, the actin and myosin have less room to overlap and develop tension. If the muscle is stretched to a point at which actin and myosin no longer overlap, no cross-bridges can be formed and no tension can develop.
4. **Types of skeletal muscle fiber** (Table 1-8)
   a. **Fast-twitch**
      - Fibers that are stimulated by large, **fast-conducting nerves**
      - Mainly use stored **glycogen** and thus **anaerobic** respiration for energy; therefore, they fatigue easily due to lactic acid build-up.

- **Whitish** in color because they contain only small amounts of myoglobin
- Have relatively few mitochondria and therefore are used for **explosive high-intensity activity** (e.g., sprinting), drawing on stored glycogen

   b. **Slow-twitch**
  - Fibers that are innervated by small-diameter, **slow-conducting nerves**
  - Use both **fats** and **carbohydrates** as an energy source and are resistant to fatigue
  - Rich in **myoglobin,** which makes them **red**
  - Muscles controlling **posture** are mainly composed of slow-twitch fibers. These muscle fibers are adapted for **continual low-intensity activity** (e.g., walking).

> **Clinical note: Strength training** causes an increase in the number of myofilaments in each muscle fiber. This increases the force that the muscle is able to generate and increases the mass of the muscle even though the number of muscle fibers is unchanged. **Endurance training** usually does not increase the mass of muscle but instead increases the number of blood vessels (for delivery of more oxygen and glucose) and mitochondria (for delivery of ATP) in the muscle.

V. **Smooth Muscle**
  A. **Structure**
  - Smooth muscle is arranged in **circular layers around hollow organs** (e.g., esophagus, respiratory airways) and **blood vessels** (including the aorta but not the heart); contraction reduces the size of these structures.
  - The **cells** are **spindle-shaped**.
  - The actin-myosin myofilaments are not arranged into sarcomeres, so cells are **nonstriated** in appearance.
  - The absence of sarcomeres enables smooth muscle to contract even when the cells are enormously stretched (i.e., smooth muscle contraction is not limited by the length-tension relationship).
  - The sarcoplasmic reticulum is loosely arranged within the cells, and there are **no T tubules.**
  - Cells do contain **dense bodies,** structures analogous to the Z disks found in skeletal muscle.
  B. **Types**
  1. **Single-unit (unitary or visceral) smooth muscle**
  - The **predominant type** of smooth muscle in the body, located in the gastrointestinal tract, bladder, uterus, and ureters
  - Functions as a **syncytium.** Low-resistance channels between cells (**gap junctions**) transmit nerve impulses, causing the contraction of many cells at once.
  - A unique quality of gastrointestinal smooth muscle is the rhythmic fluctuation of membrane potential (**slow waves**) that give rise to **spike potentials** which can cause muscle contraction (i.e., they function as a **pacemaker**) (see Chapter 7, Extrinsic Regulation of the Gastrointestinal Tract).

- Although slow waves are the primary regulator of single-unit smooth muscle, activity can be modified substantially via the autonomic nervous system.

2. **Multiunit smooth muscle**
   - Located in the iris, ciliary muscle of the lens, arrector pili of the skin, and vas deferens. Similar to skeletal muscle in that each muscle fiber is innervated, and therefore functions, separately.
   - Gap junctions are absent.
   - Because there is **no pacemaker activity**, regulation of multiunit smooth muscle is **dependent** on the autonomic nervous system.

C. **Mechanism of contraction**
   - Slow waves give risk to spike potentials, which stimulate cell contraction.
   - The **initial phase** of contraction is triggered by an increase in cytoplasmic calcium, released from the sarcoplasmic reticulum, as occurs in skeletal muscle.
   - **Sustained contraction** is mediated by continued influx of Ca^{2+} into the cytoplasm from the interstitium, via voltage-gated calcium channels on the cell membrane. Calcium combines with the protein calmodulin to form the **calcium-calmodulin (Ca^{2+}-CaM) complex** and activates **myosin light-chain kinase** (MLCK). MLCK in turn phosphorylates the myosin cross-bridges, exposing binding sites for actin. Actin and myosin then form cross-bridges and contract the muscle cell.
   - **Relaxation** occurs when Ca^{2+} has been pumped back into the sarcoplasmic reticulum and can no longer form the Ca^{2+}-CaM complex.

D. **Regulation of contraction**
   - Most smooth muscle has intrinsic pacemaker activity, but smooth muscle activity can be modulated by the **autonomic nervous system** (i.e., it is generally *not* under voluntary control). **Sympathetic** and **parasympathetic nerves** are distributed to all organ systems in the body and stimulate smooth muscle activity in many organs at once.
   - For example, in the **"fight or flight" response, sympathetic** stimulation causes a myriad of responses such as pupillary dilation, dilation of coronary arteries, decreased intestinal motility, and bronchial dilation. In general, parasympathetic stimulation has the opposite effects.

> **Clinical note:** In **Chagas' disease,** infection with the protozoan parasite *Trypanosoma cruzi* (found in South America) can cause destruction of the myenteric plexus of the enteric nervous system, resulting in severely impaired regulation of intestinal smooth muscle contraction, particularly in the esophagus. Clinical manifestations may include difficulty swallowing (dysphagia), chest pain from esophageal distention, and frequent bouts of pneumonia caused by aspiration of esophageal contents. The myenteric plexus of the colon may also be destroyed, causing **toxic megacolon.**

VI. **Cardiac Muscle**
   A. **Structure**
      - Similar to smooth muscle, the cells are interconnected via gap junctions and function as a syncytium (Table 1-9).

TABLE 1-9:
Comparison of Skeletal, Cardiac, and Smooth Muscle

Feature	Skeletal Muscle	Cardiac Muscle	Smooth Muscle
Location	Bone to bone	Heart	Around hollow organs (gastrointestinal tract, airways, ureters)
Cell morphology	Large diameter, multinucleated cells	Uninuclear and/or binucleated, branched cells	Small diameter
Striated	Yes	Yes	No
Gap junctions	No	Yes	Yes
Sarcomeres	Yes	Yes	No, actin inserts into dense bodies instead of Z disks
Innervation	Somatic nervous system	Autonomic nervous system	Autonomic nervous system
Type of contraction	Graded	All or none	All or none
Mechanism of contraction	Sliding filament mechanism	Sliding filament mechanism	Calcium-calmodulin–induced activation of myosin light-chain kinase
Origin of calcium	Sarcoplasmic reticulum	Sarcoplasmic reticulum and extracellular fluid	Sarcoplasmic reticulum and extracellular fluid
Troponin	Yes	Yes	No
Postsynaptic receptor	Nicotinic receptor at neuromuscular junction	Adrenergic and muscarinic receptors throughout the heart	Muscarinic receptors widely distributed along the cell surface
Action potential	Short duration	Long duration	Long duration
Resting membrane potential	Stable	Unstable	Rhythmic fluctuations (slow waves), which give rise to spike potentials
Conduction of action potentials	Restricted to that particular muscle fiber, action potential travels bidirectionally along fiber	Functional syncytium, conducted via gap junctions	Functional syncytium, conducted via gap junctions
Pacemaker activity	No	Yes	Yes
Effect of denervation	Atrophy	Will function adequately (e.g., heart transplant) but ability to exercise will be dependent on circulating catecholamines only	Still able to maintain tone
Examples of pathology	Muscular dystrophy, myositis	Congestive heart failure	CREST syndrome, achalasia, Chagas' disease

- Similar to skeletal muscle, they contain sarcomeres and are striated in appearance.

B. **Mechanism of contraction**
- Similar to skeletal muscle, contraction occurs through a sliding filament mechanism.
- In contrast to skeletal muscle, extracellular Ca^{2+} plays a substantial role in triggering contraction.
- Similar to smooth muscle, contraction occurs in an "all or none" manner.

Pharmacology note: The fact that extracellular calcium plays such an important role in stimulating cardiac muscle contraction is exploited by **calcium channel–blocking drugs** such as diltiazem and verapamil. **Calcium channel blockers** reduce heart rate and contractility without adversely affecting skeletal muscle functioning and are therefore useful for treating hypertension and a myriad of cardiac conditions.

C. **Regulation of contraction**
   - Similar to smooth muscle, cardiac cells have an unstable RMP that allows them to generate their own electrical pacemaker activity.
   - Rate of contraction (**chronotropy**), strength of contraction (**inotropy**), rate of conduction (**dromotropy**), and rate of relaxation (**lusitropy**) are further regulated by the autonomic nervous system:
     (1) Sympathetic stimulation has **positive** chronotropic, inotropic, dromotropic, and lusitropic effects through the binding of norepinephrine and epinephrine to **adrenergic receptors.**
     (2) Parasympathetic stimulation has **negative** chronotropic, inotropic, dromotropic, and lusitropic effects through the binding of ACh to **muscarinic receptors.**

Clinical note: The most common childhood-onset muscular dystrophy, **Duchenne muscular dystrophy,** is X-linked and is caused by a defect in the gene for **dystrophin**, a protein necessary for sarcolemma stability in striated muscle. Breakdown of sarcolemma results in calcium influx, enzyme activation, and muscle necrosis; fatty tissue and connective tissue fill the spaces once occupied by muscle, giving muscle a *pseudohypertrophic* appearance. Muscle weakness starts in the legs, with wide-based gait, hyperlordosis, and what appears to be hypertrophy of muscle. Patients are usually wheelchair-bound by 12 years of age. Lack of dystrophin in the brain leads to mental retardation. Mortality is 100% and is caused not by skeletal muscle defects but mostly by the **absence of dystrophin in cardiac muscle,** which results in fibrosis of the myocardium and subsequent heart failure, pulmonary congestion, and arrhythmias.

2

Neurophysiology

I. **Introduction**
  - The nervous system is unique in that it affects every other system of the body. It consists of several complex components that function in an organized fashion at extremely high speeds.
  - The human brain is a network of more than 100 billion nerve cells that, through specific pathways, communicate with each other and with various motor and sensory systems. Ultimately, these networks allow one to think, move, feel, experience, and manipulate one's environment.
  - Injury to or deficit in any part of the nervous system can lead to devastating and debilitating effects.

II. **Organization and Functional Anatomy of the Nervous System**
  - The nervous system is anatomically subdivided into
    (1) The central nervous system (CNS): the brain and the spinal cord
    (2) The peripheral nervous system (PNS): peripheral nerves that originate from the brainstem and spinal cord (cranial nerves and spinal nerves, respectively), as well as specialized clusters of neurons referred to as ganglia
  - The **PNS** is divided into two functional components, the **somatic** and **autonomic** divisions.
  A. **The somatic nervous system**
    - This controls all **voluntary actions** (i.e., intentional movements but not reflexive ones).
    - All "processing" occurs in the brain and therefore at a conscious level.
    - Anatomically, it consists of an **"afferent loop,"** comprising the **sensory nerves** leading to the brain, and an **"efferent loop,"** comprising **motor nerves** from the brain to the muscles.
  B. **The autonomic nervous system**
    - This controls all **involuntary actions** (e.g., reflexes, respiration) by regulating functioning of viscera, smooth muscle, and exocrine and endocrine glands.
    - It comprises **sensory** and **motor neurons** running between the brain and various internal organs such as the heart, lungs, viscera, and endocrine and exocrine glands.
    - It is further divided into the parasympathetic, sympathetic, and enteric nervous systems.
  C. **Protection of the brain**
    - This is ensured by two separate systems, the **blood-brain barrier** and the **blood-CSF barrier.**

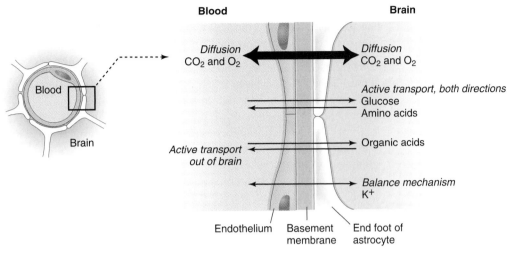

2-1: Blood-brain barrier.

1. **Blood-brain barrier (BBB)** (Fig. 2-1)
   - Composed of **endothelial cells** packed tightly together to form **tight junctions** that prevent passage of most molecules.
   - An underlying basement membrane and specialized glial cells (astrocytes), which project processes (**pedicels**) that attach to the walls of the capillary, reinforce this barrier.
   - Very few substances can cross the BBB into brain tissue:
     (1) **Water** is able to freely diffuse.
     (2) **Glucose** (the primary energy source of the brain) and amino acids require carrier-mediated transport.
     (3) **Nonpolar lipid-soluble substances** cross more readily than polar water-soluble ones.
     (4) Other **active transport systems** are present to pump weak organic acids, halides, and extracellular K^+ across the BBB.

   > **Clinical note: In vasogenic edema** (typically secondary to a brain tumor), the blood vessels are poorly developed, are leaky, and lack the transport properties of a normal BBB. This abnormal vessel permeability results in accumulation of interstitial fluid in the brain. Permeability of the BBB can also be altered in infections such as **bacterial meningitis;** although this accounts for some of the adverse neurologic effects of infection, it also permits improved delivery of antibiotics to the CNS.

2. **The blood-CSF barrier**
   - Cerebrospinal fluid (CSF) is a clear, colorless fluid that normally contains none or few cells, a small amount of protein, and a moderate amount of glucose.
   - The **blood-CSF barrier** is composed of epithelial cells of the choroid plexus—a highly vascular structure, located within the ventricles, that

produces CSF; the **tight junctions** between the cells serve to selectively allow substances access to the CSF.

- Transport mechanisms across the barrier are similar to those of the BBB.

> **Clinical note:** The composition of CSF may be altered in various disease states. Leukocytes or excess protein makes it appear cloudy; blood may make it appear red. In some diseases, the CSF has a characteristic composition. For instance, in **viral meningitis** it shows increased numbers of lymphocytes, normal to slightly elevated protein concentration, normal glucose concentration, and a normal to mildly elevated "opening pressure." In **bacterial meningitis,** there are increased numbers of polymorphonuclear leukocytes, an increased protein concentration, a decreased glucose concentration, and an increased opening pressure. In **multiple sclerosis,** the protein content, or γ-globulin content, is increased.

III. **The Autonomic Nervous System**
- The primary function of the **autonomic nervous system (ANS)** is to control and regulate the visceral functions of the body (e.g., heart rate, glandular secretions).
- These functions are regulated by **brain "centers"** in the **hypothalamus** and **brainstem.**
- For example, vasomotor, respiratory, and vomiting centers are located in the medulla. Temperature, thirst, and appetite-regulating centers are located in the hypothalamus.

A. **Organization**
- The ANS operates primarily through **visceral reflexes.** Sensory signals from visceral organs enter the **autonomic ganglia, brainstem,** or **hypothalamus.** These entities interpret the signal and reflexively send signals back to the visceral organ to control its activity.
- The **efferent** autonomic signals are transmitted to the various organs of the body through two major subdivisions, the **sympathetic nervous system** and the **parasympathetic nervous system.**
- A third subdivision, the **enteric nervous system,** controls the gastrointestinal tract intrinsically. However, the sympathetic and parasympathetic divisions also influence it, so it is not a completely stand-alone system.
- An example of a visceral reflex is the **response to cold.** Cold receptors on the skin transmit signals to the hypothalamus, which in turn causes several reflexive adjustments via autonomic efferents, including:
  (1) Stimulating muscle contraction (shivering), which increases the rate of body heat production
  (2) Promoting skin vasoconstriction to diminish loss of body heat from the skin

1. **The sympathetic division: "fight or flight"**
- The sympathetic nervous system is called the "fight or flight" system because it is most active in times of stress, fear, or excitement.

TABLE 2-1:
Effects of the Autonomic Nervous System on Target Organs

Target Organ	Sympathetic	Physiologic Mechanism	Parasympathetic	Physiologic Mechanism
Eyes	Pupil dilation (mydriasis)	Pupil dilation from contraction of dilator pupillae (radial fibers of iris)	Pupil constriction (miosis)	Contraction of sphincter pupillae (circular fibers of iris)
Bronchioles	Bronchodilation	β_2-mediated smooth muscle relaxation	Bronchoconstriction	M3-mediated smooth muscle contraction
Kidney	↓ Renal perfusion, ↑ renin secretion	α_1-mediated vasoconstriction and β_2-mediated renin secretion	Very limited innervation	No
Heart	↑ Heart rate, ↑ stroke volume, ↑ cardiac output,	↑ Permeability nodal tissue to Na^+ ions, ↑ sensitivity of cardiomyocytes to calcium ions	↓ Heart rate, ↓ stroke volume, ↓ cardiac output	Increased permeability of nodal tissue to K^+ ions
Gastrointestinal tract	↓ Digestion and motility	Stimulates sphincter muscle contraction and splanchnic vasoconstriction	Promotes digestion	Stimulates intestinal secretions and peristalsis, inhibits sphincter muscle contraction
Bladder	Urinary retention	Constricts sphincter, relaxes detrusor muscle	Stimulates urination	Relaxes sphincter, contracts detrusor muscle
Sweat glands	↑ Sweating	Postganglionic sympathetic cholinergic transmission	↑ Sweating	Postganglionic parasympathetic cholinergic transmission
Penis	Ejaculation		Erection	Vasodilation

- For example, at the exact moment a sudden fear is made conscious, the sympathetic nervous system takes over. Bodily changes include a racing heart, dilated pupils, sweating, and skeletal muscle prepared for running.
- While the body is poising itself for escape, it recruits additional energy from systems that are not vital to surviving the encounter. For instance, sympathetic output shuts down all gut and genitourinary function, to allow all efforts to be put into the escape.
- See Table 2-1 for a summary of the actions of the sympathetic division of the nervous system.

a. **Functional anatomy** (Fig. 2-2)
   - Sympathetic nerves are different from skeletal motor nerves in that each sympathetic pathway is composed of two neurons, a **preganglionic neuron** and a **postganglionic neuron** (Table 2-2).

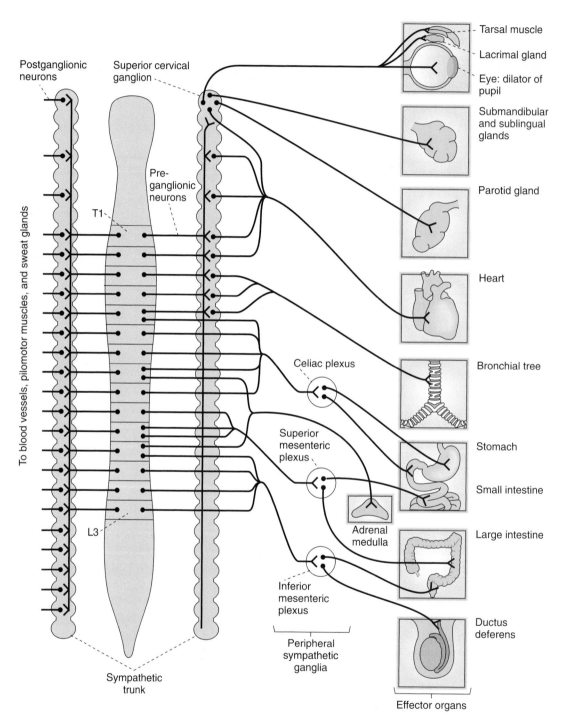

Postganglionic neurons

Superior cervical ganglion

Pre-ganglionic neurons

To blood vessels, pilomotor muscles, and sweat glands

T1

L3

Sympathetic trunk

Celiac plexus

Superior mesenteric plexus

Inferior mesenteric plexus

Adrenal medulla

Peripheral sympathetic ganglia

Tarsal muscle

Lacrimal gland

Eye: dilator of pupil

Submandibular and sublingual glands

Parotid gland

Heart

Bronchial tree

Stomach

Small intestine

Large intestine

Ductus deferens

Effector organs

2-2: *The sympathetic nervous system. L, lumbar; T, thoracic.*

TABLE 2-2:
Comparison of Neurons of the Autonomic and Somatic Nervous Systems

| Characteristic | AUTONOMIC | | SOMATIC | |
	Sympathetic	Parasympathetic	Sensory	Motor
Preganglionic neuron origin of ANS or location of cell body of 1st order neuron in somatic nervous system	Spinal cord segments T1–T12, L1–L3	Cranial nerve nuclei III, VII, IX, and X; spinal cord segments S2–S4	Dorsal root ganglia	Anterior horn of spinal cord
Preganglionic neuron length	Short	Long	—	—
Preganglionic neurotransmitter		ACh	—	—
Ganglia location	Paravertebral chain	Near effector organ	—	—
Postganglionic receptor	Nicotinic	Nicotinic	—	—
Postganglionic neuron length	Long	Short	—	—
Postganglionic neurotransmitter	Norepinephrine (except sweat glands which are acetylcholine)	Acetylcholine	Acetylcholine (at synapses in spinal cord)	Acetylcholine (in synapse at neuromuscular junction)
Effector organs	Cardiac and smooth muscle, glands	Cardiac and smooth muscle, glands	Brain and spinal cord	Skeletal muscle
Effector organ receptors	α_1, α_2, β_1, β_2	Muscarinic	Nicotinic	Nicotinic

*In the somatic nervous system there is a single neuron (rather than a preganglionic and a postganglionic neuron) that transmits an action potential either from the spinal cord to the effector or from the periphery/environment to the spinal cord.

- The **preganglionic** nerve fibers originate in the **intermediolateral horn of the spinal cord** between cord segments T1 and L2. They pass through the anterior roots of the cord via the white rami and do one of three things:
  (1) Synapse in the **paravertebral sympathetic chains of ganglia** that lie to the two sides of the vertebral column or in the two prevertebral ganglia (the **celiac** and **hypogastric ganglia**);
  (2) Pass upward or downward in the chain and synapse in one of the other ganglia;
  (3) Pass through one of the sympathetic nerves radiating outward from the chain and finally synapse in a **peripheral sympathetic ganglion.**
- The **postganglionic** fiber then exits the ganglion and projects to the **effector organ.**
- The **adrenal medulla** is a specialized ganglion of the **sympathetic division** that synthesizes and secretes **epinephrine** and **norepinephrine.** Preganglionic sympathetic fibers pass, without synapsing, from the

intermediolateral horn cells of the spinal cord, through the sympathetic chains and the splanchnic nerves, and finally to the adrenal medulla, where they synapse on the **chromaffin cells.**

- **Chromaffin cells** are modified neuronal cells that secrete **epinephrine** (80%) and **norepinephrine** (20%) into the bloodstream. These circulating hormones have almost the same effects on various organs as direct sympathetic stimulation, except that the effects last 5 to 10 times as long because of their slow removal from the bloodstream.

2. **The parasympathetic division: "rest and digest"**
   - The parasympathetic nervous system is called the "rest and digest" system because it is most active in times of rest, relaxation, and rejuvenation.
   - For instance, when a person is relaxed, his or her parasympathetic nervous system is in control. Pupils are constricted, glycogen is being stored, and digestion is occurring. Simultaneously, those organs activated in times of stress, such as skeletal and cardiac muscle, are relaxed. See Table 2-1 for a summary of the actions of the parasympathetic division of the nervous system.
   a. **Functional anatomy** (Fig. 2-3)
      - As in the sympathetic nervous system, parasympathetic pathways are composed of **preganglionic** and **postganglionic** neurons.
      - The **preganglionic** nerve fibers originate in **cranial nerve nuclei** in the brainstem and in the **intermediolateral horn of the spinal cord** between cord segments S2 and S4 (craniosacral origin).
      - These fibers pass uninterrupted all the way to the **effector organ**. In the wall of the effector organ, the preganglionic fibers synapse with very short **postganglionic fibers**, which in turn affect the function of the organ.

3. **The enteric nervous system**
   - This is contained entirely within the gut wall and is composed of the **submucosal (Meissner's) plexus** and the **myenteric (Auerbach's) plexus.**
   - Stimulation of the **submucosal plexus** promotes digestion, largely by stimulating secretions from the mucosal epithelium.
   - Stimulation of the **myenteric plexus** increases intestinal motility by stimulating peristalsis and inhibiting contraction of sphincter muscles throughout the intestinal tract.
   - The ANS can powerfully influence functioning of the enteric nervous system:
     (1) The sympathetic nervous system inhibits peristalsis and increases sphincter tone.
     (2) The parasympathetic system promotes peristalsis and relaxes the sphincters, thereby enhancing digestion.

> **Clinical note:** In **Hirschsprung's disease** (congenital aganglionic megacolon), the neural crest (ganglion) cells that form the myenteric plexus fail to migrate to the colon. The absence of these cells results in intestinal obstruction due to narrowing of the

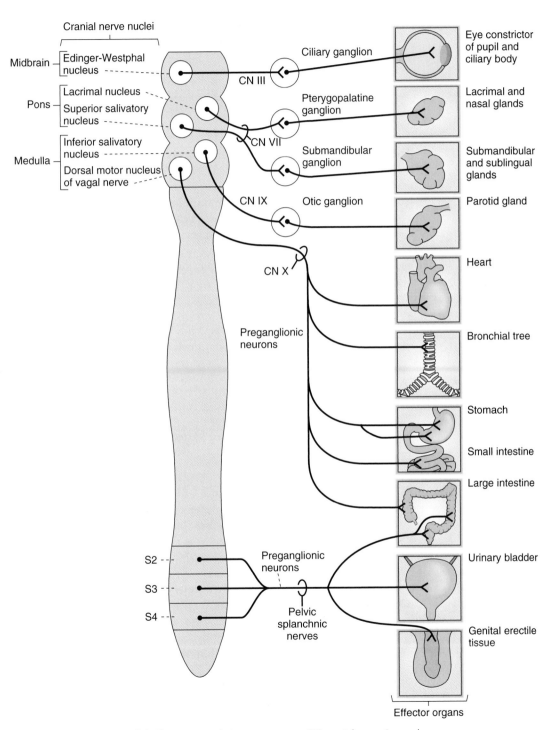

2-3: *The parasympathetic nervous system. CN, cranial nerve; S, sacral.*

affected "aganglionic" segment, causing **delayed passage of meconium** in the neonate, **abdominal distention,** and **vomiting.** The proximal portion of bowel is dilated (megacolon). Treatment involves resection of the narrow, aganglionic segment (samples are sent for pathologic analysis until ganglion cells are found in the bowel sections).

B. **Neurotransmitters of the ANS**
   - **Acetylcholine** (ACh) is a cholinergic neurotransmitter that is released from all preganglionic neurons. It is also released from postganglionic parasympathetic neurons.
   - **Norepinephrine** (NE) is an adrenergic neurotransmitter that is released from all postganglionic neurons of the sympathetic division except neurons that control the sweat glands and some blood vessels (which release ACh).
   - **Vasoactive inhibitory peptide** (VIP) and **substance P** are peptidergic neurotransmitters that are co-localized with ACh in some postganglionic parasympathetic fibers.
   - **Dopamine** is a neurotransmitter in the interneurons of the sympathetic ganglia.
   - **Nitric oxide** (NO) has a newly discovered role as a neurotransmitter, being responsible for the relaxation of smooth muscle and for penile erection.

   > **Pharmacology note:** Agents that mimic the actions of ACh (e.g., pilocarpine for contraction of ciliary muscle in glaucoma) are termed **cholinomimetics** (or **parasympathomimetics**). Agents that mimic the actions of epinephrine and norepinephrine (e.g., albuterol for bronchodilation in asthma) are termed **sympathomimetics.**

C. **Neurotransmitter receptor types**
   1. **Adrenergic receptors** (Table 2-3)
      - Located at sympathetic effector organs
      - **Norepinephrine** released from sympathetic neurons binds to these receptors, as do adrenal **catecholamines** (this is why the sympathetic nervous system is sometimes referred to as the **sympathoadrenal system**).
      - **Norepinephrine** has preferential affinity for **α-receptors** whereas **epinephrine** binds both **α-** and **β-receptors** with relatively equal affinity.
   2. **Cholinergic receptors** (Table 2-4; Fig. 2-4)
      - Located at parasympathetic effector organs (and a few sympathetic effector organs such as sweat glands), at preganglionic junctions innervated by both arms of the ANS, and on muscle cells in the somatic nervous system
      - Types: **muscarinic** and **nicotinic**
        (1) There are three well-characterized types of muscarinic receptors: **M1 (gastric, CNS), M2 (cardiac),** and **M3 (smooth muscle).**
        (2) There are two well-characterized types of nicotinic receptors: N_N **(preganglionic-postganglionic junction)** and N_M **(neuromuscular junction).**

TABLE 2-3:
Adrenergic Receptors

Receptor Subtype	Primary Locations	Normal Physiology Associated with Receptor Activation	Clinical Pharmacology
α_1	Vascular smooth muscle cells	Binding of catecholamines stimulates contraction usually via Gq subunit, causing vasoconstriction and increased blood pressure	α-Blockers (e.g., prazosin) lower blood pressure by reducing total peripheral resistance
α_2	Presynaptic	Binding of synaptic norepinephrine results in feedback inhibition via Gi subunit to regulate release of neurotransmitter	Centrally acting α_2-agonists (e.g., clonidine) inhibit sympathetic outflow. This lowers blood pressure by reducing cardiac output (by reducing heart rate and contractility) and lowering peripheral vascular resistance (by stimulating vasodilation)
β_1	Heart	Binding of catecholamines is generally stimulatory in nature, increasing cardiac contractility (positive inotropy) and heart rate (positive chronotropy)	Dopamine is indicated for hypovolemic shock (e.g., arterial hemorrhage); increases cardiac output but simultaneously stimulates renal vasodilation, thereby preserving renal perfusion
β_1-Blockers such as metoprolol lower blood pressure by reducing cardiac stroke volume and heart rate, both of which lower cardiac output
β_2	Vascular and nonvascular smooth muscle cells	Binding of catecholamines causes relaxation of muscle cells; bronchodilation and vasodilation in blood vessels of skeletal muscle during exercise (via regulation of myosin light chain kinase and myosin light chain phosphate activities)	β_2-Blockers (e.g., propranolol) are useful antihypertensives
β-Agonists (e.g., albuterol) are useful for stimulating bronchodilation in an asthmatic attack; such bronchodilation helps improve pulmonary ventilation during an asthmatic attack
β_3	Adipose	Lipolysis via stimulation of hormone-sensitive lipase (HSL)	β_3-Agonists may stimulate lipolysis and have potential role as weight-loss aids

IV. **Control of Movement**
- The control of movement is complex and involves coordinated functioning of multiple hierarchical structures within the CNS such as the motor cortices, basal ganglia, cerebellum, lower motor neurons, and the sensory system.
- Planning, initiation, and modification of movement is dependent on a proper functioning of the complicated interplay between a **CNS stimulus,** a **musculoskeletal effector,** and a **proprioceptive sensor.**
- Movements are classified as either voluntary or involuntary:
  (1) **Voluntary movements** require conscious planning, which occurs in cortical centers such as the premotor and motor cortices.
  (2) **Involuntary movements** or reflexes occur at an unconscious level; they are largely independent of cortical control and dependent on brainstem and spinal cord reflexes.
  A. **Motor neurons**
  - Muscles can be supplied by two types of motor neurons: **alpha motor neurons** and **gamma motor neurons.**

TABLE 2-4:
Acetylcholine Receptors (Cholinoceptors)

Receptor Subtype	Primary Locations	Normal Physiology Associated with Receptor Activation	Clinical Pharmacology
M1	Gastric, central nervous system	Parietal cell activity, neuronal activity	M1 antagonists (e.g., pirenzepine) are useful for treating ulcers
M2	Heart	Vagal release of acetylcholine has negative chronotropic effect on the heart and decreases blood pressure	M2 antagonists (e.g., atropine) are useful during surgery to prevent anesthetic-mediated bradycardia
M3	Smooth muscle	Contraction of smooth muscle (e.g., intestinal motility)	M3 agonists (e.g., pilocarpine) are used for contraction of ciliary muscle in glaucoma
N_N	Preganglionic-postganglionic junction	Stimulation of both arms of the autonomic nervous system	Low-level nicotine stimulation, high-level nicotine or ganglion blockers such as hexamethonium inhibit autonomic outflow
N_M	Neuromuscular junction	Generation of an end plate potential and action potential, resulting in contraction of skeletal muscle	Depolarizing neuromuscular agents (succinylcholine) and nondepolarizing neuromuscular agents (tubocurare) are used during surgeries

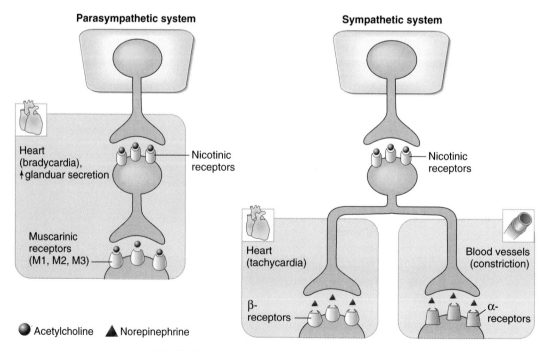

2-4: Cholinergic receptors in the autonomic nervous system.

TABLE 2-5:
Classification of Motor Nerve Fibers

Fiber Type	Diameter	Conduction Velocity	Function
Alpha (A-alpha)	Largest	Fastest	Supply extrafusal muscle fibers
Gamma (A-gamma)	Medium	Medium	Supply intrafusal muscle fibers
Preganglionic autonomic fibers (B)	Small	Medium	Control and regulate cardiac muscle, smooth muscle, and glands
Postganglionic autonomic fibers (C)	Smallest	Slowest	Control and regulate cardiac muscle, smooth muscle, and glands

- Alpha motor neurons are large, myelinated axons that innervate **extrafusal muscle fibers,** contraction of which causes movement at a joint.
- Gamma motor neurons are small, myelinated axons that innervate **intrafusal muscle fibers,** contraction of which does not result in movement but does play an important role in muscle tone and joint proprioception.
- These fibers are summarized in Table 2-5.

B. **Control of voluntary movement**
- Control of voluntary movement by the brain can be thought of as occurring in multiple stages.
  (1) The thought of performing the movement arises from the **premotor cortex.**
  (2) A specific motor plan is "selected" from the **motor cortex.**
  (3) The **basal ganglia** and **thalamus** then grant "permission" for the planned movement.
  (4) In the **motor cortex,** neurons "fire," activating descending **corticospinal fibers.**
  (5) These fibers then stimulate **alpha motor neurons,** which stimulate **muscle contraction** (performance of the movement).

C. **Role of the cerebral cortex in movement**
- The motor cortex of the frontal lobe is responsible for formation and execution of motor plans for voluntary movements.
- It comprises the premotor, supplementary, and primary motor cortices. The majority of descending corticospinal fibers originate from the motor cortices of the frontal lobe.
- Descending corticobulbar and corticospinal fibers travel through the **internal capsule** en route to their target nuclei in the brainstem and spinal cord, respectively.
- Stimulation of the primary motor cortex results in **discrete movements of contralateral muscles** (e.g., moving a finger) whereas stimulation of the association motor cortices results in more **complex, patterned movements** (e.g., waving the entire arm).

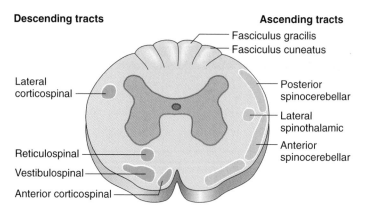

Descending tracts   **Ascending tracts**

Fasciculus gracilis
Fasciculus cuneatus

Lateral corticospinal

Posterior spinocerebellar

Lateral spinothalamic

Anterior spinocerebellar

Reticulospinal

Vestibulospinal

Anterior corticospinal

2-5: *Motor tracts of the spinal cord (also showing the sensory tracts, fasciculus gracilis, and fasciculus cuneatus).*

D. **Role of spinal cord tracts in movement** (Table 2-6)
  • Important in **rhythmic movements** such as chewing and swallowing, as well as **reflexive movements** such as withdrawal reflexes
  • Tracts can be divided anatomically into two categories, pyramidal and extrapyramidal.
    (1) The **pyramidal tracts** originate in the cerebral cortex, pass through the medullary pyramid, and terminate in the motor brainstem and spinal cord. They include the corticobulbar, lateral corticospinal, and ventral corticospinal tracts (Fig. 2-5).
    (2) The **extrapyramidal tracts** control motor activities but are not part of the pyramidal tracts. These include the rubrospinal, pontine and medullary reticulospinal, lateral and medial vestibulospinal, and tectospinal tracts.

> **Anatomy note:** The ventral horn is somatotopically organized, such that ventromedially located alpha motor neurons innervate axial and proximal muscles and dorsolaterally located alpha motor neurons control distal limb muscles.

1. **Medial descending system (MDS)**
  • The tracts of the MDS terminate in the ventromedial portion of the **anterior horn** (hence their name).
  • They influence activity of alpha motor neurons that control **axial** and **proximal muscles.**
  • They contribute to **posture control** by integrating visual, vestibular, and somatosensory information.

> **Clinical note:** Any lesion of the MDS may cause impaired control of the axial muscles, loss of balance while walking, and loss of corrective reflexes.

  a. **Lateral and medial vestibulospinal tracts**
    • Arise from **brainstem vestibular nuclei** and travel in the **anterior funiculus** of the spinal cord

TABLE 2-6:
Overview of Spinal Cord Tracts

Tract	Origin	Course	Termination	Function
Pyramidal				
Ventral corticospinal	Cerebral cortex at premotor cortex (Brodmann 6) and primary motor cortex (Brodmann 4)	Telencephalon: posterior limb of internal capsule Midbrain: crus cerebri Pons: basilar portion of pons Medulla: medullary pyramids	Spinal cord and synapse bilaterally with ventromedial cell column and adjoining portions of intermediate-zone horn motor neurons	Mediates voluntary skilled motor activity, primarily axial muscles
Lateral corticospinal	Cerebral cortex at premotor cortex (Brodmann 6), primary motor cortex (Brodmann 4), and primary sensory cortex (Brodmann 3, 1, and 2)	Telencephalon: posterior limb of internal capsule Midbrain: crus cerebri Pons: basilar portion of pons Medulla: medullary pyramids where the fibers decussate	Contralateral spinal cord, on motor nuclei in lateral part of anterior horn and to interneurons in the intermediate zone	Mediates voluntary skilled motor activity of the distal limbs and coarse regulation of the proximal limbs
Corticobulbar	Frontal eye fields (Brodmann 8 and 6), precentral gyrus (Brodmann 4), postcentral gyrus (Brodmann 3, 1, and 2)	Frontal eye field: caudal portions of anterior limb of internal capsule in telencephalon Precentral gyrus: genu of internal capsule Postcentral gyrus: rostral portions of posterior limb of internal capsule	Frontal eye field: rostral interstitial nucleus of medial longitudinal fasciculus and paramedian pontine reticular formation which project to the nuclei of III, IV, and VI Pre/post central gyrus: nuclei of cranial nerves V, VII, XI, and XII and nucleus ambiguus	Controls muscles of head and face
Extrapyramidal				
Rubrospinal	Red nucleus	Crosses to opposite side in the ventral tegmental decussation of lower brainstem and follows a course immediately adjacent and anterior to the corticospinal tracts	Interneurons in lateral columns of spinal cord	Stimulates flexors and inhibits extensors

continued

TABLE 2-6:
Overview of Spinal Cord Tracts—cont'd

Tract	Origin	Course	Termination	Function
Pontine reticulospinal	Nuclei in the pons	Descend in ventral column of spinal cord	Ipsilateral ventromedial spinal cord neurons	Stimulates flexors and extensors, with predominant effect on extensors
Medullary reticulospinal	Medullary reticular formation	Descend in ventral column of spinal cord	Spinal cord interneurons in intermediate gray area (synapses bilaterally with ipsilateral preponderance)	Inhibits extensors and flexors, with predominant effect on extensors
Lateral vestibulospinal	Dieters' nucleus	Descend in ventral column of spinal cord	Ipsilateral motoneurons and interneurons	Stimulates extensors and inhibits flexors
Tectospinal	Superior colliculus	Fibers cross in posterior tegmental decussation and descend in ventral column of spinal cord	Cervical spinal cord	Control of neck muscles

- Stimulate alpha motor neurons involved in excitation of **extensor antigravity muscles** (e.g., rectus femoris, triceps)
b. **Pontine (medial) and medullary (lateral) reticulospinal tracts**
  - Arise from the brainstem reticular formation.
  - The **pontine reticulospinal tract** descends in the anterior funiculus of the spinal cord and acts in concert with the vestibulospinal tracts, being excitatory to **extensor antigravity muscles.**
  - The **medullary reticulospinal tract** descends in the lateral funiculus of the spinal cord and is inhibitory to **extensor antigravity muscles.**
c. **Tectospinal tract**
  - Descends from **the superior colliculus** to the cervical segments of spinal cord
  - Important in **reflexive movements** of the **head** and **neck** in response to visual stimuli
d. **Ventral corticospinal tract**
  - Originates in the primary motor cortex and premotor cortex and descends in the **anterior funiculus** of the spinal cord, projecting bilaterally to the ventromedial portion of the anterior horn at the level at which it synapses
  - Important in the control of **axial** and **proximal muscles** (in contrast to the lateral corticospinal tract, which controls more distal muscles)

2. **Lateral descending system**
   - These tracts terminate in the dorsolateral portion of the anterior horn (hence their name).
   - They influence activity of the **distal limb muscles** and execution of more **complex motor plans,** especially of the arm and hand.
   a. **Lateral corticospinal tract**
      - Arises from the primary motor cortex, premotor cortex, and supplementary motor cortex.
      - After crossing sides (**decussation**) in the **caudal medulla,** these tracts descend in the **lateral funiculus** of the spinal cord and synapse on alpha motor neurons, controlling **distal limb muscles.**

      > **Clinical note:** A lesion of the **lateral corticospinal tract** can sometimes be appreciated by the presence of **Babinski's sign** on physical examination. In a healthy patient, stimulation of the plantar aspect of the foot normally results in downward movement of the big toe (plantar flexion). In a patient with a lesion of the pyramidal tract, however, the big toe may move upward (dorsiflexion) in response to plantar stimulation. When this occurs, Babinski's sign is said to be present.

   b. **Rubrospinal tract**
      - Descends in the **lateral funiculus** of the spinal cord and contributes to control of the activity of **flexor muscles.**
      - Despite its importance in other primates, it seems to play a limited role in humans.

3. **Relationship of upper and lower motor neurons**
   - The term **"upper motor neurons"** encompasses motor neurons originating (primarily) from the motor cortices that descend to synapse on lower motor neurons located in the brainstem and spinal cord.
   - The term **"lower motor neurons"** encompasses motor neurons originating in the brainstem and spinal cord and their path from their origin to the muscle they innervate.
   - **Upper motor neurons are tonically inhibitory to lower alpha motor neurons.** A lesion therefore causes *disinhibition* of lower motor neurons, resulting in spasticity and hyperreflexia (Table 2-7).

   > **Clinical note: Amyotrophic lateral sclerosis** (ALS) is a neurodegenerative disease characterized by loss of pyramidal cells in the motor cortex as well as loss of ventral horn cells throughout the spinal cord. The dysfunction of both upper and lower motor neurons results in clinical signs of both types of lesions occurring simultaneously (e.g., hyperreflexia in one limb with hyporeflexia in another).

E. **Role of the basal ganglia in movement**
   - The basal ganglia comprise subcortical (**basal**) clusters of nuclei (**ganglia**). They are important in the initiation of **voluntary movements,** becoming activated just before initiation of the movement.

TABLE 2-7:
Lesions of Upper and Lower Motor Neurons

Parameter	Upper Motor Neuron Lesion	Lower Motor Neuron Lesion
Cause	Lesion of cortex or corticospinal tract	Damage to lower motor neurons
Examples	Amyotrophic lateral sclerosis	Poliomyelitis and Werdnig-Hoffman disease
Clinical signs		
Babinski's sign	Present	Absent
Paralysis	Spastic	Flaccid
Muscle wasting	Absent or minimal	Present
Fasciculations	Absent	Present
Hyperreflexia or hyporeflexia	Hyperreflexia, clonus	Hyporeflexia
Deep tendon reflexes	Hyperactive	Absent

TABLE 2-8:
Basal Ganglia Terms

Basal Ganglia Term	Composition
Striatum	Putamen and caudate nucleus
Corpus striatum	Striatum and lentiform nucleus
Lentiform nucleus	Putamen and globus pallidus

- They include the putamen and caudate nucleus (collectively termed the "striatum"), globus pallidus, substantia nigra, and subthalamic nucleus (Table 2-8).
- **Output** of the basal ganglia is to the motor **thalamus,** which in turn projects to the **motor cortex.** Basal ganglia output is always **inhibitory** in nature.
- The basal ganglia influence movement through one of two pathways, the **direct** or the **indirect pathway.**
- Lesions of the basal ganglia give rise to **contralateral motor deficits.**
1. **The direct pathway** (Fig. 2-6)
   - Activated by binding of dopamine to **D1 receptors** in the striatum
   - **Direct inhibition** of basal ganglia output to the motor thalamus
   - Because the output is always inhibitory, the result is **_dis_inhibition** of the **motor thalamus,** thereby allowing excitatory thalamocortical projections to stimulate the motor cortex to **promote movement.**
2. **The indirect pathway** (see Fig. 2-6)
   - Inhibited by binding of dopamine to **D2 receptors** in the striatum
   - **Indirect stimulation,** via the subthalamic nucleus, of basal ganglia output to the motor thalamus
   - Because the basal ganglia output is always inhibitory, the result is **inhibition** of the **motor thalamus,** and hence **inhibition of movement.**

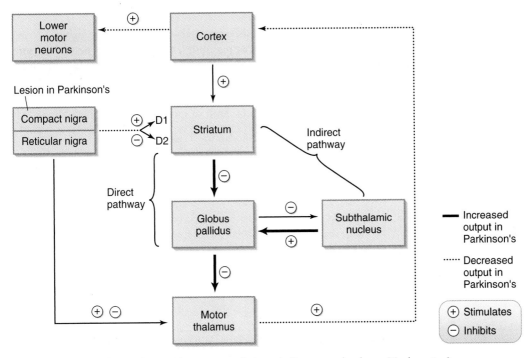

2-6: *The direct and indirect pathways. Changes seen in Parkinson's disease are also shown. D1, dopamine-1 receptor; D2, dopamine-2 receptor.*

Clinical note: Parkinson's disease is a degenerative disease involving the **loss of dopaminergic neurons** in the **substantia nigra.** The loss of dopaminergic transmission (see Fig. 2-6) causes a relative deficiency of dopamine and excess of ACh in the striatum. Gross specimens show a loss of pigmentation in the substantia nigra. Histology shows Lewy bodies (intracytoplasmic, round, eosinophilic inclusion bodies). Patients present with a resting, "pill-rolling" tremor that disappears with movement, slowing of all voluntary movements, expressionless face, cogwheel rigidity of limbs, and a wide-based shuffling gait. Treatment consists of **dopamine agonists** (or precursors such as levodopa) and **anticholinergics** such as atropine.

F. **Role of the cerebellum in movement**
   - The cerebellum is important in coordinating **speed, trajectory,** and **force** of movements *as they occur.* It is also important in the maintenance of **posture** and **equilibrium.**
   - To perform these functions, the cerebellum must process *in real time* an enormous amount of information received from the body's muscles, joints, and limbs.
   - In functional terms, the cerebellum is divided into three divisions: pontocerebellum, spinocerebellum, and vestibulocerebellum.

1. **Pontocerebellum (neocerebellum, cerebrocerebellum)**
   - Consists of the lateral zones of the cerebellar hemispheres, is highly developed, and is crucial to the **planning** and **timing** of **sequential motor movements**
   - Receives large input from **motor cortex**
   - Efferent output from **dentate nucleus** to **red nucleus** and **thalamus**
   - Lesions of the pontocerebellum result in incoordination of the limbs.

   > **Clinical note: Lateral cerebellar lesions** cause a defect known as **"decomposition of movement."** The result is a disruption in the timing of the components of a movement, which appear to take place sequentially rather than being coordinated smoothly. However, remaining portions of the motor control system are often able to compensate. Serious and permanent damage occurs when lesions affect the deep cerebellar nuclei—the dentate, interposed, and fastigial nuclei—in addition to the cerebellar cortex.

2. **Spinocerebellum (paleocerebellum)**
   - Responsible for smooth **coordination** of **movements** of the distal limbs (especially the hands and fingers) for the performance of precise and purposeful movements
   - Receives input from two areas when a movement is performed:
     (1) **Direct information** from the **motor cortex and red nucleus** informing the cerebellum of the intended plan of movement
     (2) **Feedback information** from the peripheral parts of the body (via **muscle spindles** and **Golgi tendon organs**) indicating what actual movement resulted

   > **Clinical note:** Lesions of the **interposed nuclei,** which is located in the **spinocerebellum,** result in dysmetria (inability to control range of movement), ataxia (loss of coordination of movements), terminal tremor (attempts to correct abnormal movement result in a tremor), and pendular reflexes (limb oscillates instead of returning to original position and stopping).

3. **Vestibulocerebellum (archicerebellum)**
   - Important in **posture, equilibrium,** and **control of eye movements**
   - Receives input directly from the **vestibular apparatus** via the eighth cranial nerve (CN VII) and indirectly via the vestibular nuclei
   - Efferent output is largely from the **fastigial nucleus** to the **vestibular nuclei** and influences the ascending medial longitudinal fasciculus (coordination of eye movements) and the descending medial and lateral vestibulospinal tracts.
   - Lesions result in pendular **nystagmus** and truncal **ataxia** (Table 2-9).

   > **Clinical note:** The cerebellum plays an important role in maintenance of equilibrium. It achieves this by receiving sensory information from the eye and the vestibular apparatus of the inner ear and proprioceptive input from the muscles and joints via the spinocerebellar tracts.

TABLE 2-9:
Motor Deficits Associated with Cerebellar Lesions

Sign	Description
Nystagmus	Rapid back-and-forth movements of the eye (e.g., pendular vs vestibular nystagmus), with the fast phase of nystagmus pointing toward the lesion (i.e., direction of eye gaze in fast phase "points" to the lesion)
Dysarthria	Difficulty in producing coherent speech because of inability to coordinate laryngeal muscles (not to be confused with aphasias, caused by damage to the cerebral cortex)
Ataxia	Incoordination of movements or gait (trunkal ataxia). Patients typically fall to side of lesion (recall that cerebellar lesions produce ipsilateral deficits)
Intention tremor	Tremor appears only during a voluntary movement
Dysdiadochokinesia	Inability to coordinate rapidly alternating movements, such as rapid pronation and supination at the wrist
Dysmetria	Inability to properly judge distances: overshooting (hypermetria) or undershooting the target (hypometria)

*Cerebellar lesions typically give rise to ipsilateral effects (in contrast to lesions of the basal ganglia and cerebral cortex).

Cerebellar disease can be detected by the **Romberg test.** While performing the Romberg test, the patient is asked to close the eyes and stand with the feet close together. Closing the eyes leaves only vestibular and proprioceptive input to the cerebellum, which is sufficient to maintain balance if they are fully functional. However, in the presence of vestibular disease (e.g., vestibulitis) or sensory deficits (e.g., diabetic neuropathy), the cerebellum may not be able to function effectively, and the patient will be unable to maintain appropriate balance. If vestibular disease and sensory deficits can be ruled out by examination or history, then a positive Romberg test implies primary cerebellar disease.

V. **The Sensory System**
- The sensory system comprises touch, proprioception, vibration, temperature, vision, olfaction, taste, and audition.
  A. **Sensory receptors**
    - **Sensory receptors** are specialized **nerve cells** that detect environmental stimuli and transduce them via neural signals. There are several different types (Table 2-10).
    - A **receptive field** is an area of the sensory surface (e.g., skin) to which the application of appropriate stimuli causes a response in a sensory receptor. These receptive fields allow the body to be topographically mapped (by their receptors) throughout the whole nervous system, from the skin to the brain.

TABLE 2-10:
Classification of Sensory Nerve Fibers

Fiber Type	Diameter	Conduction Velocity	Function
Ia (A-alpha)	Largest	Fastest	Muscle spindles/proprioception
Ib (A-alpha)	Largest	Fastest	Golgi tendon organs/proprioception
II (A-beta)	Medium	Medium	Touch, pressure, and vibration
III (A-delta)	Small	Medium	Slow pain and temperature
IV (C)	Smallest	Slowest	Slow pain and temperature, unmyelinated

- Some signals need to be transmitted to the CNS rapidly, whereas others can be transmitted more slowly; therefore, different types of sensory fibers have different sizes and velocities.

B. **Sensory transduction**
  - A process whereby a stimulus is detected, amplified, and "conducted" to its ultimate target
  - Signal transduction typically occurs through changes in membrane potential.
  - All sensory receptors have one feature in common: once stimulated, the immediate effect is to change the membrane electrical potential of the receptor. This change is called a **receptor potential.**
  - The receptor potential is achieved by opening ion channels, allowing current to flow. In most cases, the flow is **inward** and the receptor is **depolarized.** If the receptor potential is large enough, the membrane potential reaches or exceed **threshold,** and **action potentials** fire.
  - The **signal intensity** (e.g., intensity of pain) can be conveyed by using increased numbers of parallel fibers or by sending increased numbers of "nerve impulses" (action potentials):
    (1) **Spatial summation:** Increased signal strength is transmitted by using progressively greater numbers of fibers.
    (2) **Temporal summation:** Increased signal strength is transmitted by increasing the frequency of action potentials in each fiber.

C. **Adaptation**
  - A special characteristic of all sensory receptors is that they **adapt,** either partially or completely, to any constant stimulus after a period of time.
  - **Slowly adapting (tonic)** receptors continue to transmit impulses to the brain as long as the stimulus is present. Thus, they keep the brain constantly aware of the status of the body and its relation to its surroundings. They include **muscle spindles, pressure receptors,** and **slow pain** receptors.
  - **Rapidly adapting (phasic)** receptors rapidly adapt to a constant stimulus by decreasing their action potential frequency over time. They are stimulated by changes in stimulus strength and primarily alert the brain to the start and stop of a stimulus. They include **light touch receptors** (e.g., Meissner's corpuscles) and **deep pressure receptors** (e.g., Pacinian corpuscles).

D. **Sensory pathways**
- A **sensory pathway** is a group of neurons linked synaptically that share a common function and course.
- The **sensory receptor** is stimulated and a **receptor potential** is created (i.e., electrical energy).
- The signal from the receptor is received by **first-order neurons (primary afferent neurons),** the cell bodies of which are located in the **dorsal root ganglia.**
- The **second-order neurons,** located in the spinal cord or brainstem, receive signals from the first-order neurons and transmit them to the **thalamus.** It is important to note that the axons of these neurons **cross the midline** at a relay nucleus in the spinal cord before synapsing in the thalamus; therefore, **sensory information originating on one side of the body communicates with the contralateral thalamic nuclei.**
- The **third-order neurons** are located in the relay nuclei of the thalamus, the ventral posterior nucleus, and send the signal to the cerebral cortex.
- The **fourth-order neurons,** located in the cerebral cortex, confer **conscious perception** of the stimulus. The orientation of these neurons in the cortex creates a **sensory homunculus,** which is essentially a map of the body on the brain (Fig. 2-7).

E. **Specific pathways of the somatosensory system**
   1. **Dorsal column system (DCS): medial lemniscal pathway**
      - The DCS processes the sensations of fine touch, pressure, proprioception, two-point discrimination, and vibration.
      - **Primary afferents** travel ipsilaterally up the spinal cord to synapse on the **nucleus gracilis** and **nucleus cuneatus** in the medulla.
      - The **second-order neurons** decussate in the medulla via the internal arcuate fibers and ascend via the **medial lemnisci** to the **contralateral ventral posterolateral nucleus** of the thalamus. Here, **third-order neurons** project to the cortex to synapse with **fourth-order neurons,** and the sensation is made conscious.

> **Clinical note:** A **lesion of the DCS** results in a deficit in fine touch, pressure, proprioception, two-point discrimination, and vibration on the **ipsilateral** side of the body below the level of the lesion. The damage is ipsilateral because the fibers of the DCS do not cross the midline until they reach the medulla. Damage to the DCS is also evident in several disease states. For example in **tabes dorsalis,** a late stage manifestation of syphilis, neurons in the dorsal root ganglia are destroyed, which in turn causes degeneration of the myelinated afferent fibers in the dorsal columns. Signs include an ataxic wide-based gait, paresthesias, and deficits in touch and proprioception. Damage to the DCS may also be seen in long-term **cobalamin (vitamin B$_{12}$) deficiency** secondary to pernicious anemia; this leads to demyelination, axonal degeneration, and eventual neuronal death; the DCS is usually involved, resulting in numbness and paresthesias in the extremities, weakness, and ataxia.

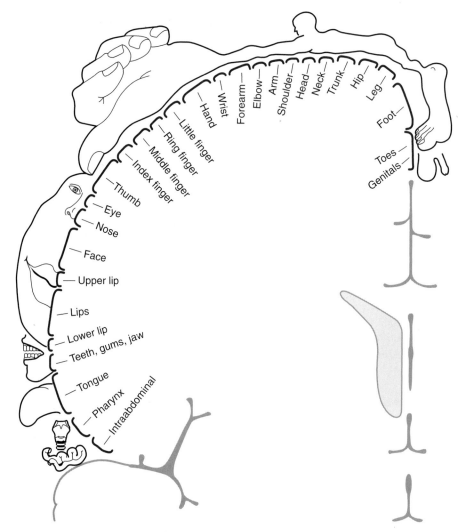

2-7: *Sensory homunculus. Note that the face, hands, and fingers—areas where precise localization is critical—represent the largest areas of the homunculus.*

2. **Anterolateral system (ALS)**
   - The ALS processes the sensations of **pain, temperature,** and **crude touch.**
   - **Primary afferents** enter the spinal cord and synapse in the **dorsal horn.**
   - The **second-order neurons** then **cross the midline in the spinal cord** at the **anterior commissure** and ascend via the anterior spinothalamic tract and lateral spinothalamic tract to the contralateral thalamus.
   - **Third-order neurons** project to the cortex and synapse with **fourth-order neurons,** as in the DCS.

> **Clinical note:** A **lesion of the ALS** results in a deficit in pain, temperature, and crude touch on the **contralateral side** of the body below the level of the lesion. For instance, a lesion at T8 affects everything below that point on the contralateral side; the upper extremity is not affected, because it is above the site of injury. In general, pain and temperature deficits secondary to ALS injury are more prominent than crude touch deficits, because the intact DCS and provides an alternative means of experiencing touch in the affected areas.

F. **Special aspects of the somatosensory system**
   1. **Thalamus**
      • Arranged somatotopically
      • Is the primary relay point between the cortex and lower-order afferents

      > **Clinical note: Destruction of thalamic nuclei** results in loss of sensation on the **contralateral** side of the body.

   2. **Physiology of pain perception**
      a. **Pain receptors**
         • Pain receptors are free nerve endings that are located in the skin, muscle, and viscera and are responsible for **nociception** (the detection and perception of pain).
         • In contrast to other receptors of the body, pain receptors adapt very little and sometimes not at all.
      b. **Pain fibers**
         • **Fast pain** is carried by **group III fibers** and is described as sharp, pricking, acute, or electric pain. It is **well localized** and has a rapid onset and offset. An example is pain experienced by stepping on a tack or stubbing a toe.
         • **Slow pain** is carried by **C fibers** and is described as burning, aching, throbbing, or chronic pain. It is **poorly localized** and sometimes vague. Examples include chronic back pain, headache pain, and aching joints.
   3. **Dermatomes** (Fig. 2-8; Table 2-11)
      • A dermatome is a localized area of skin that is innervated by a single nerve originating from a single nerve root.
      • Knowledge of dermatome distribution can help localize nerve injury with physical examination.

      > **Anatomy note:** Pain from viscera is often referred to sites on the skin; this is called **referred pain.** The pain is usually experienced in the dermatome supplied by the spinal nerve that enters the spinal cord at the same level as the visceral nerve (Table 2-12).

VI. **Special Senses**
   • A number of senses are called "special" senses because to function they employ modified and unique CNS components.

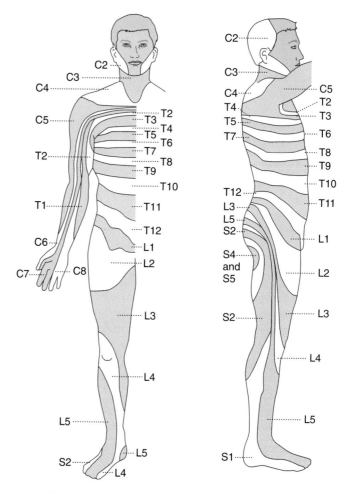

2-8: *Dermatomes. C, cranial; L, lumbar; S, sacral; T, thoracic.*

- They comprise vision, hearing (audition), equilibrium (the vestibular system), olfaction, and taste.
A. **Vision**
  - Perception of a visual stimulus occurs in several stages.
  - Light enters the eye through the **cornea,** the amount of light passing through the cornea being determined by the size of the **pupil** (Fig. 2-9).
  - It then passes through the **lens,** the shape of which is adjusted by intraocular muscles to focus light on the **retina.**
  - Photoreceptors on the retina transmit signals to the brain (through the optic nerve), at which point the visual stimulus is perceived.
  1. **Structure of the retina** (Fig. 2-10)
     - The retina is a sheet of photoreceptors on the posterior aspect of the orbit. It lies in front of epithelium that is filled with the black pigment **melanin,** which functions to absorb any light not captured by the retina.

TABLE 2-11:
Dermatomes Important in Clinical Diagnosis and
Identification of Level of Spinal Cord Injury

Dermatome	Area Innervated
C3	Front and back of neck
C6	Thumb, pointer finger, lateral forearm
C7	Middle finger
C8	Ring and little finger, medial hand
T10	Umbilicus
L1	Inguinal
L3	Knee
L5	Anterior ankle and foot, and first three toes
S1	Heel, plantar surface of foot (all toes except big toe), and fourth and fifth toes on dorsum of foot
S3/4	Genital area
S5	Perianal

TABLE 2-12:
Referred Pain

Site of Pain	Organs from Which Pain Is Referred
Lower abdomen (above pubic bone)	Large bowel, bladder
Umbilical region	Small bowel, pancreas
Upper abdomen	Duodenum, stomach
Behind sternum	Esophagus, trachea
Tip of shoulder	Diaphragm
Chest (central), arms (usually left arm), neck, abdomen (occasionally)	Heart
Back of head and neck	Meninges

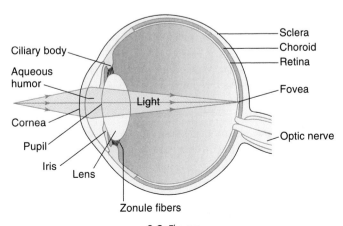

2-9: *The eye.*

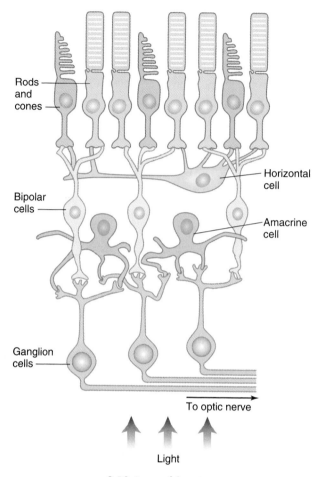

Rods and cones

Horizontal cell

Bipolar cells

Amacrine cell

Ganglion cells

To optic nerve

Light

2-10: *Layers of the retina.*

- It has several layers of different types of cells, all of which are necessary for proper vision.
- The most posterior layer is composed of photoreceptor cells, the rods, and cones.
- The **optic disc** is where the axons of the ganglion cells converge to exit the retina as the optic nerve. There are no rods or cones in the optic disc, which results in a *blind spot.*

a. **Rods**
  - These photoreceptors are very sensitive to light but do not detect color–they are responsible for low-acuity vision at night, when the light supply is poor.
  - They are more numerous than cones and are located diffusely throughout the retina but not in the macula.
  - Their photosensitive element is **rhodopsin,** which is composed of **11-*cis*-retinal** and **scotopsin.**

- When exposed to light, rhodopsin decomposes to **all-*trans*-retinal** and then to other intermediate compounds; this triggers an electrical impulse that is sent to the occipital lobe of the brain.

> **Clinical note:** Vitamin A is needed to form retinal, which is part of the rhodopsin molecule. In vitamin A deficiency, there is not enough vitamin A to form sufficient amounts of rhodopsin, resulting in poor night vision.

  b. **Cones**
  - These photoreceptors are less sensitive to light but do detect color—they are responsible for high-acuity color vision during the day, when the light supply is good.
  - They are less numerous than rods and are concentrated in the fovea centralis of the macula.
  - Their photosensitive elements are **color pigments.**

2. **Visual pathways** (Fig. 2-11)
  - Once light stimulates rods and cones, they stimulate the next layer of cells, the **bipolar cells.** In turn these stimulate **ganglion cells,** which lie in the most anterior layer of the retina and the axons of which form the **optic nerve.**
  - The optic nerve (CN II) receives the image and projects to the **optic chiasm.** The optic tract projects from the optic chiasm and synapses with the **lateral geniculate body** (LGB).
    (1) Ganglion cells from the **nasal hemiretina** project to the **contralateral LGB,** whereas cells from the **temporal hemiretina** project to the **ipsilateral LGB.** This concept is important in understanding lesions and the visual defects that result.
    (2) The **optic radiation (geniculocalcarine tract)** then projects from the LGB via an upper and lower division to the **visual cortex (Brodmann's area 17).** The **visual cortex** is retinotopically organized in that the posterior area receives **macular input** (central vision), the intermediate area receives **perimacular input** (peripheral vision), and the anterior area receives monocular input. It is in the visual cortex that the signals are finally interpreted and the image is ultimately "seen."
  - Two accessory cell types in the retina also aid in vision: **horizontal cells** transmit signals horizontally in the outer layer from the photoreceptors to the bipolar cells; **amacrine cells** transmit signals between the bipolar cells and ganglion cells in the inner layer.

3. **Ocular reflexes**
  a. **Pupillary light reflex**
  - This reflex prevents excessive radiation from entering the eye when light intensity is high.
  - It can be elicited by shining light in one eye. A normal response is constriction of both pupils. Constriction of the pupil the light is directed at is termed the **"direct response,"** and constriction of the other eye is termed the **"consensual response."**

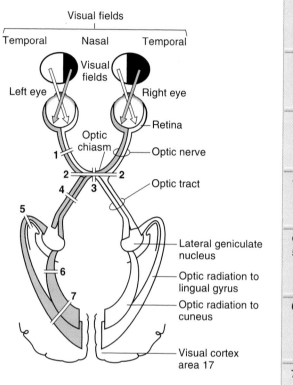

Lesion	Visual defect
1. Optic nerve	Ipsilateral blindness
Optic chiasm 2. Bilateral lateral compression	Binasal hemianopia
3. Midsagittal transection/pressure	Bitemporal hemianopia
4. Optic tract (left)	Right hemianopia
Optic radiation (left) 5. Lower division	Right upper quandrantanopia
6. Upper division	Right lower quandrantanopia
7. Both divisions	Right hemianopia with macular sparing

2-11: *The visual pathways, showing the consequences of lesions at various points.*

- The **consensual response** occurs because
  (1) Impulses from the retina of the eye into which the light is shone pass via the optic nerve (CN II) to the **pretectal area** of the midbrain.
  (2) Cells in the pretectal area relay the impulse to the **Edinger-Westphal** (accessory oculomotor) **nuclei** of both eyes.
  (3) Each nucleus contains preganglionic parasympathetic neurons that in turn send the signal to the **ciliary ganglion** of the corresponding eye via the oculomotor nerve (CN III).
  (4) Postganglionic parasympathetic neurons in the ciliary ganglia innervate the smooth muscle of the pupillary sphincters. Thus, pupil **constriction is bilateral.**

Clinical note: Deficits in the pupillary light reflex are evident in several different CNS diseases, including neurosyphilis, alcoholism, and encephalitis. Any damage to either Edinger-Westphal nucleus results in an abnormal or absent reflex. An **Argyll Robertson pupil,** often a sign of neurosyphilis, is one that constricts with accommodation but not in response to light.

    b. **Accommodation reflex**
- This brings nearby objects into proper focus.
- When a distant object is brought close to the eyes, the focal point is initially behind the retina, resulting in a blurred image. In the **accommodation reflex,** parasympathetic outflow from the Edinger-Westphal nuclei causes contraction of the **ciliary muscle,** resulting in less tension in the **suspensory ligaments.** This causes the lens to take on a more convex shape, increasing its **refractive power** so that the image is accurately focused on the retina.
- Parasympathetic outflow also contracts the radial fibers of the **iris (sphincter pupillae),** decreasing the amount of light that enters the pupil; this results in better **focusing** of the light and less scattering.
- There is simultaneous contraction of the **medial recti,** which results in **convergence** of the eyes onto the near object.

B. **Audition**
    1. **Structure of the ear** (Fig. 2-12)
- The **outer ear** consists of the pinna and the external auditory canal.

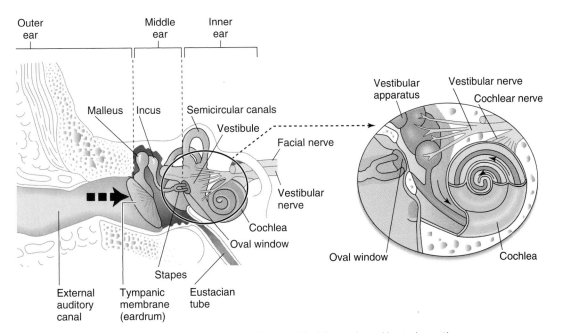

2-12: Structure of the ear (anterior view). In the inset, the direction of fluid flow in the cochlea is shown. The shaded areas of the vestibular system (inset) are the areas that bear hair cells.

- The **middle ear** comprises the tympanic membrane and three **ossicles** (small bones): malleus, incus, and stapes.
- The **inner ear** is fluid filled and consists of
  (1) The bony labyrinth: semicircular canals, cochlea, and vestibule
  (2) A series of ducts called the **membranous labyrinth.** Fluid is located both inside the ducts (**endolymph**) and outside the ducts (**perilymph**).
- The **cochlea** (Fig. 2-13) consists of three tubular canals, the **scala vestibuli** and **scala tympani,** both of which contain perilymph (high Na^+), and the **scala media,** which contains endolymph (high K^+).
- The cochlea is bordered by the **basilar membrane**, which houses the **organ of Corti** (see Fig. 2-13).
- The **organ of Corti** contains the receptor cells necessary for audition: the **inner** and **outer hair cells.** These have **cilia** that are embedded in the **tectorial membrane** of the organ of Corti.
  (1) **Inner hair cells** are the **primary sensory elements;** they are arranged in single rows and are few in number. They synapse with myelinated neurons, axons of which comprise 90% of the **cochlear nerve.**
  (2) **Outer hair cells** serve to **reduce the threshold of the inner hair cells.** They are arranged in parallel rows and are greater in number than the inner cells. They synapse with dendrites of unmyelinated neurons, axons of which comprise 10% of the **cochlear nerve.**

2. **Perception of sound**
- The outer ear directs sound waves into the external auditory canal.
- The waves travel until they reach the air-filled middle ear, where they cause **the tympanic membrane** to vibrate.
- This vibration causes the ossicles to vibrate, resulting in **amplification** of the sound energy and **displacement of the fluid** in the inner ear.

> **Clinical note: Conduction deafness** results from impairment of external or middle ear structures that conduct sound into the cochlea. Common causes are cerumen impaction (obstruction), otitis media, and otosclerosis.

a. **Auditory transduction**
- This is the process in which a sound wave is turned into an electrical message; it occurs in the **organ of Corti.**
- The external and middle structures of the ear collect sound, amplify it, and transmit it to the inner ear, specifically the organ of Corti. This transmission causes vibrations of the **basilar membrane.**
- Vibrations of the basilar membrane stimulate the cilia of the inner and outer hair cells, causing the **hair cells to bend** by a shearing force as they push against the tectorial membrane.
- Bending of the cilia causes **changes in the K^+ conductance** of the hair cell membrane. Bending in one direction causes **depolarization;** in the other, **hyperpolarization.** The bending back and forth also causes a **cochlear microphonic potential,** which results in intermittent **firing of the cochlear nerves.**

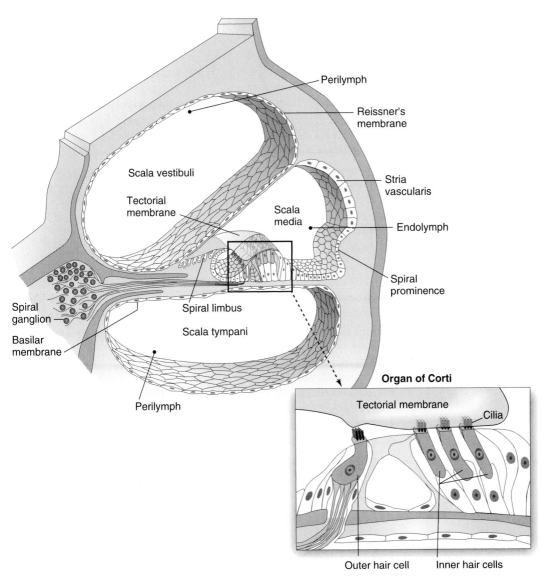

Perilymph

Reissner's membrane

Scala vestibuli

Stria vascularis

Tectorial membrane

Scala media

Endolymph

Spiral prominence

Spiral ganglion

Spiral limbus

Basilar membrane

Scala tympani

Perilymph

Organ of Corti

Tectorial membrane

Cilia

Outer hair cell   Inner hair cells

2-13: The cochlea.

- On depolarization, the hair cells activate the **bipolar cells** of the **spiral (cochlear) ganglion.** This ganglion projects centrally as the **cochlear nerve (CN VIII).**
  (1) The **cochlear nerve** enters the brainstem at the **cerebellopontine angle** and synapses with the **cochlear nuclei.**

(2) Axons from the cochlear nuclei then project **contralaterally** to the **superior olivary nucleus** (sound localization) and then to the **lateral lemniscus.**

(3) Axons project from the lateral lemniscus to the **nucleus of the inferior colliculus.**

(4) These axons then project to the **medial geniculate body.**

(5) Axons of the medial geniculate body then travel through the internal capsule as the **auditory radiation**, which synapses with the **primary auditory cortex (Brodmann's areas 41 and 42).**

> **Clinical note: Sensorineural deafness** is caused by damage to the inner ear, auditory nerve, or central auditory pathway. In **presbycusis,** a common condition in older adults associated with high-frequency (4000–8000 Hz) hearing loss, degenerative disease of the base of the basilar membrane and loss of hair cells in the organ of Corti are the primary reasons for the hearing loss.

b. **Sound encoding**
- Different frequencies of sound stimulate different hair cells, depending on their location along the basilar membrane of the cochlea. This is **sound encoding.**
- **High frequencies** cause hair cells at the **base** of the basilar membrane, near the oval and round windows, to vibrate.
- **Low frequencies** cause hair cells at the **apex** of the basilar membrane, near the helicotrema, to vibrate.
- Thus, when evaluating hearing loss, the location of damage can be identified on the basis of whether the loss is low or high frequency.

> **Clinical note: Rinne's test** is used to compare bone and air conduction. The base of a vibrating tuning fork is placed on the mastoid process until the patient can no longer hear the bone-conducted vibration; at this point, the vibrating end of the fork is repositioned about 1 cm from the external meatus, and the patient is asked if anything can be heard. Normally and in sensorineural deafness, air conduction is better than bone conduction in both ears; in conduction deafness, bone conduction is better (Table 2-13).

> **Clinical note: Weber's test** is performed by placing a vibrating tuning fork on the vertex of the skull and asking the patient if the sound is the same in both ears. Normally, the sound is heard equally on both sides (see Table 2-13). In **conduction deafness** the sound is heard better in the ear most affected by deafness, and in **sensorineural deafness** it is heard better in the unaffected ear.

C. **The vestibular system (vestibular organ)**
- The vestibular system maintains posture and equilibrium (balance) and coordinates head and eye movements.

TABLE 2-13:
Interpretation of Auditory Tests

Finding	Rinne's Test—Comparison of Air and Bone Conduction	Weber's Test—Sound Lateralizes to
Normal findings	Air > bone, both ears	(No lateralization)
Left ear		
Conduction deafness	Bone > air on *left* Air > bone on *right*	*Left* ear
Partial sensorineural deafness	Air > bone, both ears	*Right* ear
Right Ear		
Conduction deafness	Bone > air on *right* Air > bone on *left*	*Right* ear
Partial sensorineural deafness	Air > bone, both ears	*Left* ear

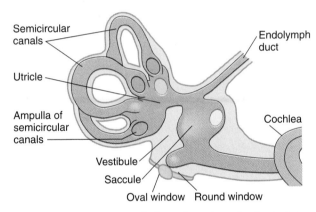

2-14: *The vestibular system (anterior view). The hair cells are located in the shaded areas (maculae).*

1. **Structure of the vestibular organ** (Fig. 2-14)
   - The **vestibular organ** is a membranous labyrinth consisting of three perpendicular semicircular canals, a utricle, and a saccule, all interconnecting and filled with endolymph.
   - The **semicircular canals** detect **rotation** or angular acceleration.
   - The **utricle** and the **saccule** detect **linear acceleration.**
   - Each semicircular canal contains **hair cells (receptor cells).** Each hair cell has two types of cilia that are embedded in a gelatinous structure called the **cupula:** a **kinocilium,** the longest cilium on each hair cell, and other smaller cilia called **stereocilia.**
   - The hair cells are innervated by peripheral processes of **bipolar cells,** which are housed in the **vestibular ganglion** of the internal auditory meatus. The central projecting portions of the bipolar cells form the **vestibular portion of CN VIII,** which projects to the **vestibular nuclei** and **flocculonodular lobe** of the **cerebellum.**

- The **vestibular nuclei,** which receive input from both the hair cells and the flocculonodular lobe, project fibers to
  (1) The flocculonodular lobe and CNs III, IV, and VI via the **medial longitudinal fasciculus** (MLF)
  (2) The spinal cord via the lateral vestibulospinal tract
  (3) The ventral posteroinferior and posterolateral nuclei of the thalamus (both of which project to the postcentral gyrus)

2. **Vestibular transduction**
   - The process of vestibular transduction is similar to that of auditory transduction in that the bending of hair cells "translates" movement into a change in electrical potential.
   - With rotation, the cupula rotate in the same direction as the movement.
   - Initially, the cupula moves faster than the endolymph, which results in the cilia's being bent.
     (1) If the **stereocilia** bend **toward** the **kinocilium,** the hair cell is **depolarized** and excited.
     (2) If the **stereocilia** bend **away** from the **kinocilium,** the hair cell is **hyperpolarized** and inhibited.
   - Once the endolymph "catches up" with the cupula, the cilia return to an upright position, at which point the hair cells are no longer depolarized or hyperpolarized.

> **Clinical note:** Injury to the vestibulocerebellar pathway results in a staggering ataxic gait with a tendency to fall toward the side of the lesion. Injury to this system also results in a spontaneous nystagmus, as discussed later, and vertigo. Nystagmus is normally a corrective reflex.

3. **Vestibular-ocular reflexes**
   - The vestibular-ocular reflexes stabilize visual images by compensating for head movement.
   - The reflexes are mediated by the vestibular nuclei, MLF, ocular motor nuclei, and CNs III, IV, and VI.
   - **Nystagmus** is a repetitive pattern of eye movement that results from the slow and quick phases of eye movement and is the reflex used to compensate for head movement; it can be clinically relevant, as noted earlier in vestibulocerebellar injury. The direction of nystagmus is defined as the direction of the fast (rapid eye) movement. The vestibular system drives the slow phase of eye movement, and the brainstem generates the quick phase.
   a. **Vestibular (horizontal) nystagmus**
      - Resets eye position during sustained rotation of the head
      - The fast phase of nystagmus is in the direction of rotation.
      - The slow phase is in the opposite direction.
   b. **Postrotatory (horizontal) nystagmus**
      - Stabilizes the visual image once the head stops rotating

CONSCIOUS PATIENT UNCONSCIOUS PATIENT

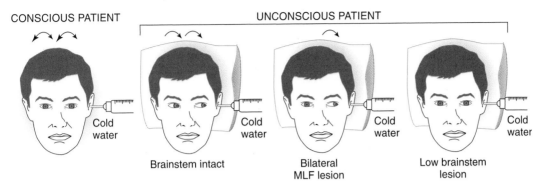

2-15: *Caloric nystagmus. The arrows show the direction of eye movement. MLF, medial longitudinal fasciculus.*

- The fast phase of nystagmus is in the opposite direction to that of rotation.
- The slow phase of nystagmus is in the direction of rotation.

c. **Caloric nystagmus**
- The normal response to cold water irrigation of the external auditory meatus is nystagmus to the opposite side.
- The normal response to warm water irrigation of the external auditory meatus is nystagmus to the same side.

> **Clinical note:** In comatose patients, the nature of the nystagmus elicited by cold water irrigation can help determine the location of a lesion (Fig. 2-15).

D. **Olfaction**
1. **Structure of olfactory apparatus** (Fig. 2-16)
   - Smell is detected by **olfactory receptor cells,** which are situated in mucus-coated **olfactory epithelium** that lines the posterodorsal parts of the nasal cavities.
   - Olfactory glands (Bowman's glands) secrete a fluid that bathes the cilia of the receptors and acts as a solvent for odorant molecules.
   - Olfactory receptor cells (first-order neurons) are stimulated by the binding of odor molecules to their cilia.
   - The axons of the olfactory receptor cells form **CN I (olfactory nerve);** these project through the **cribriform plate** at the base of the cranium to synapse with the **mitral cells of the olfactory bulb.**
   - The **mitral cells** of the olfactory bulb are excitatory, second-order neurons. The output axons of the mitral cells form the **olfactory tract** and **lateral olfactory stria,** both of which project to the **primary olfactory cortex** and the **amygdala.** It is at these locations that smell is perceived.
   - Olfactory receptor cells are the only neurons in the adult human that are regularly replaced.

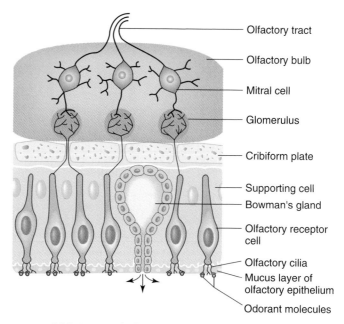

2-16: *Structure of olfactory epithelium and the olfactory bulb.*

Anatomy note: Because CN I passes through the cribriform plate on its way to the olfactory bulb, **cribriform plate fractures** may result in **hyposmia** (reduced olfaction) or **anosmia** (no olfaction).

2. **Olfactory transduction**
   - Odoriferous molecules bind to cilia on the olfactory receptor cells. Activation of receptors leads to the **stimulation of G proteins** and, in turn, activation of **adenylate cyclase.**
   - The activation of adenylate cyclase leads to an **increase** in **intracellular cyclic adenosine monophosphate (cAMP),** which **opens Na^+ channels** in the olfactory receptor membrane and results in **depolarization** of the receptor.
   - Depolarization leads to the generation and propagation of action potentials that eventually reach the **primary olfactory cortex** and culminate in the perception of smell.

E. **Taste**
   1. **Functional anatomy**
      - Taste is detected by **taste receptor cells** (Fig. 2-17), which are located on specialized **papillae** of the taste buds and are stimulated by taste chemicals.
      - Different areas of the tongue consist of different types of taste buds and communicate with the taste center of the brain via different cranial nerves.
        (1) The taste buds on the **anterior two-thirds** of the tongue have **fungiform papillae** and primarily detect **sweet** and **salty** tastes. They

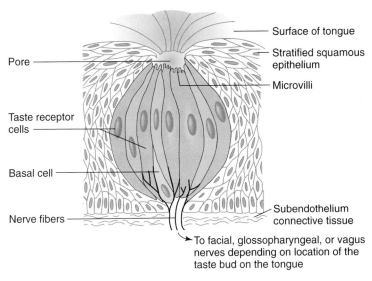

Pore

Taste receptor
cells

Basal cell

Nerve fibers

Surface of tongue

Stratified squamous
epithelium

Microvilli

Subendothelium
connective tissue

To facial, glossopharyngeal, or vagus
nerves depending on location of the
taste bud on the tongue

2-17: *Taste bud.*

send signals centrally via the **lingual nerve** to the **chorda tympani** and
finally into **CN VII (facial).**

(2) Taste buds on the **posterior one-third** of the tongue have
circumvallate papillae and **foliate papillae,** which detect **bitter** and
sour tastes. Most of them send signals centrally via **CN IX
(glossopharyngeal).** However, some located in the back of the throat
and epiglottis send signals centrally via **CN X (vagus).**

- CNs VII, IX, and X synapse with the tractus solitarius (solitary nucleus).
- Second-order neurons leave the solitary nucleus and project **ipsilaterally** to
the **ventral posterior medial nucleus of the thalamus.** Neurons from the
thalamus project to the taste cortex located in the **primary somatosensory
cortex.**

2. **Taste transduction**
- The binding of taste chemicals to the taste receptors causes a
depolarization of the receptor membrane. The depolarization results in an
action potential that is propagated centrally until the taste sensation (sweet,
sour, salty, or bitter) is perceived.

VII. **Higher Functions of the Cerebral Cortex**
A. **Learning and memory**
- Physiologically, memories are caused by changes in the sensitivity of synaptic
transmission between neurons as a result of previous neural activity. These
changes result in **memory tracts,** which are facilitated pathways developed for
the transmission of signals through the neural circuits of the brain, providing
for memory.

- **Short-term memories** last for **seconds or minutes** unless they are converted into longer-term memories. The basis of short-term memory involves **synaptic changes.**
- **Intermediate long-term memories** last for **days to weeks** but then are forgotten. Intermediate long-term memories result from **temporary chemical** and/or **physical changes.**
- **Long-term memories** can be recalled **years later.** The formation of long-term memories involves **structural changes** in the nervous system and the formation of stable memory tracts.

> **Clinical note: Bilateral lesions** of the **hippocampus** prevent the formation of new long-term memories, though the exact mechanism of damage of memory control is not known.

B. **Language**
  - The major area for **language comprehension** is located behind the primary auditory cortex in the posterior part of the superior gyrus of the temporal lobe and is called **Wernicke's area.**

> **Clinical note:** Lesions to this area of the brain result in a fluent, **receptive aphasia** which consists of the inability to comprehend spoken language. The deficit is characterized by fluent verbalization that lacks meaning.

  - The major area for **articulating language** is located in the prefrontal and premotor facial region of the cortex and is called **Broca's speech area.**

> **Clinical note:** Damage to this area of the brain results in a nonfluent, **expressive aphasia,** which reflects a difficulty in piecing together words to produce speech. Patients can understand written and spoken language but are unable to express themselves verbally.

  - In 95% of people, **Wernicke's** and **Broca's areas** for language comprehension and speech production, respectively, are located in the **left hemisphere.**
    (1) The brain's **left hemisphere** is dominant with respect to language, even in most left-handed people.
    (2) The **right hemisphere** is dominant with respect to facial expression, intonation, spatial tasks, and body language.

C. **Brain waves**
  - Waves of electrical activity that are large enough to be electrically recorded from the outer surface of the head with an **electroencephalogram (EEG)**
  - Their **intensity** is determined by the number of neurons that fire in synchrony: the EEG records them only when thousands or millions of neurons fire synchronously.
  - Both the **intensity** and the **pattern** of electrical activity are determined by the level of excitation of the brain during sleep and wakefulness or in disease states such as epilepsy (Fig. 2-18).
    (1) **Alpha waves** (8–13 per second) are observed in normal adults when they are **awake** and in a **quiet, resting** state.

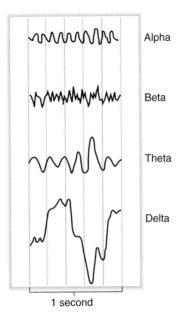

Alpha

Beta

Theta

Delta

1 second

2-18: *Electroencephalogram (EEG) patterns showing electrical activity during sleep.*

(2) **Beta waves** (14–80 cycles per second) are observed in **awake, alert** individuals.

(3) **Theta waves** (4–7 per second) are observed normally in children. They are also observed in adults with brain disorders or during emotional stress.

(4) **Delta waves** include all waves with a frequency of less than 3.5 per second; they are found in very deep sleep, in infants, and in patients with serious organic brain disease.

D. **Sleep**
- The sleep-wake cycle is a **circadian** (i.e., 24-hour) rhythm. This cycle is driven by the suprachiasmatic nucleus of the hypothalamus (which receives input from the retina).
- Sleep is divided into two broad types: non–rapid eye movement (NREM) sleep and rapid eye movement (REM) sleep.
- NREM and REM occur in alternating cycles, with the majority of time being spent in NREM sleep.
- On the basis of EEG changes, NREM sleep can be further divided into four stages:
  (1) **Stage 1** consists of very light sleep with low-voltage EEG waves.
  (2) **Stage 2** is the primary sleep stage during a normal night's sleep. The EEG is characterized by sleep spindles—multiple small waves in rapid succession—and K complexes—a negatively deflecting wave immediately followed by a positively deflecting wave.
  (3) **Stage 3** is a deeper sleep pattern, with decreased EEG activity and muscle tone. Sleep spindles and K complexes may still be seen on the EEG.

(4) **Stage 4** is an even deeper sleep with delta waves on the EEG recording and a further reduction in muscle tone.
- In **REM sleep,** the EEG resembles that of an awake, resting person or a person in stage 1 sleep. Sleep spindles and K complexes should not be present on the EEG.

> **Clinical note:** Aging, alcohol, and benzodiazepines decrease the duration of REM sleep.

VIII. **Cerebral Blood Supply** (Fig. 2-19)
- The brain is highly vulnerable to anoxia and ischemia for a variety of reasons (e.g., high metabolic rate, primary dependence on glucose as a fuel source).
- However, the cerebral vasculature is structured to provide protection from circulatory compromise as well as to efficiently deliver nutrients and remove waste.
- There are two main systems that ensure proper blood flow to the brain: **the internal carotid system** and the **vertebrobasilar system.**
- The **Circle of Willis** connects these two major circulatory systems and also provides an alternative blood supply if circulation is compromised in one of them (see Fig. 2-19).

A. **Internal carotid system**
- Primarily perfuses the cerebral hemispheres, with the exception of the visual cortex and the posterior inferior surface of the temporal lobe.

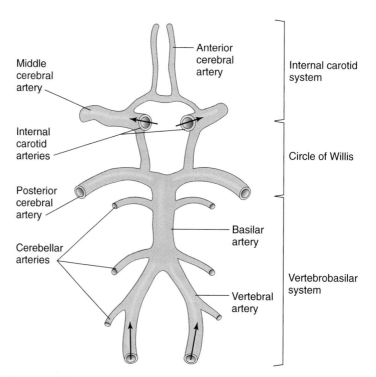

2-19: *Cerebral blood supply, showing the arteries at the base of the brain (viewed from below).*

- The **anterior cerebral arteries** supply blood to the inferior frontal lobes, the medial surfaces of the frontal and parietal lobes, and the anterior corpus callosum. Small penetrating branches supply the limbic structures, the head of the caudate, and the anterior limb of the internal capsule.

  > **Clinical note:** Occlusion or infarction of the anterior cerebral artery (ACA) may cause weakness and sensory loss of the distal contralateral leg, because the ACA supplies blood to area of brain that controls the distal contralateral leg, as seen in Figure 2-7.

- The **middle cerebral arteries** (MCA) supply blood to the majority of the cortex and white matter, including the frontal, parietal, temporal, and occipital lobes and the insula. Small penetrating branches of the MCA supply the posterior limb of the internal capsule, the putamen, the outer globus pallidus, and the body of the caudate.

  > **Clinical note:** The most common **stroke** syndrome occurs from **infarction of tissue in the distribution of the MCA.** Infarction damages the cortex and white matter and results in contralateral weakness, sensory loss, homonymous hemianopsia, and, depending on the hemisphere involved, either language disturbance or impaired spatial perception. The weakness and sensory loss affect the face and arm more than the leg (ACA supply), because the MCA supplies blood to the areas of brain that control the contralateral face and upper extremity, as seen in Figure 2-7.

B. **Vertebrobasilar system**
  - This originates as a branch of the **subclavian artery.**
  - The **posterior cerebral arteries** (PCA) supply the posterior inferior surface of the temporal lobes, medial occipital lobes, midbrain, and cerebellum.

  > **Clinical note: Circulatory compromise of the PCA** may result in a homonymous hemianopsia (see Fig. 2-7) as a result of injury to the visual cortex. Macular vision is spared, because the occipital pole receives its blood supply from the MCA. If the blockage or infarction is in the proximal portion of the PCA, the thalamus may be affected, which would result in contralateral sensory loss.

Endocrine Physiology

I. **Hormones**

- The primary function of hormones is to **maintain homeostasis** (e.g., regulate plasma glucose and electrolyte balance) and coordinate physiologic processes such as **development, metabolism,** and **reproduction.**
- Hormones typically act slowly relative to the nervous system and maintain homeostasis by using various **feedback mechanisms.**

A. **Mechanism of action of hormones**

- All hormones must interact with a **cellular receptor,** which then transduces a signal and generates a cellular response. The effectiveness of a given hormone therefore depends on the concentration of **free hormone** (that which is available for binding), the concentration of **hormone receptor,** and the **effectiveness** of the **transduction mechanism.**
- **Note:** All endocrine diseases are due to a quantitative or qualitative **defect in hormone synthesis** or **altered tissue sensitivity** to circulating hormone, usually manifesting as a disruption of a well-characterized homeostatic control system.

B. **Types of hormones and their individual effector mechanisms**

1. **Steroid hormones**

- Steroid hormones are **lipid-soluble** compounds derived from **cholesterol** that are able to enter all cells of the body by diffusing through the lipid-rich plasma membrane. They produce their effects by binding to receptors in either the cytosol or the nucleus of cells in target tissues, and this hormone-receptor complex then activates **transcription** of specific **genes** (Fig. 3-1).
- Because steroid hormones can diffuse freely through lipid membranes, they **cannot be stored** within intracellular vesicles. They are therefore **produced continually,** and synthesis and secretion increase on demand.
- Additionally, because steroid hormones are lipid soluble, they must circulate bound to plasma proteins. They are therefore **not freely filtered** by the kidney, which contributes to their long half-life relative to most peptide hormones, and they are typically **metabolized by the liver.**
- The principal steroid hormones include the **sex steroids**—testosterone, progesterone, and estrogen—and the **adrenal steroids**—cortisol and aldosterone.

2. **Thyroid hormones**

- Thyroid hormones are unique in that they are derived from the amino acid **tyrosine** rather than cholesterol, yet have a **mechanism of action similar to steroid hormones** (i.e., they diffuse into a cell, bind to a receptor, and activate gene transcription).

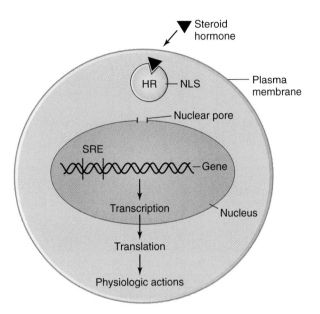

3-1: *After diffusing through the plasma membrane, most steroid hormones bind to a cytoplasmic receptor. This hormone-receptor complex then undergoes a conformational change which uncovers a nuclear localization site that allows access to the nucleus. The complex then binds to and activates genes that contain the appropriate steroid response element within their sequence. HR, hormone receptor; NLS, nuclear localization sequence; SRE, steroid response element.*

3. **Proteoglycans, proteins, peptide hormones, and amino acids**
    - These **polar compounds** bind to membrane-associated receptors on target cells. The signal transduction mechanism used by these agents varies, depending on the receptor type. Because they are **hydrophilic,** they **can be stored** in cytoplasmic granules of endocrine cells and **released on demand.**
    - Some travel "free" as soluble compounds in the blood, whereas others travel mainly "bound," associated with specific binding proteins. In general, the free hormones that are not associated with carrier proteins have shorter half-lives than the bound hormones.
    - There are four primary classes of membrane-spanning receptors to which these hormones can bind: tyrosine and serine **kinase receptors, ligand-gated ion channels, receptor-linked kinases,** and **G protein–coupled receptors.** Figure 3-2 shows the mechanism underlying G protein signal transduction.
C. **Hormone-binding proteins**
    - Certain hormones circulate bound to hormone-binding proteins. These binding proteins serve several important physiologic functions.
    - First, they **provide a reservoir of hormone** which exists in equilibrium with the free hormone and **buffers** any moment-to-moment changes in free hormone concentration.
    - Second, they **extend** the **half-life** of the bound hormone considerably, because it is the free hormone that is metabolized by the liver or excreted by the kidney. All steroid hormones and a few peptide hormones have binding proteins (Table 3-1).

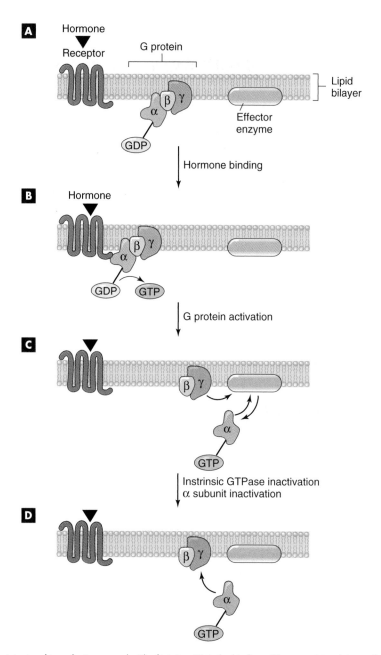

3-2: *G protein signal transduction cascade. The first step (**A**) is the binding of hormone (triangle) to a G protein–associated membrane receptor. This hormone binding stimulates the receptor to undergo a conformational change (**B**), which causes the α-subunit of the G protein to release guanosine diphosphate (GDP) and bind guanosine triphosphate (GTP). This causes the α-subunit to dissociate from the β-γ complex. The α-subunit and the β-γ complex are then free to diffuse laterally within the lipid bilayer and activate or inhibit the activity of various effector molecules, such as adenylate cyclase (**C**). After several seconds, intrinsic GTPase activity of the α-subunit degrades the GTP to GDP. The GDP-bound α-subunit is inactive and also binds to the β-γ complex (**D**), restoring the system to its original condition. The intrinsic adenosine triphosphatase (ATPase) activity of the α-GTP complex limits the duration of the response.*

TABLE 3-1:
Hormone Binding Action of Some Plasma Proteins

Plasma Protein	Hormone
Albumin	Multiple lipophilic hormones
Transthyretin	Thyroxine (T_4)
Transcortin	Cortisol, aldosterone
Thyroxine-binding globulin	Triiodothyronine (T_3), thyroxine
Sex-steroid–binding globulin	Testosterone, estrogen

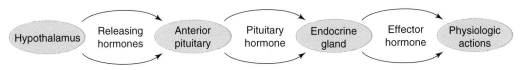

3-3: *Hierarchical control of hormone secretion.*

TABLE 3-2:
Effect of Hormones Released by the Hypothalamus on the Anterior Pituitary

Hormone	Effect on Anterior Pituitary
Growth hormone–releasing hormone (GHRH)	Stimulates growth hormone (GH) secretion
Prolactin-inhibitory factor (dopamine)	Inhibits prolactin secretion
Somatostatin	Inhibits GH secretion
Gonadotropin-releasing hormone (GnRH)	Stimulates luteinizing hormone (LH) and follicle-stimulating hormone (FSH) secretion
Corticotropin-releasing hormone (CRH)	Stimulates adrenocorticotropic hormone (ACTH) secretion
Thyrotropin-releasing hormone (TRH)	Stimulates thyroid-stimulating hormone (TSH) secretion

D. **Hierarchical control of hormone secretion**
- For several hormonal control systems, a hierarchical axis exists consisting of the hypothalamus, the anterior pituitary (adenohypophysis), and a specific endocrine gland (Fig. 3-3).
- The **hypothalamus,** at the top of the axis, secretes **"releasing hormones"** into a capillary bed that converges on the **pituitary** and then reexpands into another capillary bed within the **anterior pituitary** (hypothalamic-hypophyseal portal system) (Table 3-2; Fig. 3-4). The releasing hormones then stimulate specific cell types of the anterior pituitary and stimulate (or inhibit) pituitary hormone secretion. The pituitary hormone, in turn, may either act directly on target

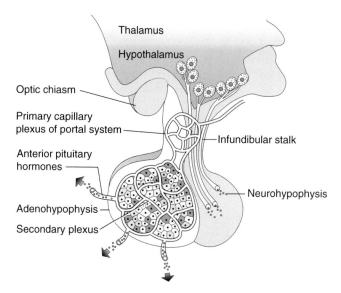

3-4: *Hypothalamic-hypophyseal portal system.*

tissues (e.g., prolactin) or stimulate an endocrine gland to produce an effector hormone (e.g., thyroid-stimulating hormone).
- The hypothalamus also controls the secretion of the hormones of the **posterior pituitary** (neurohypophysis), but in a different fashion. Posterior pituitary **hormones** are **synthesized by neurons in the hypothalamus** and transported along axons into the posterior pituitary. There they are **released** into the bloodstream **as neurosecretory granules** in response to appropriate stimuli.

E. **Classification of endocrine diseases**
- A hormone deficiency or excess can occur as the result of a defect anywhere along the hypothalamic–pituitary–target organ axis; therefore, it is important to determine the **location of the defect** in order to make an accurate diagnosis. **In primary endocrine diseases, the defect is in the endocrine organ.** For example, if a defect renders the **thyroid** gland unable to produce thyroid hormone effectively, the disease is known as **primary hypothyroidism.** If the defect is in the **pituitary gland,** the disease is known as **secondary hypothyroidism;** if the defect is in the **hypothalamus,** the disease is known as **tertiary hypothyroidism.**

II. **Hormonal Control Systems of the Anterior Pituitary**
A. **Hypothalamic-pituitary-adrenal axis**
- The primary function of the hypothalamic-pituitary-adrenal axis is to maintain physiologically appropriate levels of the hormone cortisol in the blood.
- Corticotropin-releasing hormone (**CRH**) from the hypothalamus stimulates the secretion of adrenocorticotropic hormone (**ACTH**) from the anterior pituitary (via activation of corticotroph cells). ACTH then acts on the **adrenal cortex** to stimulate the synthesis and secretion of **glucocorticoids** and **androgens** (but not

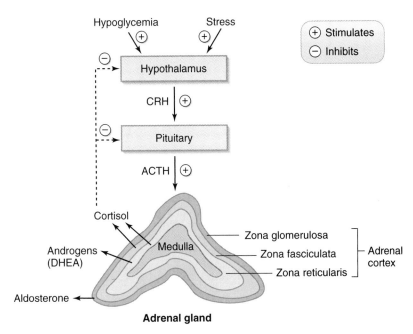

3-5: *Main determinants of hypothalamic-pituitary-adrenal axis. ACTH, adrenocorticotropic hormone; CRH, corticotropin-releasing hormone; DHEA, dehydroepiandrosterone.*

mineralocorticoids). The primary glucocorticoid is **cortisol,** and the primary adrenal androgen is dehydroepiandrosterone (**DHEA**), a precursor of testosterone.

1. **Regulation of the hypothalamic-pituitary-adrenal axis**
   - As shown in Figure 3-5, **cortisol** secretion is stimulated by **hypoglycemia** or **stressful conditions** (e.g., surgery), when the sympathetic nervous system is also activated. This is why cortisol is sometimes referred to as the **"stress hormone."** Cortisol secretion is normally inhibited by increased plasma levels of cortisol because of the negative feedback effect of cortisol, which inhibits hypothalamic CRH and pituitary ACTH secretion.
   - Note from the figure that **androgens do not negatively feedback** and **inhibit CRH or ACTH secretion,** a fact that takes on added importance when trying to understand the signs and symptoms associated with adrenal disorders such as **congenital adrenal hyperplasia** (discussed later).

   > **Pathology note: A tumor of the adrenal gland** that autonomously hypersecretes cortisol causes negative feedback on the hypothalamus and pituitary and decreases the secretion of ACTH. In this circumstance, the patient may have an increased cortisol level and a decreased ACTH level.

   - Cortisol has a **diurnal** pattern of secretion that is based on the daily pattern of ACTH secretion from the pituitary. Cortisol levels are highest in the early morning because of the nocturnal surge of ACTH (Fig. 3-6).

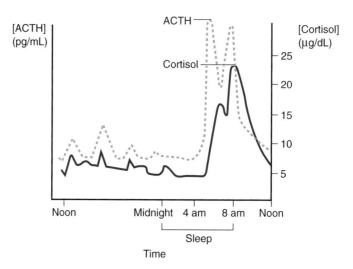

3-6: *Diurnal secretion of adrenocorticotropic hormone and cortisol. ACTH, adrenocorticotropic hormone.*

   2. **Biosynthetic pathway of adrenal corticosteroids**
- The **rate-limiting step** in adrenal steroid synthesis is the **conversion of cholesterol to pregnenolone** (see Fig. 3-10). The synthetic pathway for each adrenal steroid occurs in a specific region of the adrenal gland: mineralocorticoid synthesis occurs in the zona **glomerulosa,** cortisol synthesis in the zona **fasciculata,** and androgen synthesis in the zona **reticularis.** Although the principal mineralocorticoid aldosterone is synthesized in the adrenal cortex, its synthesis is only slightly affected by ACTH.
- **Note:** The gonads and the adrenals are the only tissues that convert cholesterol to steroid hormones.

   3. **Mechanism of action of cortisol** (see Fig. 3-1)
- As a steroid hormone, cortisol is able to diffuse through the plasma membrane of cells and bind to a cytoplasmic receptor. This hormone-receptor complex then enters the nucleus, binds specific DNA sequences, and regulates the expression of various "steroid-responsive" genes.

   4. **Physiologic actions of cortisol** (Fig. 3-7)
    a. **Fuel metabolism**
- In the **fasting state,** cortisol helps maintain adequate plasma levels of glucose for **glucose-dependent tissues** such as the **central nervous system** (CNS). It accomplishes this by **inhibiting the peripheral utilization of glucose** by muscle and adipose tissue while simultaneously **stimulating hepatic gluconeogenesis.**
- Cortisol exerts catabolic actions on most tissues, with the exception of the liver, on which it exerts anabolic actions.
- Cortisol stimulates hepatic gluconeogenesis in several ways. It promotes **muscle breakdown,** which releases amino acids into the gluconeogenic pathway; it stimulates the **synthesis** of hepatic **gluconeogenic enzymes;**

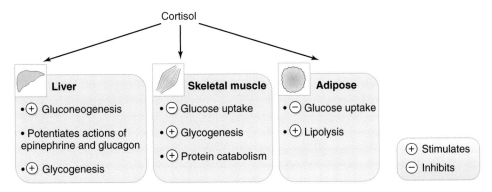

3-7: *Metabolic actions of cortisol.*

and it potentiates the actions of **glucagon** and the **catecholamines** on the liver.

- Cortisol additionally **stimulates lipolysis in adipose tissue,** which helps maintain plasma levels of **glycerol** and **fatty acids** during the fasting state. These substrates can then be used as an **alternative fuel source** in various tissues, thereby **sparing plasma glucose.** In the liver, these substrates can be used as an energy source to support gluconeogenesis.

> **Clinical note:** Because of cortisol's propensity to increase plasma glucose levels, prolonged exposure to supraphysiologic levels of cortisol will often cause **glucose intolerance** and may lead to frank **diabetes mellitus** in a significant number of patients.

  b. **Effects on blood pressure and plasma volume**
  - Cortisol increases blood pressure in several ways. It facilitates activity of the sympathetic nervous system by **increasing** the expression of α- and β-adrenergic receptors in multiple tissues. Stimulation of α_1-adrenergic receptors on vascular smooth muscle results in **vasoconstriction.** In contrast, stimulation of β_2-adrenergic receptors on vascular smooth muscle cells results in **vasodilation.**
  - β-Receptor agonism is also important in mediating sympathetic stimulation of the heart, **bronchodilation, stimulation of renin secretion,** and metabolism, including **lipolysis** and **glycogenolysis.**
  - At **increased levels,** cortisol exerts **mineralocorticoid actions** on the kidneys because it is similar in structure to aldosterone. This stimulates renal sodium reabsorption and causes **plasma volume expansion.**
  - **Note:** Ordinarily, cortisol is degraded by intracellular enzymes in the cells of mineralocorticoid-responsive tissues. However at higher levels, these enzymes become saturated, at which point cortisol may **bind to mineralocorticoid receptors** and exert physiologic effects.
  c. **Effects on inflammatory and immune responses**
  - Cortisol has powerful anti-inflammatory effects.

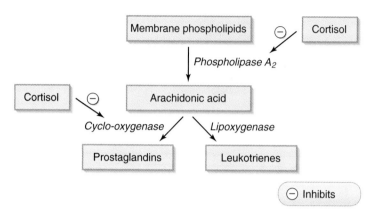

3-8: *Anti-inflammatory action of cortisol.*

- It **inhibits** activity of the enzyme **phospholipase** and also **inhibits** the transcription of various inflammatory **cytokines.** As shown in Figure 3-8, inhibition of phospholipase leads to **decreased arachidonic acid production** and therefore to decreased production of **prostaglandins** and **leukotrienes,** both potent inflammatory mediators.

d. **Effects on bone**
- At supraphysiologic levels, cortisol weakens bones by inhibiting bone-forming cells (osteoblasts) and stimulating bone-degrading cells (osteoclasts).
- In addition, cortisol reduces intestinal absorption of calcium, which can precipitate a compensatory increase in parathyroid hormone (PTH) secretion, causing further bone breakdown.

> **Pathology/Pharmacology note:** Increased levels of glucocorticoids can severely compromise the blood supply to certain susceptible bones, resulting in **avascular necrosis** of the bone. Avascular necrosis most commonly occurs in the **femoral head** of the hip joint in patients treated with glucocorticoids.

5. **Pathophysiology of the CRH-ACTH-cortisol axis**
   a. **Hypercortisolism (Cushing syndrome)**
   - "Cushing syndrome" refers to the constellation of signs and symptoms associated with hypercortisolism, whether the source of the cortisol is exogenous or endogenous. Recall that cortisol promotes hyperglycemia, muscle breakdown, destruction of bone, and plasma volume expansion. Hypercortisolic states may therefore result in **diabetes mellitus, muscle wasting, osteoporosis,** and **hypertension.**
   - Hypercortisolism is most commonly physician-induced (**iatrogenic**). The most common endogenous source of elevated cortisol is an ACTH-hypersecreting **tumor of the pituitary,** a condition referred to as **Cushing disease.** Other causes of Cushing syndrome (Fig. 3-9) include cortisol-

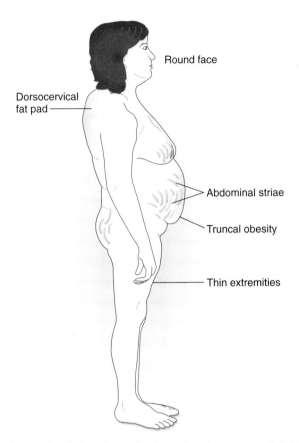

Round face

Dorsocervical fat pad

Abdominal striae

Truncal obesity

Thin extremities

3-9: *Classic physical features of Cushing syndrome. The classic physical presentation of Cushing syndrome is central obesity that spares the extremities (extremity wasting may even occur), a rounded face ("moon facies"), abdominal striae, and a dorsocervical fat pad ("buffalo hump"). Although glucocorticoids are lipolytic, they cause fat deposition on the trunk and face. In addition to hyperglycemia, osteoporosis, hypertension, and muscle wasting, hirsutism may be present in the ACTH-dependent forms of Cushing syndrome due to stimulation of adrenal androgen production by the excess ACTH. Oligomenorrhea, acne, and deepening of the voice can also occur in females as a result of increased levels of androgens.*

hypersecreting adrenal tumors and ectopic production of ACTH by a tumor (e.g., **small cell lung cancer**).

> **Clinical note:** The **dexamethasone suppression test** can be used to differentiate between Cushing disease and ectopic ACTH production in a patient with hypercortisolism and elevated ACTH. In **Cushing disease,** the pituitary still retains some responsiveness to feedback inhibition by cortisol or by synthetic glucocorticoids such as dexamethasone (high doses of dexamethasone significantly decrease plasma cortisol). In contrast, **ectopic ACTH secretion by a tumor** is not controlled via feedback inhibition by cortisol or dexamethasone (dexamethasone does not affect plasma cortisol).

b. **Hypocortisolism**
- The principal pathologic consequences of inadequate cortisol levels include **weakness, fatigue, hypotension, hypoglycemia,** and **hyponatremia.**
- As with hypercortisolism, the most common cause of hypocortisolic states is iatrogenic, because many patients with various conditions (often autoimmune in nature) are treated with glucocorticoids on a long-term basis.

> **Clinical note:** The exogenous administration of glucocorticoids on a long-term basis normally suppresses the hypothalamic-pituitary-adrenal axis. If steroid therapy is abruptly stopped, patients are susceptible to developing **acute adrenal insufficiency.** Therefore, whenever steroid therapy is to be stopped, it should be a gradual weaning process, which allows the hypothalamic-pituitary-adrenal axis to recover by the time the steroids are completely stopped.
>
> Adrenal insufficiency (**Addison's disease**) also develops when the adrenal cortex is destroyed. Usually, the cause is **autoimmune destruction** of the adrenals, but sometimes it is **tuberculosis** or **metastatic cancer** involving the adrenals. Signs and symptoms of adrenal insufficiency reflect deficiencies in glucocorticoids and mineralocorticoids and include **hypotension** and **salt wasting.** Reduced feedback inhibition of the hypothalamic-pituitary axis from deficient cortisol synthesis results in increased ACTH secretion by the pituitary. When ACTH is cleaved from its precursor proopiomelanocortin (**POMC**), melanocyte-stimulating hormone (**MSH**) is concurrently released. MSH then stimulates melanin-containing skin cells (**melanocytes**), causing **hyperpigmentation** of the skin, which is frequently seen in Addison's disease.

6. **Hypothalamic-pituitary regulation of adrenal androgen synthesis**
- ACTH stimulates the synthesis of DHEA and androstenedione by the adrenal cortex. Both substances are androgen prohormones that are converted, mainly in the periphery, to testosterone and dihydrotestosterone (DHT).
- Note that androgens **do not cause feedback inhibition of CRH or ACTH secretion.**

7. **Pathophysiology of congenital adrenal hyperplasias (CAH)**
- This group of rare disorders is characterized by **defects in the cortisol biosynthetic pathway.** In CAH, the impaired cortisol synthesis reduces feedback inhibition of the hypothalamic-pituitary axis, resulting in **increased ACTH secretion.** The elevated concentration of ACTH then **stimulates bilateral adrenal hyperplasia.** The continual stimulation of the adrenals by ACTH leads to "shunting" of cortisol precursors to androgens, which may cause **virilization** in male neonates or **ambiguous genitalia** in female neonates. Additionally, **salt wasting** and **hypotension** may be present if the

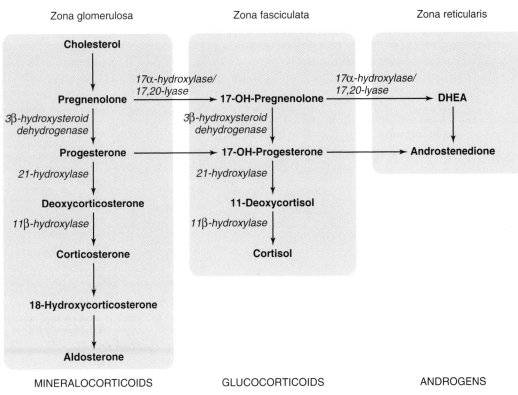

3-10: *Pathways of adrenal steroidogenesis. DHEA, dehydroepiandrosterone.*

steroidogenic pathway involved results in **impaired mineralocorticoid synthesis.**
- The most common form of CAH is caused by deficiency of the enzyme **21-hydroxylase** (Fig. 3-10).

8. **Pathophysiology of adrenal disorders** (Table 3-3)

B. **Hypothalamic-pituitary-thyroid axis**
- The primary function of the hypothalamic-pituitary-thyroid axis is to maintain physiologically appropriate plasma levels of the **thyroid hormones** triiodothyronine (T_3) and thyroxine (T_4). Thyrotropin-releasing hormone (**TRH**) from the hypothalamus stimulates thyroid-stimulating hormone (**TSH**) secretion from **thyrotrophs** within the anterior pituitary. TSH in turn stimulates the secretion of the thyroid hormones T_3 and T_4 from **follicular cells** within the thyroid gland.
- **Note:** The hormone **calcitonin** is also synthesized and secreted by **parafollicular cells** within the thyroid gland, but this activity is not under hypothalamic or pituitary control.

1. **Steps in the synthesis of thyroid hormones** (Fig. 3-11)
   a. Plasma iodide ion (I^-) is taken up by thyroid follicular cells by the iodide pump and extruded into the follicular lumen.

TABLE 3-3:
Adrenal Disorders and Commonly Associated Clinical Features

Disorder	Pathophysiology	Clinical Features	Treatment
Primary adrenal insufficiency (Addison's disease)	Autoimmune, metastatic, or tubercular destruction of adrenal cortices	↓ Aldosterone → hyperkalemic metabolic acidosis, sodium wasting, dehydration, hypotension ↓ Cortisol → hypoglycemia, weakness, vulnerability to stress ↓ Adrenal androgens → loss of pubic and axillary hair in females ↑ ACTH → hyperpigmentation	Glucocorticoid and mineralocorticoid replacement therapy
Acute adrenal insufficiency	Septicemia (e.g., *Neisseria meningitidis*), iatrogenic (e.g., sudden withdrawal from long-term steroid therapy)	Symptoms of Addison's disease (see above)	Treat underlying cause (e.g., septicemia) and initiate steroid replacement therapy
Primary hypercortisolism	Adrenal tumor	↑ Cortisol → hyperglycemia, central obesity, hypertension, osteoporosis, muscle wasting, abdominal striae	Steroid synthesis inhibitors (e.g., ketoconazole, metyrapone) or surgery
Secondary hypercortisolism	Pituitary tumor (Cushing disease) or ectopic ACTH production	↑ ACTH → hypercortisolism, hyperpigmentation ↑ Cortisol → same effects as in Cushing syndrome ↑ Androgens → hirsutism ↓ ACTH due to feedback inhibition of pituitary	Surgery

ACTH, adrenocorticotropic hormone.

b. (I^-) is oxidized to iodine (I_2) by peroxidase.

c. Iodine is attached to tyrosine residues that are attached to thyroglobulin (the major protein of the follicular colloid), forming monoiodotyrosine (MIT) and diiodotyrosine (DIT), the so-called **organification** step.

d. Coupling of MIT and DIT into T_4 and T_3

e. Endocytosis of thyroglobulin from colloid

f. Hydrolytic cleavage of T_3 and T_4 from thyroglobulin and diffusion of T_4 and T_3 into plasma

> **Pharmacology note:** Patients with **hyperthyroidism** are often treated with **propylthiouracil (PTU)** and/or **methimazole,** drugs that inhibit the synthesis of thyroid hormones. These drugs act by inhibiting the oxidation and organification of iodide within the thyroid, thereby reducing the synthesis of thyroid hormones. Because large

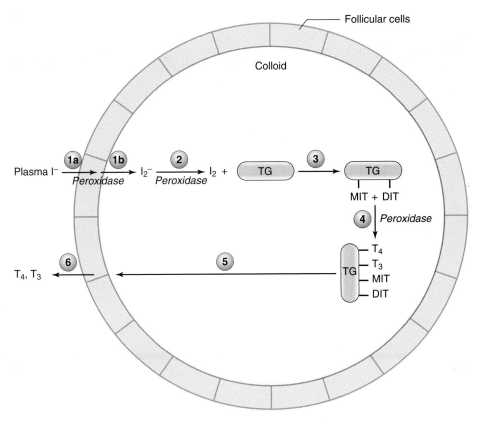

3-11: *Thyroid hormone synthesis in the thyroid follicle. (1) Uptake of plasma I⁻ by iodide pump of thyroid follicular cells (a) and extrusion into follicular lumen (b). (2) Oxidation of I⁻ to I₂ by peroxidase. (3) Organification: I₂ is attached to tyrosine residues attached to thyroglobin (TG), forming monoiodotyrosine (MIT) and diiodotyrosine (DIT). (4) Coupling of MIT and DIT to T₄ and T₃. (5) Endocytosis of TG from colloid. (6) Hydrolytic cleavage of T₃ and T₄ from TG and diffusion of T₄ and T₃ into plasma. T₃, triiodothyronine; T₄, thyroxine.*

quantities of thyroid hormones are stored in colloid, it takes **several weeks for these drugs to deplete thyroid T₄ levels** and return systemic thyroid hormone levels to normal. However, in large doses, PTU can have more rapid effects by **inhibiting** the **peripheral conversion** of T_4 to T_3.

2. **Physiologic actions of thyroid hormones** (Fig. 3-12)
   a. **Increased basal metabolic rate (BMR)**
      - Thyroid hormones increase the BMR mainly by upregulating the **expression** and increasing the **activity** of the sodium-potassium adenosine triphosphatase pump (**Na⁺,K⁺-ATPase pump**) in most tissues.
      - The increase in BMR causes **heat intolerance,** a common symptom of hyperthyroidism.

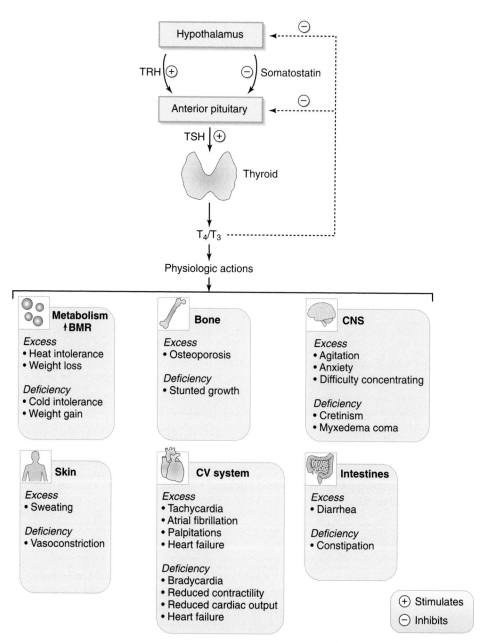

3-12: *Thyroid regulation, physiology, and pathophysiology. BMR, basal metabolic rate; CHF, congestive heart failure; CNS, central nervous system; CV, cardiovascular; T₃, triiodothyronine; T₄, thyroxine; TRH, thyrotropin-releasing hormone; TSH, thyroid-stimulating hormone.*

b. **Potentiation of catecholamine actions**
- Thyroid hormones upregulate the expression and stimulate the activity of β-adrenergic receptors in tissues, such as the heart and skeletal muscle, resulting in markedly enhanced sensitivity to circulating catecholamines. They also act **directly** on the heart to stimulate contractility and increase heart rate.
- In the heart, these effects contribute to the **increased heart rate** and **increased contractility;** in skeletal muscle, they contribute to the **muscle tremors** often associated with hyperthyroidism.

> **Pharmacology note:** By preventing catecholamines from binding to their receptors, β-adrenergic antagonists (β-blockers), such as **propranolol,** can ameliorate many of the symptoms of **hyperthyroidism** associated with excessive sympathetic activity (e.g., tachycardia, tremors).

3. **Differences between T_4 and T_3**
- The thyroid gland secretes both T_4 and T_3. T_4 is much **less potent** than T_3 but it has a **longer** plasma **half-life** than T_3. Within target cells, T_4 is converted into the more active T_3 by the enzyme **5'-monodeiodinase;** therefore, T_4 can essentially be considered a prohormone that serves as a plasma reservoir for T_3.
- Additionally, because of its prolonged half-life, plasma T_4 is much more abundant than plasma T_3. It therefore is principally responsible for the feedback inhibition of TRH secretion by the hypothalamus and TSH secretion by the pituitary.

> **Clinical note:** In **hypothyroid patients,** supplementing only T_4 (rather than T_3) usually provides adequate tissue levels of T_3 from peripheral conversion. However, certain patients respond much better to a T_4/T_3 combination. Presumably, the peripheral conversion of T_4 to T_3 may be impaired in these patients.

4. **Pathophysiology**
   a. **Hyperthyroidism**
      (1) **Signs and symptoms**
      - The increased BMR causes weight loss and heat intolerance.
      - The direct and indirect cardiovascular effects **increase the cardiac workload** and over prolonged periods may cause **heart failure.**
      - Enhanced sensitivity to catecholamines may cause **tachycardia** and **muscle tremors.**
      - Intestinal motility is stimulated, causing diarrhea.
      - Bone resorption is stimulated, which may cause osteoporosis and hypercalcemia.
      (2) **Laboratory evaluation**
      - T_3 and T_4 are always **elevated** in hyperthyroidism.
      - However, levels of TRH and TSH vary depending on the precise cause of the hyperthyroidism (Table 3-4).

TABLE 3-4:
Laboratory Values Associated with Hyperthyroidism

Type of Hyperthyroidism	Example	TRH	TSH	T₄
Primary	Graves' disease	↓	↓	↑
Secondary	Pituitary adenoma	↓	↑	↑
Tertiary	Hypothalamic tumor	↑	↑	↑

T₄, thyroxine; TRH, thyrotropin-releasing hormone; TSH, thyroid-stimulating hormone.

(3) **Differential diagnosis** (Table 3-5)
- In **Graves' disease** (also known as **diffuse toxic goiter**), the most common cause of hyperthyroidism, **stimulatory immunoglobulin G (IgG) autoantibodies** bind to TSH receptors in the thyroid. These antibodies mimic TSH and excessively stimulate, but do not destroy, the thyroid gland.
- In **toxic multinodular goiter** and in **toxic adenoma,** autonomous thyroid nodules secrete excessive levels of thyroid hormone.
- TRH-secreting or TSH-secreting **tumors of the hypothalamus or pituitary** are another cause.
- **Infections** of the thyroid gland (**viral thyroiditis**) may cause tissue inflammation and destruction, with **release of preformed thyroid hormone,** also leading to hyperthyroidism.

> **Clinical note:** The classic presentation of **Graves' disease** is **thyrotoxicosis** (e.g., tachycardia, weight loss), **diffuse goiter, ophthalmopathy** (e.g., exophthalmos), and **dermopathy** (e.g., pretibial myxedema).

b. **Hypothyroidism**
(1) **Signs and symptoms**
- The decreased BMR causes **weight gain** and **cold intolerance.**
- **Bradycardia, constipation,** and **dulled mentation**
- Congenital hypothyroidism may cause **mental retardation (cretinism)** and **short stature.**
- Hypothyroidism at any time before closure of the epiphyseal plates may also cause shorter-than-normal stature.

> **Clinical note:** Patients with a long history of untreated hypothyroidism are susceptible to the most severe manifestation of hypothyroidism, **myxedema coma;** such patients may present with profound lethargy or coma, weakness, hypothermia, and hypoglycemia. Such patients may occasionally require emergent treatment with intravenous T₃.

TABLE 3-5:
Etiology of Hyperthyroidism

Cause	Pathophysiology	Pattern of Radioiodine Uptake	Classic Presentation
Permanent Causes			
Graves' disease (diffuse toxic goiter)	Activating antibodies to TSH receptor	Diffuse uptake throughout gland	Goiter, ophthalmopathy, dermopathy
Toxic multinodular goiter	Multiple hyperactive nodules, may have mutations in genes encoding TSH receptor or G proteins	Uptake in one or a few overly active "hot" nodules Uptake in remainder of thyroid is suppressed	Older adult with history of *nontoxic* multinodular goiter May have cardiac complications such as atrial fibrillation and/or heart failure
Toxic adenoma (Plummer's disease)	Hyperactive adenoma(s); may have mutations in genes encoding TSH receptor or G proteins	Uptake in one or a few "hot" nodules Uptake in remainder of thyroid is suppressed	Younger adult with a history of a slowly growing "lump" in the neck
Pituitary adenoma	Hypersecretion of TSH	Diffuse uptake throughout thyroid	May have additional symptoms (e.g., headaches, bitemporal hemianopia, nausea and vomiting)
Transient Causes			
Autoimmune thyroiditis (e.g., Hashimoto's disease)	Autoimmune destruction of thyroid	Suppressed uptake throughout thyroid	Hyperthyroidism initially followed by hypothyroidism
Subacute thyroiditis (de Quervain's thyroiditis)	Likely secondary to viral infection of thyroid Follows upper respiratory tract infection	Suppressed uptake throughout thyroid	Thyroid exquisitely painful to palpation
Iodine-induced (jodbasedow effect)	Iodine overload may stimulate autonomous nodules, which function independently of TSH stimulation, to hypersecrete thyroid hormone	Suppressed uptake throughout thyroid	Thyrotoxicosis in patient with toxic multinodular goiter following the administration of iodine-rich radiographic contrast media and iodinated drugs such as amiodarone
Thyrotoxicosis factitia	Inadvertent or intentional ingestion of large amounts of thyroid hormone	Suppressed uptake throughout thyroid	Medical personnel who takes thyroid hormone to lose weight
Struma ovarii	Thyroid tissue forms part of ovarian germ cell tumor (teratoma) and secretes excessive thyroid hormone	Suppressed uptake throughout thyroid	Hyperthyroidism in female
Trophoblastic tumors	Malignant trophoblastic tissue secretes human chorionic gonadotropin (hCG) that stimulates the TSH receptor	Diffuse uptake throughout thyroid	Hydatidiform moles, choriocarcinoma, metastatic embryonal carcinoma of the testis

TSH, thyroid-stimulating hormone.

TABLE 3-6:
Laboratory Values Associated with Hypothyroidism

Type of Hypothyroidism	Example	TRH	TSH	T₄
Primary	Hashimoto's thyroiditis	↑	↑	↓
Secondary	Pituitary lesion	↑	↓	↓
Tertiary	Hypothalamic lesion	↓	↓	↓

T_4, thyroxine; TRH, thyrotropin-releasing hormone; TSH, thyroid-stimulating hormone.

TABLE 3-7:
Etiology and Differential Diagnosis of Hypothyroidism

Cause	Pathophysiology	Presentation	Treatment
Endemic cretinism	Dietary iodide insufficiency at early developmental stages	Severe mental retardation; innocent (Christ-like) appearing	Iodide replacement; mental retardation may be permanent
Endemic goiter	Dietary iodide insufficiency in adulthood	Goiter; common in mountainous areas such as the Andes, Himalayas, and Alps	Iodide replacement
Hashimoto's thyroiditis (autoimmune thyroiditis)	Autoimmune destruction of thyroid gland. Often occurs after a viral illness	Initially may present as hyperthyroidism but ultimately causes hypothyroidism	Thyroxine replacement
Iatrogenic	Most commonly caused by thyroidectomy. Also may occur after radiotherapy for hyperthyroidism	Hypothyroidism	Thyroxine replacement
Riedel's thyroiditis	Chronic fibrosis of thyroid gland	"Woody" thyroid	Steroids. Thyroxine
Subacute granulomatous thyroiditis (de Quervain's thyroiditis)	Viral in nature; often develops after upper respiratory tract infection	Thyroid gland is painful and tender on palpation. Often preceded by hyperthyroidism	Usually resolves gradually on its own

      (2) **Laboratory evaluation** (Table 3-6)
      (3) **Differential diagnosis** (Table 3-7)
  C. **Hypothalamic-pituitary-gonadal axis**
    • This hormonal axis is responsible for the development and maintenance of primary and secondary **sexual characteristics, menstrual cycles** in females, and **spermatogenesis** in males.
    1. **Male reproductive axis** (Fig. 3-13)
      a. **Mechanism of action of testosterone**
        • Testosterone is a steroid hormone that produces its effects by **stimulating protein synthesis.**

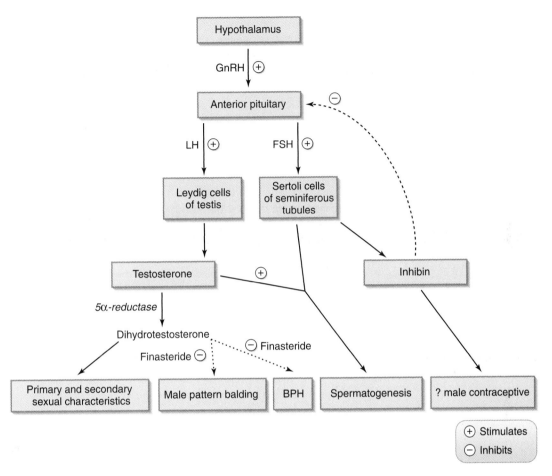

3-13: *Male axis. BPH, benign prostatic hyperplasia; FSH, follicle-stimulating hormone; GnRH, gonadotropin-releasing hormone; LH, luteinizing hormone.*

- In some tissues, especially the prostate and skin, testosterone is converted to a more potent form, **DHT,** by the enzyme **5α-reductase** before affecting cellular function.

> **Pharmacology/Pathology note:** In elderly men, the prostate gland often enlarges and compresses the urethra as it passes through the prostate, limiting urine flow rates and causing retention of urine in the bladder. One of the most commonly used drugs to treat this condition is **finasteride,** which inhibits the enzyme **5α-reductase,** thereby limiting the influence of DHT on the prostate and **shrinking it.** DHT is partly responsible for **male pattern baldness;** thus, finasteride is also modestly effective at restoring hair growth in men.

b. **Physiologic actions of testosterone**
- During embryologic development, **testosterone** is responsible for the development of the **male sexual organs,** including the penis, scrotum, prostate, epididymis, vas deferens, and seminal vesicles. In the absence of testosterone or tissue responsiveness to it, female sexual organs develop, even if the fetus is genetically male.

> **Clinical note:** In **androgen insensitivity syndrome,** the most common cause of **male hermaphroditism,** genetic males (46,XY) appear phenotypically female. This syndrome is caused by **mutations** in the **androgen receptor gene** located on the X chromosome. The testes produce testosterone, but male sexual characteristics do not develop because the **tissues are not responsive to the testosterone.** The testes also produce müllerian-inhibiting substance, which dissolves the müllerian ducts that give rise to the internal genitalia of the female, so no uterus is formed. Instead, there is typically a vagina that ends in a blind pouch.

- Testosterone is also responsible for the development of numerous **male secondary sexual characteristics.** These include increasing both **lean muscle mass** and **bone density.** Although testosterone stimulates bone growth, it causes fusion of the epiphyseal plates, so excessive levels during the growing stages may result in short stature. **Testosterone** stimulates hair growth in a male pattern (face, chest, abdomen) and is also largely responsible for **male pattern baldness.**
- The lengthening of the larynx with deepening of the voice is also due to testosterone. Testosterone increases the rate of secretion by most of the body's sebaceous glands; thus, it predisposes to acne in pubescent males. Finally, testosterone **increases** the concentration of **red blood cells,** accounting for the differences in hemoglobin and hematocrit levels between males and females.

> **Clinical note:** During fetal development, testosterone is necessary for the **normal descent** of the testes from the abdomen to the scrotum. Undescended testes (**cryptorchidism**) is more likely to occur in the **absence of testosterone** and represents a significant risk factor for **testicular cancer.** Testosterone may be given to these to stimulate testicular descent.

c. **Regulation of testosterone secretion**
- Testosterone secretion by the Leydig cells is regulated by the hypothalamic pituitary axis.
   (1) Gonadotropin-releasing hormone (**GnRH**) secretion by the hypothalamus stimulates the pituitary to secrete luteinizing hormone (**LH**) and follicle-stimulating hormone (**FSH**).
   (2) LH then stimulates testosterone secretion by the Leydig cells, whereas FSH is important in spermatogenesis (discussed later).

(3) Testosterone then cause feedback inhibition of GnRH secretion by the hypothalamus and LH secretion by the pituitary.

> **Pharmacology note: Leuprolide** is a synthetic GnRH agonist that, when exogenously administered in a continuous **nonpulsatile** manner, **inhibits** the **secretion of FSH** and **LH** by the pituitary gonadotrophs. The result is reduced synthesis of testicular androgens in males and reduced ovarian estrogens and progestins in females. In patients with prostate cancer, a reduction in androgen synthesis is desirable, because the growth of the prostate cancer may be androgen dependent.

d. **Puberty in males**
  - At the onset of puberty, the hypothalamus begins secreting **increasing amounts of GnRH,** which causes increased pituitary secretion of LH and consequently increased Leydig cell secretion of testosterone.
  - The increased testosterone levels stimulate expression of male secondary sexual characteristics and enlargement of male primary sex organs.

e. **Spermatogenesis**
  - Spermatogenesis occurs in the **seminiferous tubules** of the testicles. Testosterone is important in stimulating the growth and division of testicular germinal cells, the ultimate source of sperm cells.
  - FSH, which is secreted by the anterior pituitary in response to GnRH, stimulates the **Sertoli cells** of the seminiferous tubules to facilitate maturation of sperm. The Sertoli cells also produce a substance called **inhibin,** which inhibits the secretion of FSH by the anterior pituitary.

> **Clinical note:** FSH is required for sperm maturation within the testes. By inhibiting FSH secretion by the pituitary, **inhibin** might be able to **prevent spermatogenesis** and could therefore be used as a **male contraceptive.** Indeed, clinical trials using inhibin are currently underway.

2. **Female reproductive axis** (Fig. 3-14)
  a. **Physiologic actions of estrogen and progesterone**
    - Unlike testosterone, estrogen and progesterone are both *unnecessary* for the development of female primary sexual characteristics.
    - **Estrogen** is responsible for the development of female secondary sexual characteristics and also plays a critical role in the menstrual cycle. With the onset of puberty, the increased estrogen levels induce **breast maturation** by causing proliferation of stromal tissue, development of the ductule system, and deposition of fat. Estrogen stimulates fat deposition, particularly on the hips and buttocks and in the subcutaneous tissues. Estrogen is also critical in skeletal maturation, causing **increased bone density** and **fusion of the epiphyseal plates** in adolescent females.
    - The principal functions of **progesterone** are to **stimulate** breast development, to help regulate the **menstrual cycle,** and to help maintain

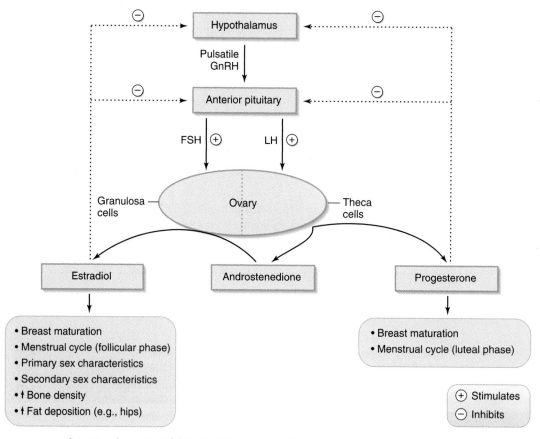

3-14: Female axis. FSH, follicle-stimulating hormone; GnRH, gonadotropin-releasing hormone; LH, luteinizing hormone.

a pregnancy. Both estrogen and progesterone **antagonize** the effects of prolactin on the breast.

b. **Regulation of secretion of estrogen and progesterone**
  • A complex cyclical pattern of FSH and LH secretion occurs in females. Hypothalamic release of GnRH causes the **gonadotrophs** in the anterior pituitary to **secrete FSH** and **LH. FSH** stimulates **estrogen** synthesis by ovarian follicles, and **LH** stimulates **progesterone** synthesis. Both estrogen and progesterone control FSH and LH secretion by feedback inhibition. As occurs in males, females reach puberty when the hypothalamus begins secreting increased levels of GnRH.

c. **Menstrual cycle** (Fig. 3-15)
  (1) **Follicular (proliferative) phase**
    • The menstrual cycle begins with the first day of **uterine bleeding** (day 1; **menses**). At this point, **estrogen** and **progesterone levels are low,** so **FSH levels** begin to gradually **increase** because of reduced negative feedback.

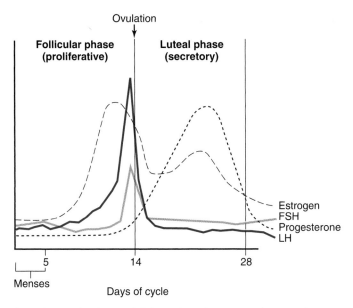

3-15: *Menstrual cycle. FSH, follicle-stimulating hormone; LH, luteinizing hormone.*

- FSH stimulates multiple follicles to develop, resulting in increased estrogen secretion. Eventually a single dominant follicle emerges and the remaining follicles undergo atresia. Although increasing levels of estrogen then begin to inhibit FSH secretion, the enlarging follicles or dominant follicle becomes increasingly sensitive to FSH, and estrogen levels continue to increase.
- When plasma estrogen levels reach a certain point, they paradoxically cause a surge in LH and FSH secretion through a positive feedback mechanism at the pituitary. The **LH surge** causes **ovulation.**
- After ovulation, the cells that lined the ovarian follicle form the **corpus luteum,** which **secretes estrogen** and **progesterone.** If an ovum is not fertilized, the corpus luteum degenerates, menses begin, and the cycle begins again. The time between the first day of menses and ovulation is referred to as the follicular phase, because the follicles are developing.

> **Pharmacology note: Estrogen-containing oral contraceptives** function by inhibiting the LH surge that is responsible for ovulation. Contraceptives provide a constant level of estrogen that maintains a continual negative feedback on pituitary gonadotropin secretion, thereby stabilizing FSH and LH secretion.

(2) **Luteal (secretory) phase**
- The time between ovulation and menses is referred to as the luteal phase (because the corpus luteum is present).
- During the follicular phase, the estrogen secreted by the ovaries stimulates **proliferation of the uterine endometrium.** When ovulation

occurs, the progesterone secreted by the corpus luteum causes the endometrium to become more secretory, preparing it for implantation of the ovum. If fertilization and implantation of the ovum do not occur, the corpus luteum degenerates and stops secreting estrogen and progesterone. Menses occurs when estrogen and progesterone levels drop, although menses is triggered primarily by the drop in progesterone.

> **Clinical note:** In some reproductive-aged females, normal menses do not occur **(amenorrhea).** This is often the result of a **failure to ovulate.** To determine if anovulation is the cause, these females are given a 10-day course of progesterone; if they begin menstruating shortly after the course of progesterone, there is compelling evidence that anovulation is causing the amenorrhea. The main source of progesterone in females is the corpus luteum; therefore, if ovulation does not occur, the corpus luteum is not formed, and consequently there is negligible progesterone synthesis. Because it is the drop in progesterone secretion that is mainly responsible for menses, lack of progesterone secretion means that menses cannot occur.

3. **Pathophysiology of reproductive disorders** (Table 3-8)
D. **Prolactin**
1. **Physiologic actions**
   • The major role of prolactin is in **breast maturation** and **lactogenesis** in pregnant females. Although prolactin secretion increases substantially during pregnancy, actual lactation is inhibited because of the simultaneously high levels of estrogen and progesterone secreted by the placenta.
   • After delivery and expulsion of the placenta, there is a drop in maternal estrogen and progesterone, and prolactin is able to **stimulate lactation** in response to **suckling** by the infant. In addition, elevated levels of prolactin serve as a "natural contraceptive" for breast-feeding females by inhibiting the hypothalamic secretion of GnRH. This explains why it is more difficult for mothers who breast-feed to become pregnant.

> **Clinical note:** Prolactin plays a more limited role in the male than in the female. However, hyperprolactinemia in males also inhibits hypothalamic GnRH secretion; causing **impotence** and **loss of libido.** Therefore, hyperprolactinemia should always be considered in the differential diagnosis of impotence.

2. **Regulation of secretion**
   • Prolactin secretion is strongly **inhibited by dopamine** (prolactin-inhibitory factor, PIF) secreted by the hypothalamus and is weakly stimulated by TRH.

> **Pharmacology note: Antipsychotic drugs** used to treat schizophrenia function largely by blocking dopamine receptors. Consequently, these drugs can block the inhibitory effect that dopamine has on prolactin secretion, resulting in **hyperprolactinemia** and its attendant consequences.

TABLE 3-8:
Pathophysiology of Some Reproductive Disorders

Disorder	Genetics	Pathophysiology	Clinical Comments
Precocious puberty	Normal karyotype	Premature maturation of arcuate nucleus in hypothalamus	Treat with GnRH agonists (e.g., leuprolide)
5α-Reductase deficiency	Normal karyotype	Insufficient conversion of testosterone to active dihydrotestosterone form	Female develops external male genitalia during puberty
Klinefelter's syndrome	47,XXY karyotype	Meiotic nondisjunction of X chromosome	Male with eunuchoid body and gynecomastia
Androgen insensitivity syndrome (male pseudohermaphroditism)	XY karyotype	Androgen receptor defect; male internal genitalia but incompletely virilized, ambiguous, or female external genitalia	Typically presents clinically with inguinal mass or absence of menarche
Female pseudohermaphroditism	46,XX karyotype	Gonads are ovaries but virilization of external genitalia	Congenital adrenal hyperplasia (21-hydroxylase deficiency)
True hermaphroditism	46,XX karyotype, most common, followed by 46,XX/46,XY mosaicism	Presence of both ovarian and testicular tissues	Ovulation and spermatogenesis may both occur
Turner's syndrome	45,XO karyotype with absent Barr body	Meiotic nondisjunction	Streaked ovaries, amenorrhea, short stature, webbed neck, aortic coarctation

GnRH, gonadotropin-releasing hormone.

3. **Pathophysiology** (Fig. 3-16)
   - Prolactin stimulates lactation and inhibits GnRH secretion; therefore, **elevated levels of prolactin** (hyperprolactinemia) in nonpregnant females can result in abnormal milk discharge from the nipples (**galactorrhea**) and **anovulatory infertility.**

   > **Pharmacology note:** Dopamine agonists such as **bromocriptine** (used in the treatment of Parkinson's disease) can be used to treat **hyperprolactinemia.** Schizophrenia is believed to be related to excess dopamine activity, and dopamine agonists such as bromocriptine can precipitate psychotic symptoms.

E. **Growth hormone (GH)**
   1. **Anabolic actions**
      - GH exerts strong **anabolic actions** that promote tissue growth, particularly of the musculoskeletal system.
      - GH mainly stimulates the liver to secrete insulin-like growth factor I (IGF-I), which mediates many of the anabolic actions of GH (Fig. 3-17).

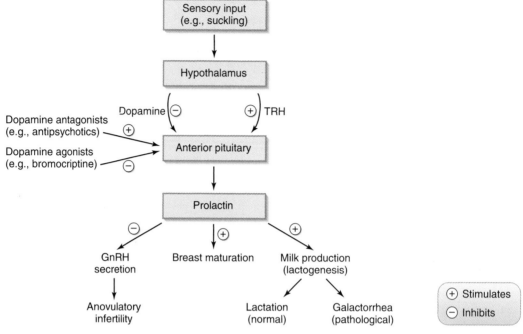

3-16: Physiologic actions of prolactin. TRH, thyrotropin-releasing hormone.

Pathology note: Excess GH levels may cause abnormal increased longitudinal bone growth before epiphyseal plate closure and may result in **gigantism,** whereas a deficiency of GH may cause **pituitary dwarfism.** After closure of the epiphyseal plate, longitudinal bone growth does not occur. However, transverse bone growth (i.e., thickening) in response to GH can continue throughout adulthood, and occurs in **acromegaly.**

2. **Metabolic actions**
   - GH acts on muscle, adipose tissue, and liver to promote fat metabolism, enhance protein synthesis, and preserve body carbohydrate. It **stimulates lipolysis** in **adipose tissue,** which increases the delivery of "combustible" fatty acids to the cells of the body. It simultaneously **inhibits protein breakdown** and **stimulates new protein synthesis** in skeletal muscle. Finally, it conserves body stores of carbohydrate by **stimulating hepatic gluconeogenesis** and **preventing glucose utilization** by the peripheral tissues, which forces them to burn fats (see Fig. 3-17).
   - These actions are helpful in stressful conditions such as fasting or starvation. Plasma glucose is preserved for the insulin-independent tissues, such as the CNS (to maintain consciousness), and skeletal muscle protein is preserved as much as possible.
   - Notice that these actions essentially are antagonistic to those of insulin. Prolonged exposure to excessive levels of GH may therefore cause

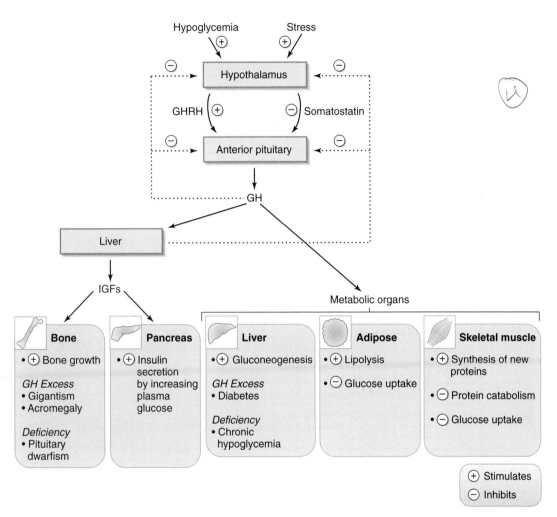

3-17: *Physiologic actions of growth hormone. GH, growth hormone; GHRH, growth hormone–releasing hormone; IGF, insulin-like growth factor.*

hyperglycemia and even overt **diabetes mellitus;** which is why GH is considered a **diabetogenic** hormone.

- **Note:** In rare states of GH deficiency (e.g., **panhypopituitarism**), chronic **hypoglycemia** may develop.

3. **Regulation of secretion**
   - GH is secreted from **pituitary somatotrophs** mainly during sleep but also in response to other stimuli, such as various forms of stress caused by fasting or hypoglycemia.
   - Secretion is regulated by hypothalamic growth hormone–releasing hormone (**GHRH**), which stimulates GH release, and by **somatostatin,** which inhibits GH release. The IGF-I that is produced in response to GH stimulation of the

liver also influences the hypothalamus and anterior pituitary by feedback inhibition.

> **Clinical note:** GH is a diabetogenic hormone that acts to increase plasma glucose levels. GH secretion is in turn suppressed by increased plasma glucose levels, a fact that can be exploited clinically when evaluating patients with suspected **hyperpituitarism.** In the **growth hormone suppression test,** an oral load of glucose (typically 75–100 g) is rapidly administered. This will increase plasma glucose levels, which should inhibit GH secretion in a healthy adult. If plasma levels of GH do not decrease substantially (to less than 2 ng/mL) in response to the glucose load, pituitary hypersecretion of GH is indicated, which may facilitate a diagnosis of **gigantism** or **acromegaly.**

> **Pharmacology note: Octreotide,** a synthetic somatostatin analogue, is used to treat GH-secreting tumors of the anterior pituitary.

III. **Hormonal Control Systems of the Posterior Pituitary**
- The posterior pituitary is composed of axonal extensions from **several** of the **hypothalamic nuclei.** The axonal terminals of these neurons secrete posterior pituitary hormones, and their activity is independent of hypothalamic releasing hormones.
  A. **Hormones of the posterior pituitary**
     1. **Antidiuretic hormone (ADH, vasopressin)**
        a. **Physiologic actions**
           - The primary physiologic action of ADH is to **stimulate water reabsorption by the kidneys,** which increases plasma volume and decreases plasma osmolarity.
           - At higher levels, ADH also **stimulates systemic vasoconstriction.**
        b. **Regulation of secretion**
           - ADH secretion depends on functioning **osmoreceptors** within the hypothalamus.
           - These specialized cells either shrink or swell in response to changing plasma osmolarity, respectively triggering or inhibiting ADH secretion. Although ADH secretion occurs in response to only slight increases in plasma osmolarity, marked reductions in plasma volume (see Fig. 4-27 in Chapter 4), as might occur during hemorrhage, are necessary to trigger substantial ADH secretion.
        c. **Pathophysiology**
           (1) **Diabetes insipidus**
              - Diabetes insipidus is caused by a **deficiency** of functional **ADH** or by **tissue insensitivity** to circulating ADH. It is characterized by the production of large volumes of **dilute urine** as the result of an impaired ability of the kidneys to concentrate urine by reabsorbing water.
              - If hypothalamic ADH secretion is compromised, the condition is known as **central diabetes insipidus;** if the kidneys are unresponsive to ADH, it is known as **nephrogenic diabetes insipidus.**

> **Clinical note: Central diabetes insipidus** can be caused by **head trauma,** hypothalamic lesions, neoplasms, gene mutations in the vasopressin gene, and exposure to various drugs. Patients with central diabetes insipidus will be responsive to exogenously administered ADH, because there is nothing wrong with their kidneys. In contrast, patients with nephrogenic diabetes insipidus *will not* respond to ADH. This difference in responsiveness serves as the **basis for clinical differentiation** between these two etiologies.

    (2) **Syndrome of inappropriate ADH secretion (SIADH)**
- In certain pathologic situations, the posterior **pituitary** may secrete **excessive** amounts of ADH. Alternatively, ectopic secretion of ADH can occur from tumors such as **small cell lung cancer.**
- Regardless of the cause, increased levels of ADH will cause **excessive water reabsorption by the kidneys,** resulting in **reduced plasma osmolarity** and **hyponatremia.**

2. **Oxytocin**
- The posterior pituitary hormone oxytocin is important in producing **uterine contractions** in response to **dilation of the cervix** during labor.
- It is also important in stimulating contraction of myoepithelial cells of the breast in response to **suckling** during breast-feeding.
- Oxytocin secretion also can be stimulated simply by the sight and sounds of the neonate.

> **Pharmacology note: Oxytocin** is often administered during labor to **augment labor.** It is also given to **reduce postpartum hemorrhage,** because the uterine contractions it stimulates clamp down on the uterine blood vessels, thereby minimizing blood loss.

IV. **Hormonal Control Systems That Do Not Involve the Pituitary**
  A. **Endocrine pancreas**
- The endocrine pancreas comprises the **islets of Langerhans,** a cluster of specialized endocrine cells that secrete various hormones important in metabolism.
- The main specialized cell types are the **α cells** that secrete glucagon, the **β cells** that secrete insulin, and the **δ cells** that secrete somatostatin (Table 3-9).

    1. **Insulin**
      a. **Mechanism of action**
- As a peptide hormone, insulin acts by binding to a cell surface receptor, the **tyrosine kinase receptor.**
- Insulin stimulates a wide variety of intracellular events, such as the **insertion of glucose transporters (GLUT4) into cell membranes** of skeletal muscle and adipose tissue and the transcriptional stimulation of genes involved in glycolysis. Onset of the effects of insulin is immediate for some (e.g., GLUT4 insertion into membranes) but can take hours or days for others (e.g., new protein synthesis).

TABLE 3-9:
Physiologic Actions of Pancreatic Hormones

Cell Type	Hormone Secreted	Primary Actions	Primary Stimulators
α	Glucagon	Stimulates hepatic glycogenolysis and gluconeogenesis to increase plasma glucose	Hypoglycemia, amino acids
β	Insulin	Anabolic actions via stimulation of glucose and amino acids in tissues; decreases levels of plasma glucose	Glucose, amino acids
δ	Somatostatin	Inhibits insulin and glucagon secretion; has inhibitory effects on all digestive processes	Glucose, amino acids, fatty acids

TABLE 3-10:
Actions of Insulin on Target Tissues

Target Tissue	Stimulates	Inhibits
Adipose	Fatty acid uptake, triglyceride synthesis and storage	Lipolysis
Liver	Glycolysis, glycogenesis, amino acid and glucose uptake, fat synthesis, cholesterol synthesis	Gluconeogenesis, β-oxidation of fatty acids, ketogenesis
Muscle	Glucose uptake, glycogenesis, glycolysis, protein synthesis	Protein catabolism

b. **Metabolic actions** (Table 3-10; Fig. 3-18)
- The principal role of insulin is to **maintain plasma glucose levels** within normal ranges. The major **stimulus** for insulin secretion is **plasma glucose,** with increasing plasma glucose levels stimulating proportionally more insulin secretion. The major **inhibitor** of insulin secretion is **low plasma glucose.**
- Insulin stimulates glucose uptake in various target tissues, especially the liver, skeletal muscles, and adipose tissue. Insulin also stimulates glycolysis and various anabolic pathways, including the synthesis of glycogen (**glycogenesis**), fat (**lipogenesis**), cholesterol, and protein.
- Certain tissues, such as the CNS, utilize glucose as their primary energy source and are able to take up glucose without the assistance of insulin. This ability becomes critically important during the fasting state, when plasma levels of insulin (and sometimes glucose) are low. When insulin levels are low, the skeletal muscles, adipose tissue, and liver do not take up

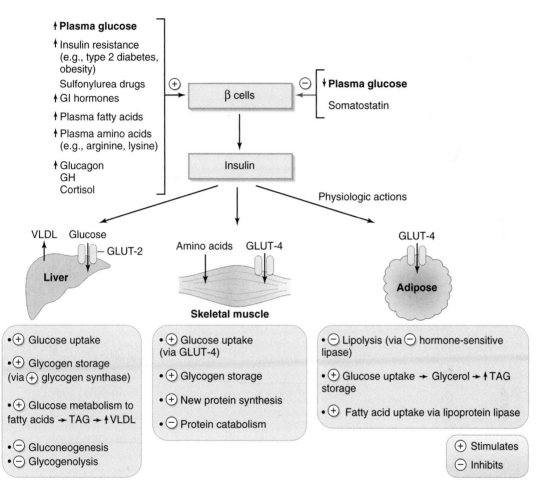

↑Plasma glucose

↑Insulin resistance
(e.g., type 2 diabetes,
obesity)

Sulfonylurea drugs

↑GI hormones

↑Plasma fatty acids

↑Plasma amino acids
(e.g., arginine, lysine)

↑Glucagon
GH
Cortisol

⊕ → β cells ← ⊖ **↓Plasma glucose**

Somatostatin

Insulin

Physiologic actions

VLDL   Glucose

GLUT-2

Liver

Amino acids   GLUT-4

Skeletal muscle

GLUT-4

Adipose

- ⊕ Glucose uptake

- ⊕ Glycogen storage
(via ⊕ glycogen synthase)

- ⊕ Glucose metabolism to
fatty acids → TAG → ↑VLDL

- ⊖ Gluconeogenesis
- ⊖ Glycogenolysis

- ⊕ Glucose uptake
(via GLUT-4)

- ⊕ Glycogen storage

- ⊕ New protein synthesis

- ⊖ Protein catabolism

- ⊖ Lipolysis (via ⊖ hormone-sensitive
lipase)

- ⊕ Glucose uptake → Glycerol → ↑TAG
storage

- ⊕ Fatty acid uptake via lipoprotein lipase

⊕ Stimulates

⊖ Inhibits

3-18: Regulation of insulin secretion and physiologic actions of insulin. GH, growth hormone; GI, gastrointestinal; GLUT, glucose transporter; TAG, triacylglycerides; VLDL, very low density lipoprotein.

significant amounts of glucose; this preserves glucose for insulin-independent tissues such as the CNS.

- In adipose tissue, insulin stimulates the expression of the enzyme **lipoprotein lipase** (LPL), which liberates free fatty acids from very low density lipoproteins (VLDL) and allows these fatty acids to enter adipocytes, where they are **stored as triglycerides.**

Pharmacology note: A class of drugs known as the **fibric acid derivatives** (e.g., clofibrate, gemfibrozil) reduce plasma **triglyceride levels** by stimulating **lipoprotein lipase** in adipose tissue. This is important because elevated triglycerides, like low-density lipoprotein (LDL) cholesterol, are a risk factor for development of **coronary artery disease.** Extremely high levels of triglycerides are also a risk factor for **pancreatitis.**

> **Clinical note:** Because glucose and potassium are simultaneously cotransported into cells, insulin **stimulates potassium uptake.** This effect is often exploited therapeutically in patients with **hyperkalemia,** in whom injection of insulin can reduce the plasma potassium level significantly.

c. **Pathophysiology of type 1 diabetes mellitus**
- The primary defect in type 1 diabetes mellitus (previously termed "insulin-dependent diabetes mellitus," or IDDM) is a deficiency of insulin, typically caused by autoimmune destruction of the pancreatic β cells. This deficiency causes hyperglycemia. The resulting increased glucose "load" delivered to the kidneys may result in loss of glucose in the urine, which causes an osmotic diuresis, termed "polyuria." This diuresis with loss of body fluids in turn stimulates thirst, termed "polydipsia."
- In addition, because insulin is a potent **anabolic hormone,** a catabolic state characterized by weight loss and muscle wasting occurs in the absence of insulin. This causes an increase in appetite (polyphagia). Together, these phenomena account for the clinical presentation of type 1 diabetes mellitus: polyuria, polydipsia, and weight loss with polyphagia.

> **Clinical note: Diabetic ketoacidosis** (DKA) is characterized by hyperglycemia, dehydration, and acidosis. It is caused by an absolute or relative **deficiency** of the anabolic hormone **insulin.** DKA can occur in type 1 diabetics who are noncompliant with their insulin regimen, or it can be triggered by stressors such as infection.
>
> In the absence of insulin, "runaway" lipolysis and β-oxidation occur in adipose tissue and liver, respectively. Moreover, the lipolysis in adipose tissue continues to "feed" β-oxidation precursors to the liver, which metabolizes these fatty acids to ketone bodies. Several of these ketone bodies are **acids** that reduce the plasma pH, resulting in an acidosis. This acidosis is further exacerbated by the **hyperglycemia,** because the hyperglycemia causes an **osmotic diuresis** that results in dehydration. With plasma volume contraction, the glomerular filtration rate (GFR) drops and the kidneys are **less able to excrete acid.**

d. **Pathophysiology of type 2 diabetes mellitus**
- The primary defect in type 2 diabetes mellitus (previously termed non–insulin-dependent diabetes mellitus, or NIDDM) is the **abnormal resistance of target tissues** (e.g., muscle, adipose tissue, liver) to circulating insulin **(insulin resistance).** This resistance is particularly common in obese persons. Insulin levels may be elevated in these patients, although it should be realized that they are still **relatively deficient** given the degree of hyperglycemia.
- As type 2 diabetes mellitus progresses, a secondary defect, β **cell dysfunction with impaired insulin secretion,** begins to play a greater

role. There are various speculations as to why this happens, including pancreatic exhaustion, glucotoxicity, and amylin deposition.

- **DKA** occurs much less frequently than in type 1 diabetes, perhaps because the insulin that is present is capable of inhibiting hepatic ketogenesis. However, if the diabetes is poorly managed or a major illness (e.g., pneumonia) ensues, plasma glucose and plasma osmolarity may become pathologically elevated, resulting in signs and symptoms. This is termed a **"hyperosmolar hyperglycemic nonketotic coma"** (HHNC).

- HHNC is caused by severe dehydration that is caused by a prolonged **hyperglycemic diuresis** in which compensatory fluid intake is inadequate. Elderly patients are particularly susceptible to HHNC because of **inadequate fluid intake** and **preexisting renal disease** (i.e., renal glucose clearance is already compromised).

> **Clinical note:** Insulin is **co-secreted** with **C peptide** by pancreatic β cells. Plasma levels of C peptide are typically **low in type 1 diabetes,** because these patients have few functional β cells. In contrast, plasma levels of C peptide are typically **high in the early stages of type 2 diabetes,** because type 2 diabetes is characterized by **insulin resistance** and **hyperinsulinemia.** Therefore, plasma levels of C peptide can help distinguish between type 1 and type 2 diabetes. However, this is an imperfect test, given that fairly high levels of C peptide may be present in type 1 diabetics diagnosed very early, and fairly low levels in type 2 diabetics diagnosed very late, after the β cells have started "failing."

> **Clinical note:** Plasma C peptide levels can also help determine the cause of **hypoglycemia.** For example, in a **malingering** patient who **injects insulin** to cause hypoglycemia, plasma levels of C peptide will be very low. In contrast, a patient with a rare insulin-secreting tumor (**insulinoma**) will have high plasma levels of C peptide.

> **Pharmacology note:** One way to reduce plasma glucose is to stimulate the β cells to secrete more insulin. The sulfonylurea drugs (e.g., tolbutamide, glyburide) stimulate insulin secretion by closing membrane-spanning K^+ channels on pancreatic β cells, resulting in depolarization, followed by calcium influx that triggers insulin secretion. These drugs are primarily useful in type 2 diabetes, because their mechanism of action is dependent on the presence of functional β cells. However, these drugs carry a significant risk of hypoglycemia, and their misuse often leads to a visit to the emergency department.

2. **Glucagon**
   - Like insulin, glucagon is a primary regulator of plasma glucose homeostasis. Glucagon functions primarily to increase plasma glucose levels, thereby opposing the actions of insulin.

a. **Regulation of secretion**
- Paradoxically, the primary stimulus for glucagon secretion from islet cells is **amino acids** rather than low plasma glucose. However, glucagon secretion is also stimulated by low plasma glucose levels and inhibited by high levels.

b. **Physiologic actions**
- At physiologic concentrations, glucagon primarily promotes hepatic glycogenolysis and gluconeogenesis. Glucagon further stimulates β-oxidation of fats by the liver, which liberates energy that can be used to support hepatic gluconeogenesis.
- Glucagon exerts only minimal metabolic actions on adipose tissue and muscle. These actions include **stimulation of lipolysis** in adipose tissue and **inhibition of glucose utilization** by the peripheral tissues. These extrahepatic actions also contribute to increased plasma glucose levels.

> **Pathology note:** Given its secretion directly into the portal circulation, **glucagon** normally has minimal extrahepatic actions because of the **first-pass effect,** whereby it is largely inactivated by the liver. Increased glucagon levels may be associated with a rare tumor of the islet α cells termed a **glucagonoma.** At higher glucagon levels, the extrahepatic effects may become **very** significant, and many of these patients will present with hyperglycemia.

B. **Adrenal mineralocorticoids**
- Aldosterone is the primary mineralocorticoid secreted from the adrenal gland. The main function of aldosterone is to maintain intravascular volume and thereby **maintain arterial blood pressure.**
  1. **Physiologic actions of aldosterone**
     - Aldosterone acts on the kidneys to stimulate **sodium** (and therefore water) **reabsorption, potassium secretion,** and **hydrogen ion secretion.**
     - The net effect is an increase in blood pressure via stimulation of plasma volume expansion. If high levels of aldosterone are present, this may also result in pathologically elevated blood pressure, hypokalemia, and a metabolic alkalosis.
  2. **Regulation of aldosterone secretion**
     - Aldosterone is primarily secreted in response to increasing plasma levels of angiotensin II and potassium.
     - ACTH has only a minimal effect on aldosterone synthesis.

C. **Adrenal catecholamines**
- The adrenal catecholamines include **epinephrine, norepinephrine,** and **dopamine,** which are all synthesized from the amino acid tyrosine in the **adrenal medulla.** These agents are responsible for the physiologic manifestations of the **"fight or flight" response,** in which a severe threat to life elicits a coordinated physiologic response to counter that threat. All catecholamines have short half-lives (seconds), so their effects are short lived.

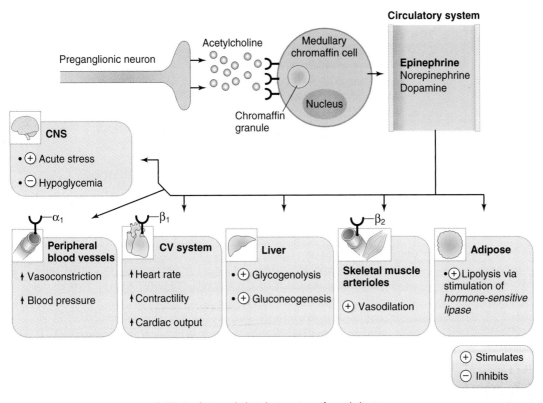

3-19: *Synthesis and physiologic actions of catecholamines.*

- **Epinephrine** is synthesized and secreted by the adrenal gland in much larger amounts than either norepinephrine or dopamine, and it is responsible for the major catecholamine-mediated physiologic responses resulting from sympathetic stimulation of the adrenal medulla.
- **Note:** Norepinephrine is the catecholamine released by postganglionic nerves of the sympathetic nervous system.
1. **Physiologic actions of catecholamines** (Fig. 3-19)
   a. **Cardiovascular effects**
      - Blood pressure is increased, because the catecholamines **increase heart rate** and **cardiac contractility** by stimulating β_1-adrenergic receptors.
      - Catecholamines also cause **peripheral vasoconstriction** by stimulating α_1-adrenergic receptors, which increases peripheral vascular resistance and further increases the arterial pressure. Catecholamines simultaneously **stimulate vasodilation in skeletal muscle** by stimulating β_2-adrenergic receptors, allowing greater blood flow to active muscles.
      - In addition, catecholamines cause **bronchodilation** by stimulating β_2-adrenergic receptors in the bronchioles, allowing greater oxygen delivery to the lungs (Table 3-11).

TABLE 3-11:
Functions of Adrenergic Receptors

Receptor Type	Location	Function
α_1	Vascular smooth muscle	Mediates vasoconstriction
α_2	Presynaptic terminals	Reduces sympathetic activity
β_1	Heart	Mediates increases in heart rate and contractility
β_2	Vascular smooth muscle within skeletal muscle	Mediates vasodilation
	Bronchiolar smooth muscle	Mediates bronchodilation

b. **Metabolic effects**
   • Catecholamines are like other "stress" hormones such as cortisol and function to **maintain adequate levels of plasma fuels** such as glucose and free fatty acids.
   • For example, epinephrine potently **stimulates glycogenolysis** and **gluconeogenesis** in the liver, as well as **lipolysis** in adipose tissue.
2. **Regulation of secretion of epinephrine**
   • The secretion of epinephrine by the adrenal medulla is under the control of the CNS. Preganglionic fibers of the sympathetic division of the autonomic nervous system synapse on **chromaffin cells** of the adrenal medulla and stimulate them to synthesize and release catecholamines.
   • A major stimulus of epinephrine secretion is hypoglycemia. The surge in epinephrine stimulates **glycogenolysis** and **gluconeogenesis** in the liver.

> **Clinical note: Chromaffin cell tumors** of the adrenal medulla, or of sites along the tract by which neural crest cells migrate to form the adrenal medulla, can arise and secrete large quantities of catecholamines. These tumors often release catecholamines in spurts, causing symptomatic episodes of hypertension, tachycardia, palpitations, sweating, and headache. Catecholamines are degraded to metanephrines and vanillylmandelic acid; therefore, increased urine levels of these metabolites may be used to diagnose a **pheochromocytoma.** Definitive treatment of a pheochromocytoma is surgical excision.

V. **Calcium and Phosphate Homeostasis: Parathyroid Hormone, Vitamin D, and Calcitonin**
   A. **Calcium homeostasis**
      • The body maintains plasma calcium levels within a narrow range because of the adverse effects caused by abnormally reduced or elevated levels of calcium. The endocrine regulation of calcium depends mainly on the actions of **PTH** and **calcitriol.** A third hormone, **calcitonin,** contributes minimally to calcium homeostasis.

- Most **calcium** (~99%) is found in the **bones.** Aside from playing an important structural role, this calcium serves as a large reservoir to replenish and maintain plasma calcium levels. Within the plasma, calcium exists either as free **ionized calcium** or as **bound calcium** associated with plasma proteins such as albumin. The ionized calcium is biologically active, and it is this portion of total body calcium that is tightly regulated by the hormones PTH, calcitriol, and calcitonin.
- Calcium stabilizes membrane potentials; therefore, **hypocalcemia** can lead to various manifestations of enhanced membrane excitability, including **muscle spasms, cardiac arrhythmias,** and **seizures. Hypercalcemia,** on the other hand, reduces membrane excitability, leading to such manifestations as **muscle weakness** and **stupor.**

> **Clinical note:** The percentage of plasma calcium that exists as free ionized calcium can be altered by changes in **plasma pH** and **plasma protein** levels. **Alkalosis** tends to decrease free ionized calcium, mainly because of greater calcium binding to negatively charged sites on albumin, and **acidosis** tends to increase ionized calcium. Changes in plasma protein levels are more likely to affect **total plasma calcium** than ionized calcium. For example, total plasma calcium levels are decreased in hypoalbuminemia, but the levels of free ionized calcium may still be normal. Therefore, before making a diagnosis of hypocalcemia or hypercalcemia, levels of plasma proteins such as albumin should be measured.

B. **Parathyroid Hormone** (Fig. 3-20)
- PTH functions to **increase plasma calcium** and to **decrease plasma phosphate.**
- PTH is released by parathyroid **chief cells,** mainly in response to hypocalcemia.
- PTH causes bone resorption, which liberates calcium into the plasma, and stimulates renal calcium reabsorption. PTH further stimulates the synthesis of 1,25-dihydroxyvitamin D by the kidneys, and it is this active form of vitamin D that increases calcium absorption in the intestines.

> **Pathology note:** Hyperparathyroidism can result in several adverse manifestations. Excessive bone resorption can cause osteoporosis as well as cysts in areas of extensively demineralized bone; this latter condition is referred to as **osteitis fibrosa cystica.** Hypercalcemia can cause renal calculi, as well as weakness and mental status changes. These manifestations are responsible for the clinical description of hyperparathyroidism: "stones, bones, groans, and psychological overtones." An adenoma of one of the parathyroid glands is the most common cause of hyperparathyroidism.

C. **1,25-Dihydroxyvitamin D** (Table 3-12)
- 1,25-Dihydroxyvitamin D is the metabolically active form of vitamin D. Vitamin D ingested in the diet or formed in the skin from exposure to sunlight must first be converted to 25-hydroxyvitamin D in the liver and then to its metabolically active form, 1,25-dihydroxyvitamin D, in the kidneys. PTH

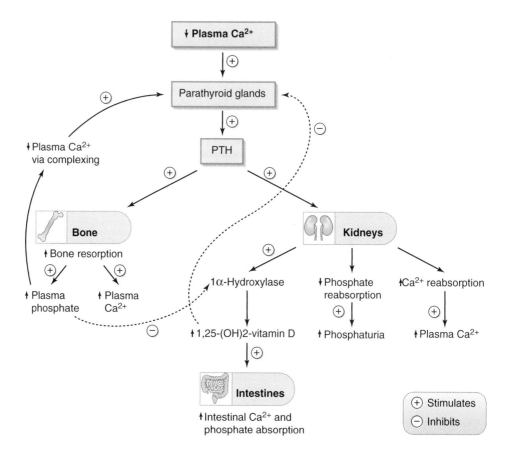

3-20: *Parathyroid hormone (PTH) overview.*

TABLE 3-12:
Organ Effects of Parathyroid Hormone and 1,25-Dihydroxyvitamin D

Hormone	Kidney	Intestine	Bone
Parathyroid hormone	Stimulates calcium reabsorption and phosphate excretion	Stimulates calcium absorption via increasing synthesis of active vitamin D	Stimulates bone resorption
1,25-Dihydroxyvitamin D	Stimulates calcium and phosphate reabsorption	Stimulates calcium and phosphate absorption	Stimulates bone resorption directly by activating osteoclasts
			Stimulates bone formation indirectly by increasing plasma calcium levels

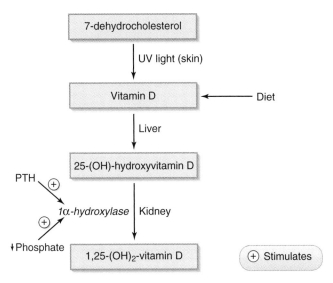

3-21: *Vitamin D synthesis. PTH, parathyroid hormone; UV, ultraviolet.*

stimulates the synthesis of 1,25-dihydroxyvitamin D in the kidneys by increasing the expression of the enzyme 1α-hydroxylase (Fig. 3-21).

- 1,25-Dihydroxyvitamin D affects calcium homeostasis in several ways: Most importantly, it stimulates **calcium absorption** in the intestine. To a lesser extent, it stimulates calcium reabsorption in the kidneys. It also directly stimulates calcium mobilization from bone.

> **Pathology note:** Although vitamin D stimulates bone resorption, its indirect effects on stimulating bone mineralization appear to outweigh its direct effects on stimulating bone resorption, given that vitamin D deficiencies result in conditions associated with impaired bone mineralization. For example, inadequate vitamin D levels in children leads to **rickets,** in which the bones are inadequately mineralized and the weight placed on them causes bowing. In adults, vitamin D deficiency weakens the bones, predisposing to fractures; in this case, the disease is referred to as **osteomalacia.** Vitamin D probably stimulates bone mineralization because of its actions to increase plasma calcium levels, which facilitates plasma calcium deposition into newly formed bone.

D. **Phosphate homeostasis**
- Phosphate levels are less tightly controlled than plasma calcium levels, because similar shifts in plasma phosphate do not tend to produce serious adverse effects.
1. **PTH and phosphate** (see Table 3-12)
   - By stimulating bone resorption, PTH causes both **calcium** and **phosphate** to be released into the plasma. The released phosphate can complex with calcium and decrease plasma calcium levels.

- Hypocalcemia does not typically result, however, because PTH also inhibits phosphate reabsorption by the proximal tubules, thus causing greater renal excretion of phosphate.
2. **1,25-Dihydroxyvitamin D and phosphate** (see Table 3-12 and Fig. 3-21)
   - 1,25-Dihydroxyvitamin D stimulates intestinal absorption of both calcium and phosphate and further stimulates renal phosphate reabsorption, in contrast to PTH.
   - In turn, increased levels of phosphate inhibit renal 1,25-dihydroxyvitamin D synthesis via a negative feedback mechanism.
   - In addition, the active form of vitamin D inhibits further vitamin D synthesis, another negative feedback mechanism.

> **Clinical note: Hypocalcemia** often develops in patients with **renal failure** because of disruptions in several mechanisms. When renal tissue is destroyed, less 1,25-dihydroxyvitamin D is synthesized by the kidney, resulting in less calcium absorption in the intestine. In addition, less phosphate is excreted because of the impaired filtration function of the kidneys, causing phosphate to accumulate. This phosphate can complex with plasma calcium and decrease ionized calcium levels. The increased plasma phosphate further inhibits an already compromised renal synthesis of 1,25-dihydroxyvitamin D.
>
> Parathyroid secretion of PTH is **strongly** stimulated because of the hypocalcemia. When PTH is secreted at excessive levels in response to hypocalcemia, it is referred to as **secondary hyperparathyroidism.** The excess PTH can cause severe bone wasting in patients with renal disease. The reduced vitamin D synthesis in renal failure and its attendant hypocalcemia contribute to bone wasting. Both of these processes contribute to **renal osteodystrophy.**

Cardiovascular Physiology

I. **Cardiac Mechanics**
  A. **Cardiac cycle: composed of systole and diastole**
    1. **Systole**
       - Systole is that part of the cardiac cycle in which the **heart contracts** and **blood is ejected.** In **atrial systole,** the atria pump blood into the relaxed ventricles, whereas in **ventricular systole,** the ventricles pump blood into the blood vessels.
       - **Blood pressure is greatest during systole** and is referred to as the **systolic blood pressure** (SBP).
    2. **Diastole**
       - Diastole is that part of the cardiac cycle in which the heart relaxes and fills with blood. **Blood pressure is lowest during diastole** and is referred to as the **diastolic blood pressure** (DBP).
       - The **pulse pressure** is the difference between the systolic and diastolic pressures:

       $$\text{Pulse pressure} = \text{SBP} - \text{DBP}$$

  B. **Heart valves: function to establish one-way flow of blood in the heart** (Fig. 4-1)
    1. **Atrioventricular valves: mitral and tricuspid valves**
       - The atrioventricular (AV) valves prevent blood from flowing back into the atria during ventricular systole.
       - The **mitral (bicuspid) valve** prevents backflow from the left ventricle into the left atrium.
       - The **tricuspid valve** prevents backflow from the right ventricle into the right atrium.
    2. **Semilunar valves: aortic and pulmonic valves**
       - The semilunar valves prevent blood from flowing back into the ventricles during ventricular diastole.
       - The **aortic valve** separates the left ventricle from the aorta.
       - The **pulmonic valve** separates the right ventricle from the pulmonary artery.
       - Both valves **normally have three cusps.**
  C. **Principal heart sounds: reflect valve closure and/or pathologic states**
    1. **S_1: closure of AV valves**
       - Closure of the AV valves in early ventricular systole produces S_1.
       - These valves close in early systole because of the rapidly increasing ventricular pressure.

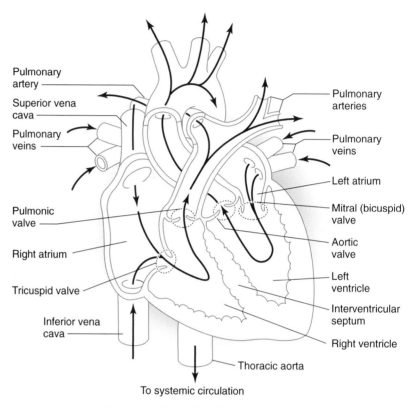

Pulmonary artery

Superior vena cava

Pulmonary veins

Pulmonic valve

Right atrium

Tricuspid valve

Inferior vena cava

Pulmonary arteries

Pulmonary veins

Left atrium

Mitral (bicuspid) valve

Aortic valve

Left ventricle

Interventricular septum

Right ventricle

Thoracic aorta

To systemic circulation

4-1: *One-way flow of blood through the heart valves.*

2. **S$_2$: closure of semilunar valves**
   - Closure of the semilunar valves in early diastole produces S$_2$.
   - Diastolic pressures in the aorta and pulmonary artery exceed the pressures in the relaxing ventricles.
3. **S$_3$: ventricular gallop**
   - An S$_3$ is sometimes heard in **early to middle diastole,** during rapid ventricular filling.
   - An S$_3$ may be caused by a sudden limitation of ventricular expansion.

   > **Clinical note:** An **S$_3$** is normal in children and young adults, but it may represent disease in older adults. An S$_3$ may be caused by rapid ventricular expansion associated with regurgitation of blood across an incompetent valve, which increases the rate of ventricular filling during diastole (e.g., **aortic regurgitation**).

4. **S$_4$: atrial gallop**
   - An S$_4$ is sometimes heard in **late diastole** and is caused by **atrial contraction against a stiffened ventricle.**
   - An S$_4$ almost always indicates **cardiac disease** and should be further evaluated.

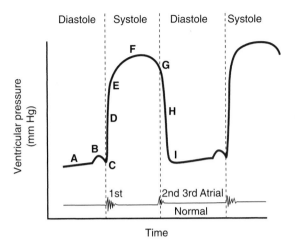

4-2: *Ventricular pressure changes during the cardiac cycle.*

> **Clinical note:** An **S₄** usually indicates decreased ventricular compliance (i.e., the ventricle does not relax as easily), which is commonly associated with ventricular hypertrophy or scarring. An S₄ is **almost always present after an acute myocardial infarction.**

D. **Ventricular pressure changes during the cardiac cycle** (Fig. 4-2)
- During diastole, the ventricles gradually increase in volume, causing **ventricular pressures to gradually increase (A).**
- The slight "hump" before systole **(B)** represents **atrial contraction** in the final "topping off" phase of ventricular filling.
- When systole begins, the increasing ventricular pressures **close the AV valves (C).**
- Pressure continually builds until the ventricular pressure exceeds that of the aorta (left ventricle) or the pulmonary artery (right ventricle) **(D).**
- The aortic valve (left ventricle) or the pulmonic valve (right ventricle) then opens **(E).**
- **Blood is ejected into the circulation (F).**
- After the ventricles have finished contracting, they begin to relax, and **intraventricular pressures decrease.** When the intraventricular pressure is less than the aortic pressure (left ventricle) or the pulmonary artery pressure (right ventricle), the aortic and pulmonic valves close **(G).**
- After closure of the semilunar valves, the ventricles continue to relax and intraventricular pressures continue to decrease **(H).**
- Once intraventricular pressures are less than atrial pressures, the AV valves open **(I),** and the **ventricular filling of diastole** begins again.
- **Note:** The normal phonocardiogram in Figure 4-2 parallels the ventricular pressure curve. S₁ (1st) occurs at the beginning of systole with AV valve closure **(C),** and S₂ (2nd) occurs at the beginning of diastole with semilunar valve

closure **(G).** If an S_3 were present, it would occur in early diastole, because it is caused by **rapid ventricular filling.** If an S_4 were present, it would occur in late diastole, because it is caused by **atrial contraction** against a stiff ventricle.

- **Note:** Rapid ventricular filling occurs in the early part of diastole, when the pressure gradients for blood flow between the pulmonary veins and left ventricle are greatest and the mitral valve is wide open.

II. **Cardiac Performance**
- Cardiac performance is often assessed by measuring the cardiac output, which is the volume of blood pumped out of the heart each minute.

A. **Cardiac output**
- Cardiac output (CO) is the **product of heart rate** (HR) and **stroke volume** (SV). HR is primarily under the influence of the autonomic nervous system. In a healthy adult, the CO is approximately 5 L/minute:

$$CO = HR \times SV$$
$$= 70 \text{ beats/minute} \times 70 \text{ mL/beat}$$
$$= 4900 \text{ mL/minute, or } 4.9 \text{ L/minute}$$

- Another way to measure CO is by measuring whole body **oxygen consumption.** The **Fick Principle** states that oxygen consumption by the body is a function of the amount of blood delivered to the tissues (**cardiac output,** CO) and the amount of O_2 extracted by the tissues (**arteriovenous O_2 difference**):

$$O_2 \text{ consumption} = CO \times ([O_2]_a - [O_2]_v)$$

where $[O_2]_a$ = arterial O_2 concentration (~200 mL O_2/L blood) and $[O_2]_v$ = venous O_2 concentration (~150 mL O_2/L blood).

- This equation can be rearranged to calculate the cardiac output:

$$CO = \frac{O_2 \text{ consumption}}{[O_2]_a - [O_2]_v}$$

- Oxygen consumption is monitored by analysis of **expired air.** Mixed venous blood is sampled by inserting a catheter into the pulmonary artery. Arterial blood is obtained from any peripheral artery in the body. For example, the CO for a healthy 70-kg man is calculated as follows:

$$CO = \frac{250 \text{ mL/minute}}{(200 - 150 \text{ mL } O_2/\text{L blood})}$$
$$= 5 \text{ L/minute}$$

B. **Stroke volume**
- **Stroke volume** (SV) is the volume of blood ejected from the ventricle during ventricular systole. The stroke volume is a major determinant of pulse pressure. In a healthy adult, the SV is calculated from the end-diastolic volume (EDV) and the end-systolic volume (ESV), as follows:

$$SV = EDV - ESV$$
$$= 120 \text{ mL} - 50 \text{ mL} = 70 \text{ mL}$$

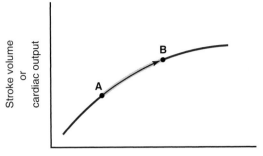

4-3: *Stroke volume versus preload. Atrial pressure at ventricular end-diastole correlates with ventricular end-diastolic volume and pressure and is often used as a surrogate marker of preload. Note that cardiac output increases from point A to point B as the preload increases.*

1. **Ejection fraction**
   - Ejection fraction (EF) is the **percentage of blood in the ventricle at the end of diastole** that is **pumped into the circulation** with each heartbeat. In other words, it is the SV divided by the EDV. In a healthy adult, the EF is calculated as follows:

$$EF = \frac{SV}{EDV}$$
$$= \frac{70\,mL}{120\,mL}$$
$$= 58.3, \text{or} \sim 60\%$$

> **Clinical note:** If the heart muscle is not contracting efficiently (e.g., after a myocardial infarction), the EF may be decreased. A decreased EF is observed in many forms of **heart failure.**

2. **Determinants of stroke volume**
   - The ventricular SV is determined by three principal factors: preload, contractility, and afterload.
   a. **Preload**
      - Preload is the **degree of tension** (load) **on the ventricular muscle when it begins to contract.** This load is mainly determined by the volume of blood within the ventricle at the end of diastole (EDV), which itself is mainly dependent on venous return. An increased EDV causes an increased SV (Fig. 4-3).
      - Precisely why an increased EDV increases SV remains controversial, but there are two prominent theories. The **Frank-Starling relationship,** also called the **length-tension relationship of the heart theory,** postulates that the increased ventricular wall tension associated with increased EDV stretches ventricular myocytes and results in a **greater overlap of actin and myosin filaments.** This greater overlap causes more forceful contractions and increases the SV.

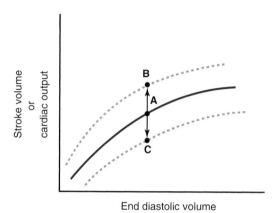

4-4: *Stroke volume versus contractility. For any given end-diastolic volume (A), addition of a positive inotropic agent (e.g., epinephrine) increases stroke volume and cardiac output by increasing contractility (B). Similarly, addition of a negative inotropic agent (e.g., antagonist of circulating epinephrine or norepinephrine) decreases stroke volume and cardiac output by decreasing contractility (C).*

- The second theory postulates that the contractile apparatus of cardiac myocytes **becomes more sensitive to cytoplasmic calcium** (Ca^{2+}) as the myocytes (and therefore sarcomeres) are stretched under conditions associated with increased preload. This concept is similar to the myogenic theory proposed to explain autoregulation of blood flow, to be discussed later.

   b. **Contractility**
   - Contractility is a measure of the **forcefulness of contractions at any given preload** (i.e., independent of myocardial wall tension at EDV) (Fig. 4-4). It is commonly referred to as the **inotropic state** of the heart.
   - **Drugs** (e.g. digitalis), **sympathetic excitation,** and **heart disease** may all affect contractility.

   c. **Afterload**
   - Afterload is the pressure or resistance **against which the ventricles must pump blood,** including systemic blood pressure and any obstruction to outflow from the ventricle, such as a **stenotic** (narrowed) **aortic valve.**
   - At a given preload and contractility, if afterload increases, then SV decreases (Fig. 4-5).

3. **Mechanical characterization of contraction**

   a. **Wall tension**
   - When pressure is increased inside a vessel, it causes a distending force. The force that opposes this distention is the **tension or stress in the vessel wall.** The **Laplace equation** relates these two forces:

$$\sigma = P \times r/2h$$

   where σ = wall tension, P = intraluminal pressure, r = intraluminal radius, h = wall thickness.

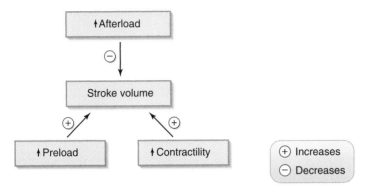

4-5: Determinants of stroke volume.

- Think of the ventricle as a very thick-walled vessel, and use the Laplace equation to determine that, if the ventricle must generate a greater intraventricular pressure to overcome an afterload, myocardial wall tension must increase.
  b. **Stroke work**
  - Stroke work is a measure of the mechanical work performed by the ventricle with each contraction. It has two main components.
  - **Pressure-volume work** is work used to push the SV into the high-pressure arterial system and is equal to the systemic arterial pressure multiplied by the SV (P × SV).
  - **Kinetic energy work** is work supplied by ventricular contraction that is used to move the ejected blood at a certain **velocity.** Under normal conditions, kinetic energy work is a minor component of the stroke work.
  - Increased stroke work is caused by increasing the SV against a constant systemic pressure (afterload) or by maintaining a given SV while afterload increases.
C. **Venous return**
  1. **Effect of venous return on cardiac output via influencing preload**
  - Increased venous return **increases preload.** The rate of venous return is determined by the **pressure gradient** between the systemic veins and the right atrium (Fig. 4-6).
  - At **increased right atrial pressures, venous return is reduced** because the pressure gradient causing venous return is less. When right atrial pressure equals systemic venous pressure, there is no pressure gradient and therefore no flow.
  - Contraction of the veins or infusion of volume **increases the systemic venous pressure** and therefore the driving force for venous return to the right side of the heart, increasing venous return (see Fig. 4-6, point B) at a given right atrial pressure. Alternatively, loss of blood or dilation of the veins **reduces systemic venous pressure** and decreases venous return (point C).

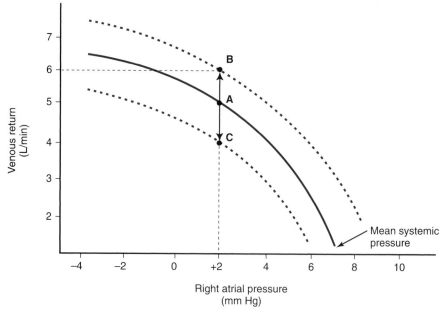

4-6: *Rate of venous return as a function of right atrial pressure.*

> **Clinical note:** Patients experiencing **massive blood loss** (e.g., **trauma patients**) are given large volumes of intravenous fluids to increase systemic venous pressure and to increase venous return, thereby increasing preload and CO.

- The situation becomes more complex when the CO curve is superimposed on the venous return curve (Fig. 4-7). Recall that as preload increases, CO increases via the **Frank-Starling relationship.** Increased preload also increases right atrial pressure, which reduces venous return and acts to reduce CO. There is, therefore, a continual balance. The right atrial pressure maintains the preload required for a given CO, but the pressure is not so great that it prevents the venous return required to maintain the CO. Thus, CO and venous return are perfectly matched!

2. **Other determinants of venous return**
   a. **Skeletal muscle pump**
      - During **physical exercise,** muscle contraction increases the pressure in the veins in the skeletal muscles, which increases the pressure gradient for venous return and thus increases the rate of venous return. This **extravascular compression** is believed to be a major force for venous return during exercise.
      - The skeletal muscle pump is particularly important in the **lower extremities,** where the force of **gravity** has a tendency to cause **venous pooling.** Muscle contraction pushes the blood through one-way valves in the lower extremities, facilitating its return to the heart.

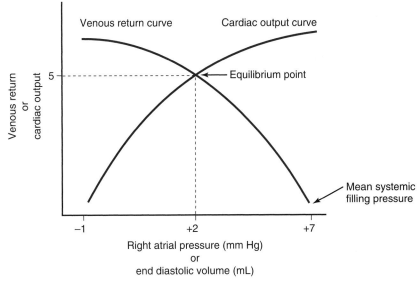

4-7: *Intersection of cardiac output curve and venous return curve.*

b. **Respiratory pump**
  • Venous return is facilitated during inspiration because of an increased venous pressure gradient associated with inspiration.
  • As the **chest wall expands outward** in inspiration, **intrathoracic pressure decreases.** At the same time, **abdominal pressure increases** (partly because of the descending diaphragm). The net result of these pressure changes is an increased pressure gradient driving increased venous return to the right atrium.

> **Clinical note:** The presence of an **inspiratory S$_2$ split** on cardiac auscultation can be explained by **increased venous return** to the right atrium **during inspiration,** which increases the EDV and necessitates a longer systole to eject the additional blood into the pulmonary artery. **Pulmonary vascular resistance also decreases** somewhat **during inspiration,** which decreases the pulmonary back pressure needed to close the pulmonic valve. These two factors delay closure of the pulmonary valve during inspiration.

D. **Ventricular pressure-volume loops**
  • Cardiac function is commonly characterized graphically by pressure-volume loops.
  • There are four phases (Fig. 4-8).
  (1) **Phase I: ventricular filling in diastole.** This phase begins with **opening of the mitral valve** and the **beginning of ventricular filling.** Notice that as ventricular volume increases, the intraventricular pressure also increases gradually, increasing preload.

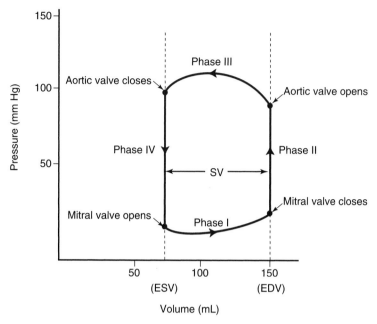

4-8: *Left ventricular pressure-volume loop. EDV, end-diastolic volume; ESV, end-systolic volume; SV, stroke volume.*

(2) **Phase II: isovolumic contraction.** This phase begins at the **onset of systole** and **closure of the mitral valve.** The ventricle is contracting, but not shrinking, because sufficient pressure must develop to exceed pressures in the aorta (pulmonary artery for the right ventricle). The greater the afterload, the more the ventricular pressure must increase to overcome it.

(3) **Phase III: ejection period.** This phase begins as pressures in the left ventricle exceed those in the aorta, causing the **aortic valve to open.** Blood is then continually ejected until the pressures in the aorta exceed those in the ventricle, and the **aortic valve closes.**

(4) **Phase IV: isovolumic relaxation.** This phase begins **immediately after closure of the aortic valve.** During this time, the ventricular muscle is relaxing, but no blood is flowing into the ventricle from the atria because the **pressures in the ventricle still exceed pressures in the atria.** The ventricular volume does not change. At the end of phase IV, the pressure in the ventricle becomes less than the pressure in the atria, causing the **AV valves to open** and allowing **ventricular filling to begin again** (phase I).

E. **Atrial pressure changes during the cardiac cycle** (Fig. 4-9)
- A slight pressure increase *(a wave)* is caused by **atrial contraction** (this and the other parts of the atrial pressure curve are marked on Fig. 4-9).
- A large pressure increase *(c wave)* is caused by **isovolumic ventricular contraction** and inward bulging of the AV valves.
- A rapid reduction in pressure *(x descent)* is caused by initiation of the **ventricular ejection** phase; sometimes referred to as the "vacuum effect."

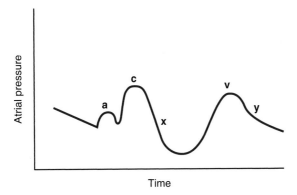

4-9: *Atrial pressure curve.*

- A gradual pressure increase *(v wave)* is caused by **atrial filling** after closure of the AV valves.
- A gradual pressure decrease *(y descent)* is caused by **ventricular filling** after opening of the AV valves.

> **Clinical note: Measurement of atrial pressures** can be helpful in determining the cause of various cardiac disorders. Elevated **right atrial** and **pulmonary artery pressures** can often be appreciated on examination by simply looking for **jugular venous distention** or by performing echocardiography. However, a more invasive procedure, using a **pulmonary wedge device** or **Swan-Ganz catheter,** is required to evaluate **left atrial pressure.** This catheter is inserted into a peripheral vein and threaded through the venous circulation until it becomes "wedged" in one of the small branches of the pulmonary artery. Equilibration of blood from the pulmonary veins then allows an indirect measurement of left atrial pressure.

F. **Pathophysiology of the major valvular diseases**
   1. **Aortic stenosis**
   - The cross-sectional area of the aortic valve becomes pathologically decreased, causing substantial resistance to ventricular ejection of blood through the valve. This increase in resistance is actually a substantial **increase in afterload,** which effectively decreases the SV and consequently decreases the CO.
   - Figure 4-10 shows a pressure-volume loop in a patient with aortic stenosis. Notice how an increased **intraventricular pressure** must be attained to overcome the significant afterload produced by the stenotic valve. The heart expends more energy developing increased pressures; therefore, less energy is available for the ejection phase, so the SV is decreased. Development of the pressure necessary to overcome the afterload also takes time, which means that it takes longer for a pulse to appear after closure of the AV valves (S_1). The combination of reduced SV (which reduces the pulse pressure) and delayed

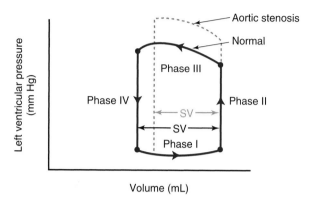

4-10: Pressure-volume changes in aortic stenosis. SV, stroke volume.

pulse from the increased afterload is responsible for the description of the pulse seen in aortic stenosis: **parvus et tardus** (weak and late).

> **Pathology note:** In some individuals, the aortic valve is **congenitally bicuspid.** These bicuspid valves are predisposed to early calcification and stenosis, often causing significant **aortic stenosis** in individuals in their late 40s or early 50s. More commonly, aortic stenosis in the elderly is caused by calcification of the normal tricuspid valve, a condition known as **senile calcific aortic stenosis.** Another cause of aortic stenosis is rheumatic fever, but this disease is becoming rare in developed nations because of the use of antibiotics.

> **Clinical note:** A **stenotic aortic valve** increases the rate of blood flow through the aortic valve, producing turbulent flow and consequently a **systolic ejection murmur** (while blood is being ejected across the valve).

2. **Aortic regurgitation** (aortic insufficiency)
   • The aortic valve does not prevent backflow of blood into the left ventricle. The *effective* SV is substantially decreased, because a significant fraction of the blood ejected into the aorta with each heartbeat returns to the left ventricle. Naturally, this also **decreases the CO.**
   • The blood that enters the aorta during systole can flow into either the systemic circulation or back into the left ventricle during diastole. The increased preload that occurs from blood regurgitating back into the ventricle may **increase the SV** (although not the *effective* SV), which helps maintain a relatively **normal systolic pressure.** However, diastolic pressure may be **substantially reduced** because of this "backward flow," thus explaining the abnormally **widened pulse pressure** commonly seen in aortic regurgitation.

> **Pathology note: Aortic regurgitation** may involve several different pathogenetic mechanisms. The most common causes are connective tissue defects that weaken the supporting aortic and valvular structures (e.g., **Marfan syndrome, Ehlers-Danlos syndrome**) and inflammatory diseases of the heart and/or aorta (e.g., **endocarditis, syphilitic aortitis**).

3. **Mitral stenosis**
   - In early diastole, the mitral valve normally opens and provides negligible resistance to blood flow from the left atrium to the left ventricle. In mitral stenosis, the **mitral valve becomes stenotic due to abnormal structural changes.** Resistance to blood flow across the mitral valve is significantly increased, and adequate ventricular filling can occur only at pathologically elevated atrial filling pressures.
   - This **increase in left atrial pressure,** and therefore pulmonary venous pressure, is responsible for many symptoms of mitral stenosis. As left atrial pressures become elevated, the hydrostatic pressures in the pulmonary veins and capillaries also become elevated, causing net **transudation of fluid into the pulmonary interstitium.** Initially, the pulmonary lymphatics can reabsorb this fluid and prevent pulmonary edema. Once the left atrial pressure exceeds 30 to 40 mm Hg, however, the compensatory capacity of the lymphatics is overwhelmed, and fluid begins to accumulate in the lungs.
   - This **fluid accumulation** causes the symptoms of mitral stenosis, such as **dyspnea** and **reduced exercise capacity.** If the degree of stenosis is moderate or severe, repair **(mitral commissurotomy)** or replacement of the mitral valve is necessary to prevent fatal progression of the disease.

> **Pathology note: Rheumatic fever** is the most common cause of mitral stenosis. Symptoms of mitral stenosis (dyspnea, exercise intolerance) usually develop about 20 years after an acute episode of rheumatic fever.

4. **Mitral regurgitation** (mitral insufficiency)
   - In early ventricular systole, ventricular contraction is normally isovolumic when both the semilunar and AV valves are closed. This allows the entire left ventricular output to move "forward" into the aorta once the aortic valve opens. In mitral regurgitation, the **mitral valve does not form a good "seal"** and allows **backward flow of blood into the left atrium** during early systole.
   - **Symptoms of mitral regurgitation** therefore may be associated with reduced forward flow CO, elevated left atrial pressures and volumes, and/or left ventricular volume overload due to the additional preload imposed on the left ventricle by the addition of the "regurgitated" blood to the normal venous return. The precise symptoms depend primarily on the **temporal course** of the mitral regurgitation.
   - In **acute settings** (e.g., **rupture of papillary muscle** in a **myocardial infarction**), severe and even fatal **pulmonary edema** may develop, because

the "unprepared" left atrium is small and relatively noncompliant, and the increase in atrial pressure is therefore rapidly transmitted to the pulmonary vasculature. Furthermore, the pulmonary lymphatics have not adapted to reabsorb more interstitial fluid.
- In **chronic settings** (e.g., **ischemic cardiomyopathy** causing gradual valvular dysfunction), the left atrium **has had time** to enlarge and become more compliant, and the pulmonary lymphatics **have had time** to augment their function. Although pulmonary complications are less likely, increasingly larger fractions of the left ventricular SV are diverted into the low-pressure left atrium, thereby decreasing forward flow SV and causing **symptoms associated with heart failure** (e.g., **fatigue, weakness**).

> **Pathology note:** Mitral regurgitation can be caused by **mitral valve prolapse,** in which the mitral leaflets billow into the left atrium during ventricular systole. Although mitral valve prolapse may give rise to a **midsystolic "click"** detectable on cardiac auscultation, it is **usually asymptomatic.**

5. **Pathophysiology of murmurs**
   - Blood flow through most of the cardiovascular system is normally **laminar** and silent. In certain circumstances, flow velocity is increased or viscosity is decreased, and nonlaminar **(turbulent) flow** occurs that can produce noise **(murmurs** or **bruits).** Turbulent flow typically occurs when the **Reynolds' number** is elevated, exceeding approximately 2500 (Fig. 4-11). The Reynolds' number (Re) can be calculated as follows:

$$Re = 2rv\rho/\eta$$

where r = radius of the vessel, v = velocity of flow, ρ = density of the fluid, and η = viscosity of the fluid.

III. **Myocardial Oxygen Supply and Demand**
  A. **Main determinants of myocardial O_2 supply**
    1. **Coronary blood flow**
       - Myocardial O_2 supply is directly related to the **rate of blood flow within the coronary arteries,** which is dependent on the length of diastole, the diastolic perfusion pressure, and the vascular resistance of the coronary arteries.
    a. **Length of diastole** (Fig. 4-12)
       - The increased extravascular pressures generated during left ventricular systole compress the coronary vessels, causing little or no myocardial blood flow during systole. Consequently, **left ventricular blood flow is largely dependent on the length of time spent in diastole,** this time being inversely proportional to HR.
       - In contrast, the right ventricle receives the majority of its blood flow during systole, because the extravascular compressive forces are much weaker in the right ventricle than in the left ventricle. Therefore, **right ventricular blood flow is largely independent of the time spent in diastole.**

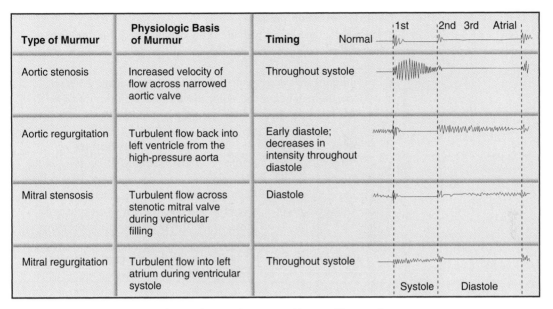

Type of Murmur	Physiologic Basis of Murmur	Timing				
				1st	2nd 3rd Atrial	
			Normal			
Aortic stenosis	Increased velocity of flow across narrowed aortic valve	Throughout systole				
Aortic regurgitation	Turbulent flow back into left ventricle from the high-pressure aorta	Early diastole; decreases in intensity throughout diastole				
Mitral stensosis	Turbulent flow across stenotic mitral valve during ventricular filling	Diastole				
Mitral regurgitation	Turbulent flow into left atrium during ventricular systole	Throughout systole		Systole	Diastole	

4-11: *Phonocardiograms from a normal heart and hearts with murmurs.*

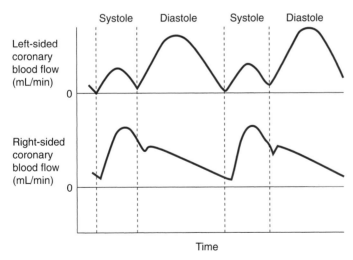

4-12: *Ventricular blood flow.*

b. **Diastolic perfusion pressure**
  • The diastolic perfusion pressure is the **driving force for coronary blood flow.** It is equivalent to the diastolic pressure within the proximal aorta.
  • In conditions that decrease diastolic pressures within the aorta (e.g., aortic regurgitation, hypotension), the diastolic perfusion pressure is decreased, and the myocardial O_2 supply is compromised.

> **Clinical note:** In severely ill patients who are **hypotensive** (e.g., after a myocardial infarction), the diastolic perfusion pressure of the aorta may be insufficient to maintain adequate coronary blood flow. The resulting **ischemia** can compromise cardiac function, and the decreased CO further decreases the diastolic perfusion pressure. To increase this perfusion pressure, an **intra-aortic balloon pump** is inserted into the distal thoracic aorta. The balloon is designed to inflate during diastole, thereby increasing the **aortic back pressure** and the **diastolic perfusion pressure.** The result is improved coronary blood flow, which improves cardiac function and increases CO.

c. **Coronary vascular resistance**
  • The resistance of the coronary vessels is governed by their radii; a **decreased radius causes greater resistance** and **reduced flow.** External compression during systole essentially halts coronary blood flow by decreasing vessel radius. During diastole, the vessels open and perfusion occurs.
  • Aside from these extravascular compressive forces, the **local production** of various **vasoactive substances** by metabolically active cardiac tissue is a major determinant of coronary vessel diameter and, hence, coronary vascular resistance and coronary blood flow. These vasoactive substances include mediators that cause vasodilation, such as **adenosine, hydrogen ions** (H^+), and **potassium** (K^+).
  • **Atherosclerotic narrowing** of the coronary vessels also **increases coronary vascular resistance.**

2. **Arterial O_2 content**
  • The arterial O_2 content mainly depends on the **O_2-carrying capacity** of the blood (i.e., amount of plasma hemoglobin) and the efficiency of gas exchange by the lungs.
  • Normally, the arterial O_2 content is constant; therefore, it does not regulate myocardial O_2 supply. In diseases such as **anemia** and **chronic obstructive pulmonary disease,** however, the decreased arterial O_2 content can severely compromise myocardial O_2 supply.

B. **Main determinants of myocardial O_2 demand**
  • **Heart rate** is most important. When the HR increases, **proportionally more time is spent in systole,** which increases the cardiac workload and therefore **increases the myocardial O_2 demand.** In addition, in conditions associated with increased HR (e.g., sympathetic activation), less time is spent in diastole,

but proportionally more time is spent in **active diastolic relaxation,** which also requires energy. Furthermore, myocardial O_2 supply is compromised, because fractionally less time is spent in diastole.

- **Myocardial wall tension:** More O_2 is consumed in the process of generating greater forces. Increased tensions may occur in the settings of increased preload, increased contractility, or increased afterload.
- **Contractility:** Myocardium in a positive inotropic state ejects a greater SV than when in a normal or negative inotropic state. Stroke work is increased, and therefore myocardial O_2 demand is increased.

> **Clinical note:** When the heart is exposed to increased afterloads, as might occur in someone with poorly controlled hypertension, it **hypertrophies.** This increase in muscle mass reduces wall tension but increases the myocardial O_2 requirement.

C. **Pathophysiology of angina pectoris**
- Angina occurs when O_2 **demand exceeds O_2 supply.** When this occurs, the ventricular myocytes begin to use anaerobic respiration, which generates lactic acid and reduces the pH. **Lactic acid accumulation** may cause the pain of angina (as it does in overworked skeletal muscles).
- **Causes of angina pectoris** include
  (1) **Atherosclerotic narrowing of coronary vessels** in coronary artery disease, which increases resistance and reduces blood flow. **Anginal pain** associated with coronary artery disease typically becomes noticeable or **more pronounced** when myocardial O_2 demand increases (e.g., in **exercise**).
  (2) **Spasm of the coronary arteries in Prinzmetal's angina,** which reduces coronary blood flow so much that the pain may occur at rest.

> **Clinical note:** Bearing in mind the determinants of myocardial O_2 supply and demand, it is clear why nitrates such as nitroglycerin are so effective in relieving anginal pain. Nitrates primarily function by **reducing wall tension generated during systole,** thus reducing the myocardial O_2 demand. They reduce wall tension by dilating both veins and arteries, which reduces preload and afterload, respectively. In addition, nitrates may prevent vasospasm of coronary arteries by causing vasodilation, thereby alleviating anginal pain in patients with **Prinzmetal's angina.**

IV. **Pathophysiology of Myocardial Adaptations**
- Cardiac muscle, much like skeletal muscle, can adapt to increased workloads.
A. **Adaptations to increased afterload** (Fig. 4-13)
- Significant afterloads (e.g., **systemic hypertension, aortic stenosis**) cause **thickening of the heart muscle.** Myocytes cannot proliferate, but they can thicken by adding sarcomeres in parallel within a myocyte, decreasing the amount of tension that each sarcomere has to generate to overcome the afterload. This process of adaptive thickening is known as **concentric hypertrophy.**

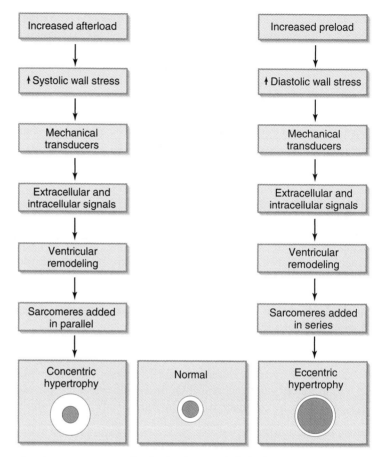

4-13: *Ventricular adaptations to increased preload and increased afterload. Note that both processes may occur simultaneously; for example, in a patient with hypertension (increased afterload) and congestive heart failure (increased preload).*

- This adaptive thickening of the myocardium occurs at the expense of **decreased ventricular compliance.** An increasingly stiff ventricle has two main adverse effects: **impaired diastolic ventricular filling,** which allows adequate filling to occur only at elevated atrial pressures, and **elevated filling pressures,** which may cause pulmonary venous congestion and pulmonary edema.

  > **Pathology note:** In a congenital cardiac disease known as **hypertrophic cardiomyopathy,** the myocardial muscle hypertrophies *without a physiologic stimulus.* This hypertrophy usually **occurs asymmetrically,** with the cardiac septum exhibiting the most hypertrophy. During systole, this enlarged septum may cause **left ventricular outflow obstruction,** resulting in a systolic murmur. This obstruction of left ventricular outflow can be so severe during intense exercise that it can cause **syncope** or even **sudden death.**

B. **Adaptations to increased preload** (see Fig. 4-13)
- **Larger-than-normal preloads** (e.g., aortic regurgitation, mitral regurgitation) **cause the heart to dilate,** and the ventricular chamber then increases in diameter with only a minimal increase in ventricular wall thickness. In contrast to concentric hypertrophy caused by increased afterload, the response to increased preload is to **add sarcomeres** within existing myocytes **in series,** rather than in parallel. This is referred to as **eccentric hypertrophy** Although the ventricular myocardium does not appreciably thicken as a result, it does elongate, which accounts for the increased ventricular chamber size. The elongation decreases preload by decreasing the amount of tension on each sarcomere at end-diastole.
- Hearts that are subject to increased preload are often referred to as **"volume-overloaded"** hearts.

> **Pathology note:** In certain pathologic situations, the heart may dilate *without being volume-overloaded*. Most commonly, this happens for unknown reasons and is known as **idiopathic dilated cardiomyopathy.** The most common known cause of dilated cardiomyopathy unrelated to volume overload is **excessive use of alcohol.**

V. **Electrophysiology of the Heart**
- Action potentials spontaneously generated by the sinoatrial (SA) node are rapidly conducted throughout the heart via the **Purkinje system** and the **intercalated disks of myocytes,** causing coordinated myocardial contraction.
- The SA node discharges at its own inherent rate (~80 times per minute) in the absence of neurohumoral input. If the SA node fails to discharge, other backup nodes become active and discharge at their own inherent rates, distribute an action potential throughout the heart, and cause myocardial contraction.
  A. **Electrophysiologic basis of spontaneous depolarization of SA node and other backup nodes** (Fig. 4-14)
  - The membrane potential in nodal tissues is never stable. The membranes gradually depolarize at rest (phase 4) because they are fairly permeable to sodium ions (Na^+).
  - When the membrane potential depolarizes to reach a certain **threshold potential,** voltage-gated **calcium channels open,** allowing a somewhat slow current of Ca^{2+} to enter the cells (phase 0) and generate an action potential.
  - After causing the action potential, the calcium channels in the nodal tissues close spontaneously, and K^+ flows out of the cells, restoring the membrane potential (phase 3). The process then begins again because of the Na^+ leak.
  - **Note:** Nodal cells do not demonstrate phases 1 and 2, which are observed in the action potentials of Purkinje fibers and cardiac myocytes.
  B. **Autonomic influence on heart rate**
  - The **rate of action potential generation by the SA node,** and thus the HR, may be influenced by several electrophysiologic mechanisms.

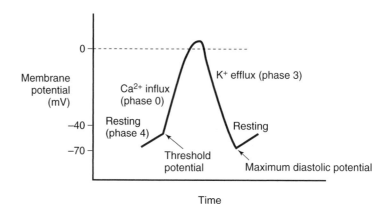

4-14: *Sinoatrial node depolarization. Ca^{2+}, calcium; K^+, potassium.*

1. **Maximum diastolic potential**
   - The maximum diastolic potential is the **most negative membrane potential of the SA node.**
   - The more negative this value, the longer the nodal cells must depolarize to reach the **threshold potential** (at which point an action potential is triggered); the result is a reduction in HR. Indeed, this is one way in which the parasympathetic nervous system, via the vagus nerve, slows the HR.
2. **Rate of depolarization in phase 4**
   - The more permeable nodal cells are to Na^+, the more rapidly they depolarize during phase 4 and reach threshold potential, increasing the HR. The less permeable nodal cells are to Na^+, the more slowly they depolarize, decreasing the HR.
   - **Catecholamines** produced by sympathetic excitation increase the HR, in part by **increasing the slope of phase 4 depolarization.** In contrast, the parasympathetic nervous system decreases the HR, in part by **decreasing the slope of phase 4 depolarization.**
3. **Threshold for generating action potentials**
   - The higher the threshold for generating action potentials, the longer phase 4 depolarization takes to reach this threshold and cause an action potential. Therefore, raising the threshold (i.e., making it less negative) decreases the HR.
   - The **sympathetic nervous system raises** the **threshold,** whereas the **parasympathetic nervous system lowers** the **threshold,** for action potential generation in nodal cells.
C. **Backup pacemakers**
   - "Backup" nodes such as the AV node are ordinarily not as permeable to Na^+ as is the SA node, so they do not spontaneously depolarize as rapidly during phase 4. An action potential initiated by the SA node typically forces the backup nodes to depolarize together with other cardiac tissue. After such depolarization, they slowly begin to depolarize again, but because their

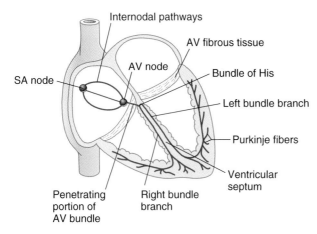

Internodal pathways

AV fibrous tissue

AV node

Bundle of His

SA node

Left bundle branch

Purkinje fibers

Ventricular septum

Penetrating portion of AV bundle

Right bundle branch

4-15: *Conduction pathways of action potentials. AV, atrioventricular; SA, sinoatrial.*

membranes are not as permeable to Na^+, the SA node depolarizes first and repeats the cycle. This process is known as **"overdrive suppression."**

- Normally, only if the SA node does not fire soon enough does one of the backup nodes initiate an action potential that is conducted throughout the heart.

D. **Conduction pathway of action potentials** (Fig. 4-15)
- After a spontaneous action potential is generated in the SA node, the action potential is distributed throughout the atria and is also rapidly conducted to the AV node through specialized internodal fibers.
- **Conduction through the AV node** then **occurs very slowly,** which gives the atria sufficient time to contract and "top off" the ventricles before ventricular systole occurs. From the AV node, impulses travel through the AV bundle as it traverses the fibrous septum that provides electrical "insulation" between the atria and the ventricles. Action potentials then travel through the right and left bundle branches of the interventricular septum and are finally distributed to the ventricular myocardium via specialized **Purkinje fibers** and **myocyte gap junctions.**

E. **Action potentials in cardiac muscle**
  1. **Phases in cardiac myocytes** (Fig. 4-16)
     a. **Phase 4: resting membrane potential**
        - In atrial and ventricular myocytes and Purkinje fibers, the resting membrane potential is maintained at a very negative level **(~−90 mV).** At this potential, the fast, voltage-gated **Na^+ channels are** generally **closed,** but they are "primed" to be opened if triggered by an incipient action potential.
        - Notice the isoelectric nature of phase 4 of the action potential in cardiac muscle, which contrasts with the upward slope of phase 4 of the nodal action potential (see Fig. 4-14).

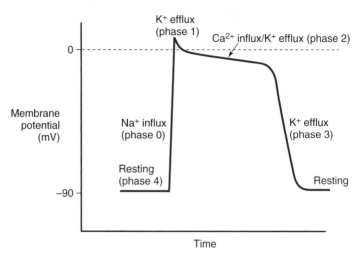

4-16: Action potential in cardiac myocytes.

  b. **Phase 0: depolarization**
- This phase is characterized by rapid cell depolarization caused by the opening of fast, voltage-gated Na^+ channels in response to action potentials coming from the cardiac conduction system.
- **Na^+,** which is much more abundant extracellularly than intracellularly, rushes into the cell and **causes the membrane potential to become increasingly positive.**

  c. **Phase 1: transient repolarization**
- This phase is caused by a transient **rapid efflux of K^+** with simultaneous **cessation of Na^+ efflux.**
- These effluxes result in a slight repolarization that is almost immediately counteracted by the opening of calcium channels and Ca^{2+} influx.

  d. **Phase 2: calcium plateau**
- This phase is characterized by a **balance** between **K^+ efflux and Ca^{2+} influx,** resulting in no net change in membrane potential.
- It accounts for the long duration of the cardiac myocyte action potential. The entry of calcium is responsible for initiating contraction of cardiac myocytes.

  e. **Phase 3: repolarization**
- This phase is characterized by a **simultaneous rapid efflux of K^+ and cessation of Ca^{2+} influx.**
- The result is repolarization and even hyperpolarization of cells.

2. **Differences in action potential generation in nodal cells and myocytes**
- The **resting membrane potential** is approximately **−70 mV in nodal cells** (see Fig. 4-14), and it is approximately **−90 mV in non-nodal cells** (see Fig. 4-16). The less negative resting membrane potential in nodal cells

effectively eliminates the contribution of the fast voltage-gated Na^+ channels to action potential generation, because at this potential they are almost all in a **conformation that cannot be triggered to open.**

- The resting membrane potential in phase 4 slopes upward and depolarizes spontaneously in nodal cells, whereas it is level in non-nodal cells.
- Notice the **slow phase 0 depolarization** due to **slow influx of Ca^{2+}** in nodal cells, compared with the steeply sloping phase 0 in non-nodal cells caused by the rapid influx of Na^+.

3. **Refractory period**
   - Immediately **after depolarization, cardiac muscle cells cannot be excited again.** The Na^+ channels responsible for phase 0 depolarization are inactivated by depolarization. There is a certain "recovery" period during which these Na^+ channels cannot be stimulated to initiate an action potential.
   - This **period of inexcitability** has two important physiologic roles. First, it **prevents tetany** (sustained contraction), which can occur in skeletal muscle from rapid stimulation, but which in the heart would cause perpetual systole. Second, it **places an upper limit on the heart rate** (approximately 180–200 beats per minute).

F. **Excitation-contraction coupling**
   - Excitation-contraction coupling reflects the "coupling" of an **increase in membrane potential (excitation) to cell contraction.** In a cardiac myocyte, the first step that occurs is the generation of an action potential at the cell surface. As this action potential spreads along the sarcolemma and transverse tubules, extracellular Ca^{2+} enters the cell, triggering Ca^{2+} release from the sarcoplasmic reticulum. This phenomenon is referred to as **Ca^{2+}-induced Ca^{2+} release.** The intracellular Ca^{2+} then stimulates contraction via a sliding filament mechanism of contraction similar to that in skeletal muscle (i.e., Ca^{2+} binds troponin, which promotes actin and myosin cross-bridge formation). The force of contraction is proportional to the intracellular Ca^{2+} level.
   - For the **ventricles to relax, Ca^{2+} must be pumped out of the cytosol back into the sarcoplasmic reticulum** or into the extracellular fluid. This process, like excitation-contraction coupling, also requires energy.
   - **Sympathetic excitation** of the heart increases contractility in large part by increasing the influx of extracellular Ca^{2+}, causing a **greater Ca^{2+}-induced Ca^{2+} release.** It also stimulates reuptake of Ca^{2+}, thereby accelerating the rate of ventricular relaxation and facilitating ventricular filling during the shortened period of diastole.

> **Pharmacology note: Calcium channel blocking drugs** (e.g., diltiazem, verapamil) have a **negative inotropic effect** on the heart by preventing the influx of extracellular Ca^{2+} during the cardiac action potential. Such a negative inotropic effect may be beneficial in patients with **chronic heart failure** (by reducing myocardial O_2 demand) and **hypertension** (by reducing CO).

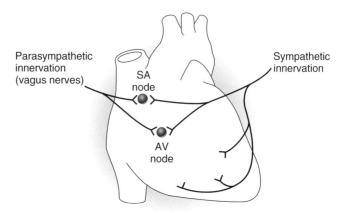

4-17: Cardiac nerves. AV, atrioventricular; SA, sinoatrial.

> **Pharmacology note: Digitalis,** a **cardiac glycoside,** has a **positive inotropic effect** on the heart because it increases cytoplasmic Ca^{2+}. It does this indirectly by inhibiting the sodium-potassium adenosine triphosphatase pump (Na^+,K^+-ATPase pump), which increases intracellular Na^+. The increased intracellular Na^+ reduces the Na^+ gradient that drives a Na^+-Ca^{2+} antiport, allowing more Ca^{2+} to accumulate in the cytosol. Because of this positive inotropic effect, digitalis may provide significant **symptomatic relief** in **patients with heart failure,** in whom cardiac contractility may be severely impaired.

G. **Autonomic innervation of the heart** (Fig. 4-17)
   1. **Sympathetic (adrenergic) innervation**
      - Sympathetic innervation to the heart is extensive, with innervation to the nodal tissues, atria, and ventricles.
      - **Norepinephrine** released from sympathetic nerves binds to adrenergic receptors in the heart, resulting in **increased heart rate** (positive **chronotropic** effect) and **increased contractility** (positive **inotropic** effect).

      > **Pharmacology note:** The β_1-receptor is the adrenergic receptor that is primarily responsible for mediating sympathetic excitation of HR and contractility. β-**Blocking drugs** such as **metoprolol** antagonize this receptor and can slow the HR and reduce contractility.

   2. **Parasympathetic (cholinergic) innervation**
      - Parasympathetic innervation of the heart is limited to the nodal tissues and the atria. There is essentially no parasympathetic innervation to the ventricles.
      - **Acetylcholine released from parasympathetic nerves** (the vagus) **binds to muscarinic receptors.** Parasympathetic stimulation decreases HR by increasing the maximum diastolic potential, raising the action potential threshold and decreasing the rate of phase 4 depolarization in nodal cells (see section V, B, 1, on maximum diastolic potential).

Clinical note: In extreme conditions (e.g., **vasovagal syncope**), marked parasympathetic outflow to the heart can cause the heart to stop beating transiently, resulting in syncope secondary to inadequate cerebral perfusion. Parasympathetic outflow can stop the heart because cholinergic stimulation impairs both action potential generation in nodal tissue and conduction of action potentials from the atria to the ventricles **(heart block).** However, because the ventricles do not receive parasympathetic input, ventricular pacemaker cells free from parasympathetic control are able to initiate de novo action potentials if they are not overdrive-suppressed by another action potential. Ventricular function is then able to resume at some level. This phenomenon is referred to as a **ventricular escape rhythm.**

Pharmacology note: The drug **atropine** blocks the muscarinic receptors in the heart and increases HR. It is therefore useful in treating patients with **acute symptomatic bradycardia.**

VI. **The Electrocardiogram**
- The **electrocardiogram (ECG)** monitors electrical activity in the heart by recording electrical changes at the surface of the body.
- The important "leads" to be familiar with are the **bipolar limb leads** (I, II, and III), the **unipolar limb leads** (aVR, aVL, and aVF), and the **precordial leads** (V1 through V6).
- The bipolar and unipolar limb leads detect electrical activity in the vertical (frontal) plane; the precordial leads detect current in the transverse plane.
  A. **The Normal ECG** (Fig. 4-18)
     - The **P wave** corresponds to **atrial depolarization.**
     - The **PR interval** corresponds to **impulse conduction through the AV node.**
     - The **QRS complex** corresponds to **ventricular depolarization.**
     - The **T wave** corresponds to **ventricular repolarization.**
  B. **Correlation of ECG with Cardiac Events**
     - Table 4-1 correlates ECG abnormalities with cardiac events and their pathophysiology.

VII. **Arterial Pressure Maintenance**
  A. **Determinants of mean arterial pressure** (MAP)
     - MAP is dependent on two variables: **cardiac output** (CO) and **total peripheral resistance** (TPR):

$$MAP = CO \times TPR$$

   - CO is a function of SV and HR (see section II, A, on cardiac output).
   - **Resistance (R)** to fluid flow through a tube (vessel) is described by the relationship:

$$R = 8\eta l/\pi r^4$$

where η = viscosity, l = length of the vessel, and r = radius of the vessel.

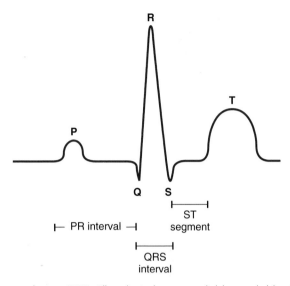

4-18: *The normal electrocardiogram (ECG). All mechanical events are slightly preceded by electrical changes on the ECG: the start of the P wave slightly precedes atrial contraction, the start of the QRS complex precedes ventricular contraction, and so on.*

TABLE 4-1:
Correlation of Electrocardiogram (ECG) with Cardiac Events

ECG Abnormality	Possible Diagnoses	Possible Pathophysiology
ST segment elevation	Acute myocardial infarction	Prolonged repolarization
Split R wave	Bundle branch block	Depolarization of right and left bundle branches no longer occurs simultaneously
PR interval >200 msec	Heart block	Excessive vagal outflow, drugs that slow atrioventricular conduction, or degenerative disease
Pathologic Q wave	"Transmural" myocardial infarction	—
Deviation of mean QRS axis	Myocardial infarction or ventricular hypertrophy	Left ventricular hypertrophy in response to increased afterload (e.g., hypertension, aortic stenosis) or right ventricular hypertrophy in response to massive pulmonary embolism
Inverted T wave	Ischemia	Prolonged ventricular depolarization and ventricular ischemia from coronary artery disease

- Because it is the fourth power of the radius that determines resistance to fluid flow, **vessel constriction** or **dilation** can have powerful effects on **fluid resistance** and **mean arterial pressure.** In the circulatory system, peripheral resistance is governed primarily by the diameters of the **arterioles,** rather than the large arteries or capillaries (Fig. 4-19). This arteriolar constriction and dilation is regulated by numerous mechanisms.

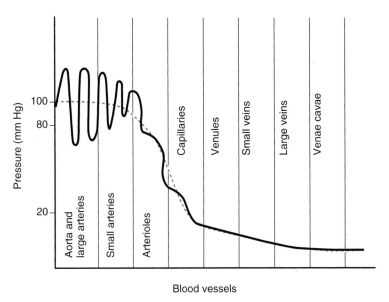

4-19: *Blood pressure oscillations throughout the vasculature. Resistance to flow dampens the pressure oscillations caused by each heartbeat and also causes the pressures to drop as blood traverses the cardiovascular system. Most of the pressure drop occurs in the arterioles, where the vascular resistance is the greatest.*

B. **Tonic sympathetic outflow via the medullary vasomotor center**
- Tonic sympathetic outflow from the medullary vasomotor center contributes to maintenance of arterial pressure by increasing TPR. It does this by maintaining normal **vasomotor tone.** When vasomotor tone is normal, the majority of the body's arterioles are at least partly constricted.
- The medullary vasomotor center is also involved in **reflex regulation of blood pressure.** It receives input regarding the arterial blood pressure from a variety of sources, including baroreceptors located in large-diameter arteries, peripheral and central chemoreceptors, and even higher brain centers such as the hypothalamus and motor cortex (Fig. 4-20).

> **Pharmacology note:** Sympathetic stimulation of vascular smooth muscle contraction is mediated by α_1-receptors. α_1-Blocking drugs such as prazosin antagonize this receptor and inhibit vasoconstriction, thereby lowering blood pressure.

C. **Rapid blood pressure control by the autonomic nervous system**
1. **Baroreceptor reflex** (Fig. 4-21)
   - This neural reflex works rapidly to **compensate for changes in arterial blood pressure** and is dependent on specialized mechanoreceptors located within the **aortic arch** and the **carotid sinuses.** When exposed to higher arterial blood pressures (point B on Fig. 4-21), the mechanoreceptors become deformed and "fire" action potentials that are relayed to the vasomotor center and other nuclei in the brainstem. This signal is inhibitory, so that medullary sympathetic outflow is blocked and parasympathetic outflow is stimulated. The decreased sympathetic outflow

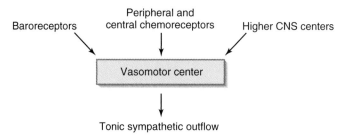

4-20: *Regulatory input to the medullary vasomotor center. CNS, central nervous system.*

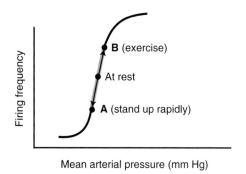

4-21: *Control of blood pressure by the baroreceptor reflex.*

causes arteriolar dilation and also decreases sympathetic drive to the heart, decreasing the HR. The parasympathetic outflow primarily affects the HR by reducing the firing frequency of the SA node. The combined result is a **rapid compensatory drop in blood pressure.**

- If the blood pressure decreases (point **A** on Fig. 4-21), the **opposite sequence of events occurs.** The baroreceptors fire less frequently, reducing inhibition of sympathetic outflow. The resulting increase in CO and peripheral vascular resistance acts rapidly to **prevent a further decline in blood pressure,** in an attempt to maintain adequate organ perfusion.

Clinical note: Pressure on the carotid sinuses, which might occur when checking for the carotid pulse, can also cause deformation of the baroreceptors. This action may be interpreted by the medullary vasomotor center and brainstem as an elevated arterial blood pressure. The resulting decreased sympathetic outflow and increased parasympathetic outflow can cause a **rapid "compensatory" drop in blood pressure** and possibly even **syncope.**

Clinical note: When a person moves rapidly from a supine to a standing position, blood pressure decreases because of venous pooling in the legs. This decline is transient only because decreased baroreceptor firing frequency stimulates sympathetic outflow, which increases the HR and causes vasoconstriction to maintain adequate blood pressure. Certain antihypertensive medications, such as the α_1-blockers (e.g., prazosin), cause marked **orthostatic hypotension,** because they block the α-adrenergic receptors required for this vasoconstriction.

2. **Central nervous system (CNS) ischemic response**
   - When blood flow to the medullary vasomotor center is compromised (e.g., severe hypotension), sympathetic outflow from the vasomotor center is strongly stimulated.
   - This stimulation occurs irrespective of the type of feedback the vasomotor center is receiving from the peripheral baroreceptors and chemoreceptors.

   Clinical note: Head injury that causes significantly increased intracranial pressure may activate the **CNS ischemic response,** decreasing blood flow to the medullary vasomotor center and causing hypertension. When this occurs and bradycardia develops, it is referred to as **Cushing's sign.**

D. **Autoregulation of local blood flow**
   - Autoregulation is the **ability of tissues to self-regulate local blood flow,** even in the face of widely varying systemic pressures. Although the primary function of autoregulation is to maintain normal tissue perfusion locally, it can have systemic effects on arterial blood pressure. For example, in response to increased extracellular fluid volume, the autoregulatory response is to cause vasoconstriction throughout the body, which increases TPR and arterial blood pressure.
   - There are two principal mechanisms of autoregulation. In the **metabolic mechanism,** local metabolism regulates local blood flow via the production of vasoactive substances, such as **adenosine** and **lactic acid.** Demand regulates supply. The **myogenic mechanism** (Fig. 4-22) is based on the differential permeability of the vascular smooth muscle cell to extracellular Ca^{2+}, which depends on the contractile state of the vascular smooth muscle cell.

E. **Vascular compliance**
   - Vascular compliance is the **ability of a vessel to withstand an increase in volume without causing a significant increase in pressure.** Mathematically, it is expressed as the volume (V) required to increase the pressure (P) by 1 mm Hg:

$$\text{Compliance} = \frac{V}{P}$$

Pathology note: If the arteries are not very compliant, as in **arteriosclerosis,** they are unable to "accept" large volumes of blood without a substantial increase in arterial pressure. This is precisely what happens in **isolated systolic hypertension** due to arteriosclerosis.

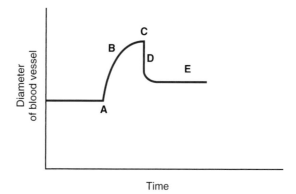

4-22: *Myogenic mechanism in autoregulation of local blood flow. If the vascular smooth muscle cell is passively stretched (**B**), which occurs with increased blood flow, Ca^{2+} permeability increases and Ca^{2+} enters the vascular smooth muscle cell (**C**). This causes contraction of the cell and a compensatory vasoconstriction (**D**). This action establishes a new blood vessel diameter (**E**), which is only slightly larger than the initial diameter (**A**), thereby maintaining a relatively constant blood flow through the capillary bed.*

- **Note: Veins are significantly more compliant than arteries,** and this increased compliance allows the veins to accept large volumes of blood without considerable increases in pressure.

F. **Long-term control via regulation of intravascular volume by the kidneys**
   - Intravascular volume is a major determinant of **blood pressure** and is **primarily under the control of the kidneys.**
   - Elevated intravascular volume increases systemic venous pressure, which in turn increases venous return. This increases preload and CO, which elevates blood pressure. Therefore, by either increasing or decreasing intravascular volume, the kidneys have a powerful effect on CO and MAP (Fig. 4-23).

   1. **Pressure diuresis**
      - In persons with normal renal function, increases in systemic blood pressure result in increased diuresis by the kidneys. This phenomenon, known as pressure diuresis, takes place because of the increased renal blood flow that occurs at elevated arterial pressures, which causes a **higher-than-normal glomerular filtration rate** (GFR) (Fig. 4-24).
      - The **increased GFR** results in increased filtration and excretion of **sodium** as well as water. The resulting loss of **sodium** and water **reduces intravascular volume,** which reduces CO and normalizes the arterial pressure. If systemic pressure decreases, the opposite sequence of events is set into motion. Decreased renal perfusion causes the kidneys to retain more sodium and water, which increases intravascular volume and restores the blood pressure. This increased excretion of sodium is referred to as **pressure natriuresis.**
      - **Note:** In theory, pressure diuresis by the kidneys can fully compensate for any increase in systemic blood pressure, thus preventing hypertension. Therefore, some clinicians believe that there is some component of renal dysfunction in most patients with hypertension.

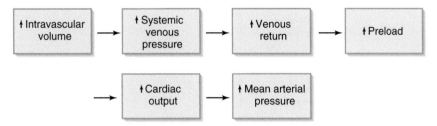

4-23: *Long-term control of intravascular volume by the kidneys.*

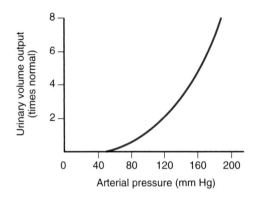

4-24: *Increased urinary output in response to arterial pressure (pressure diuresis).*

2. **Renin-angiotensin-aldosterone system**
   - The renin-angiotensin-aldosterone system is a system for **preserving intravascular volume** and **mean arterial pressure.**
   - The primary stimulus for the renin-angiotensin-aldosterone system is **reduced renal blood flow,** which typically occurs in conditions associated with reduced intravascular volume (e.g., **dehydration**). Reduced renal blood flow is sensed by a group of specialized cells located in the walls of the afferent arterioles (part of the juxtaglomerular apparatus). Renin secretion by these cells initiates an enzymatic cascade that ultimately results in the production of angiotensin II (Fig. 4-25).

   > **Clinical note:** Activation of the renin-angiotensin-aldosterone system may also occur in euvolemic and even hypervolemic states, such as **renal artery stenosis** or **congestive heart failure** (CHF). In these states, the kidney is underperfused. Activation of the renin-angiotensin-aldosterone system may not be an appropriate physiologic response; in fact, it may exacerbate the underlying disease (e.g., cause hypertension in renal artery stenosis or a more rapid decline in cardiac function in CHF).

   a. **Actions of angiotensin II**
      - Angiotensin II increases arterial blood pressure in numerous ways. Most importantly, it stimulates expansion of the intravascular volume, thus

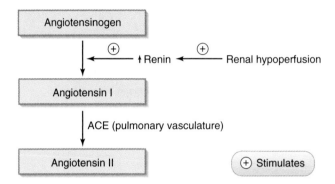

4-25: *Enzymatic cascade in the renin-angiotensin-aldosterone system. ACE, angiotensin-converting enzyme.*

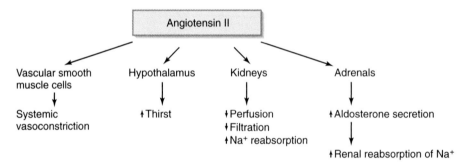

4-26: *Diagrammatic representation of physiologic actions of angiotensin II.*

maintaining adequate long-term arterial pressures. It does this in part by stimulating aldosterone secretion from the adrenal glands, and **aldosterone stimulates renal Na$^+$ retention.** Angiotensin II also stimulates Na$^+$ reabsorption in the proximal nephron and stimulates thirst (Fig. 4-26).

- Angiotensin II is a powerful **stimulator of systemic vasoconstriction,** which increases arterial blood pressure by increasing TPR. In contrast to stimulating plasma volume expansion, which can take hours to days, increased arterial vasoconstriction causes a **rapid increase in arterial blood pressure,** which may be an important protective mechanism during hemorrhage.

Pharmacology note: Blood pressure can be reduced in patients with hypertension by inhibiting the production of angiotensin II. This can be achieved by inhibiting the actions of angiotensin-converting enzyme (ACE), which converts angiotensin I to angiotensin II (see Fig. 4-25). This is precisely how ACE inhibitors function to reduce blood pressure.

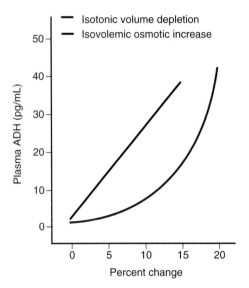

4-27: *Differential sensitivity of secretion of antidiuretic hormone (ADH) to plasma osmolarity and plasma volume status.*

3. **CNS osmoreceptors and antidiuretic hormone**
   - **Antidiuretic hormone (ADH)** is a hormone secreted from the posterior pituitary that plays an important role in the **regulation of plasma volume.** It is secreted by hypothalamic osmoreceptors in response to either slight increases in plasma osmolarity or marked reductions in plasma volume (Fig. 4-27).
   - The primary mechanism of action of ADH is to stimulate water reabsorption by the collecting tubules of the distal nephron. At higher levels, it also stimulates systemic vasoconstriction. Both of these actions are aimed at increasing MAP.
4. **Low-pressure stretch receptors that monitor venous return**
   - In contrast to the high-pressure stretch receptors in the aortic arch and carotid sinuses, low-pressure stretch receptors in the atria and vena cava are ideally positioned to monitor venous return. If large volumes of blood return to the right side of the heart, the receptors send signals via the vagus nerve and stimulate selective renal vasodilation, causing diuresis by the kidneys to decrease plasma volume.
   - Low-pressure stretch receptors also increase the HR in response to **increased venous return (Bainbridge reflex).** This action increases CO and renal perfusion, further increasing diuresis.
   - Atrial stretch from increased venous return causes the atria to secrete atrial natriuretic peptide, which further promotes diuresis.

VIII. **Fluid Exchange in the Capillaries**
   - Fluid exchange across the capillary membrane is dependent on the permeability characteristics of the capillary bed and the net filtration pressure generated across the capillary bed.

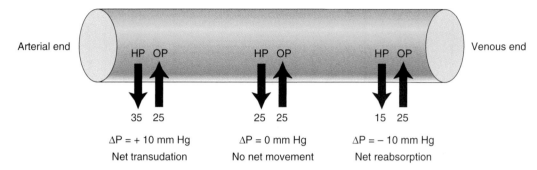

Arterial end

Venous end

HP OP

35   25

$\Delta P = + 10$ mm Hg

Net transudation

HP OP

25   25

$\Delta P = 0$ mm Hg

No net movement

HP OP

15   25

$\Delta P = - 10$ mm Hg

Net reabsorption

4-28: *Starling forces in a capillary. HP, hydrostatic pressure (mm Hg); OP, oncotic pressure (mm Hg); ΔP, difference in pressure (HP − OP).*

- The **net filtration pressure** (NFP) depends on the interaction between plasma and interstitial hydrostatic and osmotic forces, which are known as **Starling forces.** The end result of this interaction is the production of an NFP that drives fluid from the capillaries into the interstitium or from the interstitium into the capillaries, depending on the relative contribution of each force.
A. **Starling forces**
   1. **Hydrostatic pressure of the capillary (P_c)**
      - This is the outward force exerted by pressurized fluid within the blood vessel; it is greater on the arterial end of the capillary (~35 mm Hg) than it is on the venous end (~15 mm Hg).
      - This hydrostatic pressure differential along the capillary results in loss of fluid from the arterial end and reabsorption of interstitial fluid from the venous end (Fig. 4-28). In conditions such as venous obstruction, the hydrostatic pressure may become **abnormally elevated,** resulting in increased loss of fluid to the interstitium and causing edema.

      > **Pathology note:** In conditions associated with **rapid loss of intravascular volume,** such as **hemorrhage,** the hydrostatic pressure of the capillaries may become too low to cause fluid movement into the interstitium. Instead, there is **net movement of interstitial fluid into the capillaries,** which helps restore intravascular volume.

   2. **Plasma oncotic pressure or plasma colloid osmotic pressure (π_c)**
      - This is the inward force on fluid movement exerted by plasma proteins that are too large to diffuse out of the capillaries; oncotic pressure draws fluid from the interstitium into the capillaries.
      - The serum albumin level is the primary determinant of the plasma oncotic pressure. In patients with **hypoalbuminemia** (low plasma albumin), the low oncotic pressure causes fluid to move from the vascular compartment into the interstitium, resulting in edema.

> **Pathology note:** Malnutrition or liver disease can cause
> **hypoalbuminemia** and **edema,** because albumin is synthesized
> from amino acids by the liver. In addition, certain kidney diseases such
> as **nephrotic syndrome** are characterized by the loss of large
> quantities of serum protein in the urine, which also may lead to
> hypoalbuminemia and edema.

3. **Interstitial hydrostatic pressure (P_{IF})**
   - Interstitial fluid exerts an inward force.
   - The force is normally **slightly negative** because the lymphatics are
     constantly draining interstitial fluid, essentially creating a slight vacuum.
4. **Interstitial oncotic pressure (π_{IF})**
   - This is the outward force exerted by interstitial proteins.
   - The concentration of proteins in the interstitial fluid is normally much less
     than that of the plasma, so this force is less forceful than the opposing force
     of capillary oncotic pressure.

> **Pathology note:** In **inflammatory states,** the increased vascular
> permeability may result in increased levels of interstitial proteins, which
> **increases interstitial oncotic pressure** and drives fluid into the
> interstitium, causing **edema.**

B. **Starling equation**
   - The sum of the Starling forces determines the NFP across a capillary bed.
     Starling forces vary significantly in different tissues, but the driving net
     filtration in a typical capillary bed is expressed as follows:

$$\begin{aligned} \text{NFP} &= (P_c + \pi_{IF}) - (P_{IF} + \pi_c) \\ &= (17.3 + 8) - (-3 + 28) \\ &= 0.3\, \text{mm Hg} \end{aligned}$$

where NFP = net filtration pressure, P_c = hydrostatic pressure of capillary,
π_c = plasma oncotic pressure, P_{IF} = interstitial hydrostatic pressure, and
π_{IF} = interstitial oncotic pressure.
   - **Note:** The **very small NFP** (<1 mm Hg) **drives filtration across the capillary
     membrane.** This small driving pressure is sufficient because of the highly
     permeable nature of the capillary membrane. The average NFP over the entire
     capillary is very low, but at any given point it could be much higher or much
     lower (see Fig. 4-28).
C. **Pathophysiology of edema**
   - The reabsorption of fluid at the venous end of the capillary is typically slightly
     less than the loss of fluid at the arterial end of the capillary. Therefore, there is
     a constant **"leakage" of fluid** from the vascular compartment into the
     interstitial compartment.
   - One of the primary functions of the lymphatic system is to **return** this **excess
     fluid to the vascular compartment** via the thoracic duct. This capacity can be
     overwhelmed by significant alterations in the Starling forces or increased
     capillary permeability. **Dysfunction of the lymphatic system also may result
     in severe edema** (Table 4-2).

TABLE 4-2:
Starling Forces and Edema

Disorder	Physiologic Mechanism of Edema
Liver disease	↓ Plasma protein → ↓ plasma oncotic pressure
Inflammation	↑ Vascular permeability → ↑ proteins in interstitial fluid → ↑ oncotic pressure of interstitial fluid
Venous obstruction (thrombophlebitis)	Back-pressure resulting in capillary congestion → ↑ capillary hydrostatic pressure
Heart failure	Back-pressure resulting in venous congestion → increased capillary hydrostatic pressure
Myxedema	↑ Glycoproteins in interstitial fluid → ↑ oncotic pressure of interstitial fluid
Nephrotic syndrome	Proteinuria → ↓ plasma protein → ↓ plasma oncotic pressure

IX. **Pathophysiology of Heart Failure**
  A. **Inadequate cardiac output or elevated filling pressures**
    • Heart failure may be thought of as **any state in which cardiac output is inadequate to meet the body's metabolic demands** or can be maintained only at the expense of elevated ventricular filling pressures (i.e., increased preload).
  B. **Systolic heart failure:** "pump" failure
    • Approximately two thirds of cases of heart failure are systolic.
    • The pathogenesis of systolic heart failure involves either impaired ventricular contractility or pathologic increases in afterload; the end result is a decrease in SV and CO.
      (1) **Impaired contractility** may occur in association with myocardial ischemia, myocardial infarction, chronic volume-overloaded states such as aortic or mitral regurgitation, or dilated cardiomyopathy.
      (2) **Pathologic increases in afterload** may occur in association with poorly controlled hypertension and aortic stenosis.
  C. **Diastolic heart failure**
    • Approximately one third of cases of heart failure are diastolic.
    • Ventricular filling during diastole is impaired. Reduced ventricular filling occurs as the result of two distinct pathophysiologic mechanisms, either a **reduction in ventricular compliance** or an **obstruction of left ventricular filling.**
    • Reduced ventricular compliance may result from a variety of conditions:
      (1) In **left ventricular hypertrophy and hypertrophic cardiomyopathy,** the thickened myocardium "does not relax as well."
      (2) In **restrictive cardiomyopathy,** deposition of substances within the myocardium causes fibrosis, reducing compliance.
      (3) In **myocardial ischemia,** the O_2 supply is not sufficient to support the normal energy requirements of active diastolic relaxation.
    • Obstruction to left ventricular filling may occur in **mitral stenosis** and **cardiac tamponade,** in which fluid accumulates in the pericardial space and opposes

TABLE 4-3:
Compensatory Responses to Reduced Cardiac Output

Compensatory Response	Primary Triggering Stimulus	Adverse Effects
Frank-Starling relationship	Reduced renal perfusion from reduced cardiac output activates renin-angiotensin-aldosterone system and expands plasma volume	Pulmonary edema Peripheral edema
Myocardial hypertrophy	Increased myocardial wall stress	Increased myocardial oxygen demand Reduced ventricular compliance if concentric hypertrophy develops Impaired contractility if eccentric hypertrophy develops
Neurohormonal activation	Baroreceptors	Risk of arrhythmias Vasoconstriction in skeletal muscles produces weakness

ventricular filling, and in restrictive pericarditis, in which scarring of the pericardium limits ventricular expansion and filling.

> **Pathology note: Myocardial ischemia** may contribute to **both** systolic and diastolic dysfunction because ventricular contraction during systole and ventricular relaxation during diastole are both **energy-requiring processes** that depend on an adequate O_2 supply.

D. **High-output heart failure**
  - Heart failure can be precipitated by "peripheral" conditions in which the body's tissues require an ever-increasing CO.
  - For example, with **large arteriovenous fistulas** or in conditions such as **thyrotoxicosis** or severe **anemia,** the demand for CO becomes pathologically elevated. The healthy heart is initially able to meet this increased demand, but over time the strain imposed on the heart may become too great, at which point the heart begins to fail.

E. **Compensatory mechanisms**
  - The primary compensatory responses for low CO include utilization of the Frank-Starling relationship, myocardial hypertrophy, and neurohormonal activation. Table 4-3 presents the "triggers" for these compensatory responses.
  - Initially, these compensatory mechanisms may have a beneficial effect in preserving CO. However, if the underlying cause of the heart failure (e.g., hypertension, coronary artery disease, valvular disease) is not addressed, the chronic activation of these compensatory mechanisms may have deleterious effects.

X. **Circulatory Insufficiency**
  A. **Signs and symptoms**
  - Circulatory insufficiency, or shock, is a state of **inadequate tissue perfusion,** which most often occurs in hypotensive states. This inadequate tissue perfusion

TABLE 4-4:
Physiologic Basis for Signs of Shock

Signs	Physiologic Basis
Acidosis	Tissue ischemia/hypoxia → ↑ anaerobic respiration
Pale, cool, moist skin	Sympathetic-mediated peripheral vasoconstriction and sweating
Rapid, weak pulse	Reflex tachycardia in hypotension
Reduced urinary output	↓ Renal blood flow → ↓ glomerular filtration rate
Confusion	Insufficient cerebral perfusion

TABLE 4-5:
Types of Shock

Type of Shock	Pathophysiology	Examples
Cardiogenic	Failure of the heart to pump effectively (i.e., reduced ejection fraction), resulting in reduced cardiac output	Myocardial infarction, viral myocarditis
Distributive Spinal (neurogenic)	Disruption of autonomic outflow from the spinal cord, which abolishes normal tonic stimulation of arteriolar contraction by sympathetic nerves	Spinal cord injury
Septic	Bacterial infection of blood → release of bacterial toxins and cytokines → high fever and massive vasodilation → ↓ vascular resistance	Severe bacteremia
Anaphylactic	Massive IgE-mediated histamine release	Allergies
Hypovolemic	Hypovolemia → ↓ venous return → ↓ cardiac output	Hemorrhage, vomiting, diarrhea, burns, dehydration

IgE, immunoglobulin E.

invokes powerful compensatory responses from the sympathetic nervous system through diversely located baroreceptors and chemoreceptors.
- The signs and symptoms of shock, which include **cold** and **clammy skin, rapid** and **weak pulse, confusion,** and **reduced urinary output,** result as much from the inadequate tissue perfusion as from the compensatory sympathetic response.

B. **Pathophysiologic basis for classification of shock**
- In the human circulatory system, three basic pathophysiologic processes can cause circulatory insufficiency, or shock (Tables 4-4 and 4-5).
- Regardless of the precise pathophysiologic abnormality, the end result is impaired tissue perfusion.

1. **Cardiogenic shock**
- In cardiogenic shock, the heart fails as a pump; it is **unable to maintain a CO sufficient to meet the body's metabolic demands** in the presence of an adequate intravascular volume.

- The most common cause is **severe left ventricular dysfunction,** which may occur after a large left-sided myocardial infarction. Other causes include valvular disease (e.g., rupture of papillary muscle causing mitral regurgitation) and myocarditis.
2. **Distributive shock**
   - In distributive types of shock, widespread vasodilation decreases the peripheral resistance substantially, thereby lowering the blood pressure to inadequate levels. There are several causes.
   - In **neurogenic shock,** if the sympathetic tone to the vasculature is removed (e.g., by severing the spinal cord in the cervical region), massive vasodilation occurs.
   - In **septic shock,** cytokines released in response to toxins cause widespread vasodilation.
   - In **anaphylactic shock, histamine** and **prostaglandins** released in response to allergens cause widespread vasodilation and increased capillary permeability, resulting in **fluid loss into the interstitium.**
3. **Hypovolemic shock**
   - In hypovolemic shock, too little intravascular volume is present. There is simply not enough fluid within the vascular compartment to produce an effective circulating volume through no fault of the "pump" or of the "pipes."
   - Hypovolemic shock occurs mainly as a **result of hemorrhage,** but it may also may occur in conditions such as **dehydration.**

Respiratory Physiology

I. Overview

- Because it is essential for metabolism, oxygen must be provided in relatively large amounts to most cells.
- Oxygen delivery has three stages:
  - (1) **External respiration:** gas exchange between the external environment (alveolar air) and the blood (pulmonary capillaries)
  - (2) **Internal respiration:** gas exchange between the blood (systemic capillaries) and the interstitial fluid
  - (3) **Cellular respiration:** gas exchange between the interstitial fluid and the mitochondria of cells

II. Functional Anatomy of the Respiratory System

- The respiratory system is composed of large **conducting airways** which conduct air to the smaller **respiratory airways.**
- **Gas exchange** occurs in the **respiratory airways.**

> **Pathology note:** Because conducting airways do not directly participate in gas exchange, the space within them is termed **anatomic dead space.**

A. Conducting airways

- These include the nose, mouth, pharynx, larynx, trachea, bronchi, and conducting bronchioles.
- Despite their larger size, **airway resistance** is **greater** than in the respiratory airways, because the conducting airways are arranged in **series** and airflow resistance in series is additive.

1. **Bronchi** (Table 5-1)
   - The bronchi are large airways (>1 mm in diameter) that contain supportive **cartilage rings.** If not for these cartilage rings, the bronchi would be much more likely to collapse during expiration, when intrathoracic pressures increase substantially.
   - As the bronchi branch into successively smaller airways, they have fewer cartilage rings. Bronchial branches that have no cartilage and are <1 mm in diameter are termed **bronchioles.**
   - Bronchi are not physically embedded in the lung parenchyma; this allows them to dilate and constrict independently of the lung.

2. **Mucociliary tract**
   - Bronchial epithelium comprises pseudostratified columnar cells, many of which are ciliated, interspersed with mucus-secreting goblet cells.

TABLE 5-1:
Comparison of Bronchi and Bronchioles

Parameter	Bronchi	Conducting Bronchioles
Smooth muscle	Present (many layers)	Present (1–3 layers)
Cartilage	Yes	No
Epithelium	Pseudostratified columnar	Simple cuboidal
Ciliated	Yes	Yes (less)
Diameter	Independent of lung volume	Depends on lung volume
Location	Intraparenchymal and extraparenchymal	Embedded directly within connective tissue of lung

- The mucus traps inhaled foreign particles before they reach the alveoli. It is then transported by the beating cilia proximally toward the mouth, so that it can be swallowed or expectorated. This process is termed the **mucociliary escalator.**

   > **Clinical note: Primary ciliary dyskinesia** is an autosomal recessive disorder that renders cilia in airways unable to beat normally. The result is a chronic cough and recurrent infections. Cigarette smoke causes a **secondary ciliary dyskinesia.**

3. **Conducting bronchioles** (see Table 5-1)
   - In contrast to the bronchi, these small-diameter airways are physically embedded within the lung parenchyma and do not have supportive cartilage rings.
   - Therefore, as the lungs inflate and deflate, so too do these airways.

   > **Clinical note:** In **asthma,** the smooth muscle of the larger airways becomes **hypersensitive** to certain stimuli, resulting in **bronchoconstriction.** This airway narrowing produces **turbulent airflow,** which can be appreciated on examination as **wheezing.**

B. **Respiratory airways** (Table 5-2)
   - These include **respiratory bronchioles, alveolar ducts,** and **alveoli,** where gas exchange occurs.
   - Despite their smaller size, **airway resistance** is **less** than in conducting airways, because the respiratory airways are arranged in parallel, and airflow resistances in parallel are added reciprocally.
   - Similar to the smaller of the conducting bronchioles, the respiratory airways have no cartilage and are embedded in lung tissue; therefore, their diameter is primarily dependent on **lung volume.**
C. **Pulmonary membrane: the "air-blood" barrier**
   - This is a thin barrier that separates the alveolar air from the pulmonary capillary blood, through which gas exchange must occur.

TABLE 5-2:
Comparison of Conducting and Respiratory Airways

Parameter	Conducting Airways	Respiratory Airways
Histology	Ciliated columnar tissue Goblet cells (mucociliary tract)	Nonciliated cuboidal tissue No goblet cells Lacks smooth muscle
Presence of cartilage	Yes	No
Resistance	Large diameter Arranged in series High resistance	Small diameter Arranged in parallel Low resistance

- It comprises **multiple layers,** including, from the alveolar space "inward":
  (1) A **surfactant**-containing fluid layer that lines the alveoli
  (2) **Alveolar epithelium** composed of **pneumocytes** (both type I and type II)
  (3) **Epithelial** and **capillary basement membranes,** separated by a thin interstitial space (fused in areas)
  (4) Capillary endothelium

> **Pathology note:** The **alveolar epithelium** is primarily populated **by type I pneumocytes,** which play an important role in gas exchange. **Type II pneumocytes** are much less numerous but are important in producing surfactant. When the pulmonary membrane has been damaged, type II pneumocytes are able to differentiate into type I pneumocytes and effect repair of the pulmonary membrane.

III. **Mechanics of Breathing**
   - **Ventilation** is the process by which air enters and exits the lungs. It is characterized by an inspiratory phase and an expiratory phase.
   - Note that ventilation is a separate process from gas exchange.

> **Pathology note:** Gas exchange may be impaired in certain conditions in which pulmonary ventilation is nevertheless normal or even increased. Two examples are **anemia** and **high-altitude respiration.**

   A. **Inspiration**
      - An **active process** that requires substantial expansion of the thoracic cavity to accommodate the inspired air. This expansion occurs primarily as a result of **diaphragmatic contraction** and, to a lesser extent, contraction of the **external intercostal muscles** (Fig. 5-1).
      - During **forceful breathing** (e.g., exercise, lung disease), contraction of **accessory muscles** such as the sternocleidomastoid, scalenes, and pectoralis major may be necessary to assist in expanding the thorax.

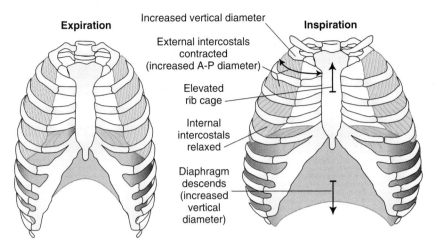

5-1: *Muscles of inspiration. Note how contraction of the diaphragm increases the vertical diameter of the thorax, whereas contraction of the external intercostal muscles results in anteroposterior (A-P) and lateral expansion of the thorax.*

Clinical note: Hypertrophy of accessory muscles may be seen when there is an increased work of breathing in patients with chronic lung disease.

Clinical note: During normal inhalation at rest, abdominal pressure increases secondary to diaphragmatic contraction. This is evident by watching a supine person's abdomen rise during quiet breathing (as long as the person is not trying to "suck in their gut"). In patients with respiratory distress, the abdomen may actually be "sucked in" while the accessory muscles of inspiration are contracting. This is known as **paradoxical breathing** and is an indicator of impending respiratory failure.

1. **Driving force for inspiration**
   - A **negative intrapleural pressure** is created by movement of the diaphragm downward and the chest wall outward. This acts like a vacuum and "sucks open" the airways, causing air to enter the lungs.
   - The relationship between intrapleural pressure and lung volume is expressed by **Boyle's law,** by which end-inspiratory lung volume (V_2) is proportional to the intrapleural pressure (P_1) and lung volume (V_1) at the beginning of inspiration and inversely proportional to the end-inspiratory pressure (P_2):

$$P_1 V_1 = P_2 V_2$$

$$V_2 = \frac{P_1 V_1}{P_2}$$

   - The pressure and volume changes that occur during the respiratory cycle are shown in Figure 5-2. Note that, as the initial intrapleural pressure decreases during inspiration, end-inspiratory lung volume increases.

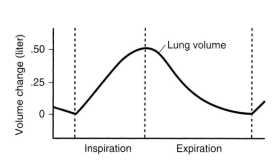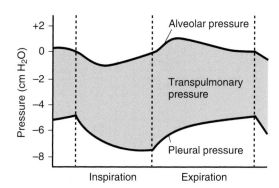

5-2: *Pressure and volume changes during the respiratory cycle. Note that alveolar pressure equals zero at the end of a tidal inspiration (when there is no airflow). In contrast, at the end of a tidal inspiration, the pleural pressure has decreased to its lowest value (approximately $-7.5\,cm\,H_2O$). The difference between pleural and alveolar pressures is referred to as the transpulmonary pressure.*

    2. **Sources of resistance during inspiration**
- **Airway resistance:** friction between air molecules and the airway walls, caused by inspired air coursing along the airways at high velocity
- **Compliance resistance:** intrinsic resistance to stretching of the alveolar air spaces and lung parenchyma
- **Tissue resistance:** friction that occurs when the pleural surfaces glide over each other as the lungs inflate

B. **Expiration**
- Usually a **passive process** in which relaxation of the diaphragm, combined with elastic recoil of the lungs and chest wall, forces air from the lungs
- During **forceful breathing** (e.g., exercise, lung disease), expiration becomes an **active process** employing **accessory muscles** such as the internal intercostals and abdominal wall muscles (e.g., rectus abdominis). Contraction of these helps to depress the rib cage, which compresses the lungs and forces air from the respiratory tree.

    1. **Driving forces for expiration**
- An **increase in intrapleural pressure** is created by movement of the diaphragm upward and the chest wall inward. This increase is then transmitted to the terminal air spaces (alveolar ducts and alveoli) and compresses them, causing air to leave the lungs. In addition, the recoil forces from the alveoli that were stretched during inspiration promote expiration.
- During **forced expiration,** this elastic recoil of the diaphragm and chest wall is accompanied by contraction of the abdominal muscles, all of which increase the intrapleural pressure.

    2. **Sources of resistance during expiration**
- As the volume of the thoracic cavity decreases during expiration, the intrathoracic pressure increases (recall Boyle's law—the inverse relationship of pressure and volume).
- The increased pressure **compresses** the airways and **reduces airway diameter.** This reduction in airway diameter is the primary source of resistance to airflow during expiration.

Clinical note: If the lung were a simple pump, its **maximum** attainable transport of gas in and out would be limited by exhalation. During expiration, the last two-thirds of the expired vital capacity is largely **independent of effort.** The best way to appreciate this is to do it yourself. No matter how hard you try, you cannot increase flow during the latter part of the expiratory cycle. The reduction in **small airway** diameter with resultant increase in airway resistance is the major determinant of this phenomenon. In contrast, **large airways** are mostly spared from collapse by the presence of cartilage. One can imagine the difficulty asthmatics face during exhalation with the addition of **bronchoconstriction.**

C. **Work of breathing**
- This is the **pressure-volume work** performed in moving volumes of air into and out of the lungs. Because expiration is usually passive, the vast majority of this work is done during inspiration. Work must be performed to overcome the three primary sources of resistance encountered during inspiration.
1. **Airway resistance**
   - As inspired air courses along the airways, **friction** and therefore airway resistance is generated **between air molecules and the walls of conducting airways.** Airway resistance normally accounts for approximately 20% of the work of breathing.
   - Because air is essentially a fluid of low viscosity, airflow resistance can be equated to the resistance encountered by a fluid traveling through a rigid tube. **Poiseuille's equation** relates airflow resistance (R), air viscosity (η), airway length (l), and airway radius (r):

$$R = 8\eta l/\pi r^{4}$$

   - In the lung, air viscosity and airway length are basically unchanging constants, whereas airway radius can change dramatically. Even slight changes in **airway diameter** have a dramatic impact on airflow resistance.

Pathology note: Airway diameter can be reduced (and airway resistance thereby increased) by a number of mechanisms. For example, airway diameters are reduced by smooth muscle contraction and excess secretions in **obstructive airway diseases** such as **asthma** and **chronic bronchitis.** Work caused by airway resistance increases markedly as a result.

Note that this description is a simplification, because Poiseuille's equation is based on the premise that airflow is laminar. Although this is true for the smaller airways, in which the total cross-sectional area is large and the airflow velocity is slow, airflow in the **upper airways** is typically **turbulent,** as evidenced by the **bronchial sounds** heard during **auscultation.**

a. **Contribution of large and small airways to resistance**
  • Under normal conditions, most of the total airway resistance actually comes from the **large conducting airways.** This is because they are arranged in series, and airflow resistances in series are **additive,** such that

$$R_{Total} = R_1 + R_2 + R_3 + \ldots + R_n$$

  • By contrast, the **small airways** (terminal bronchioles, respiratory bronchioles, and alveolar ducts) provide relatively little resistance. This is because they are arranged in parallel, and airflow resistances in parallel are added **reciprocally,** such that

$$1/R = 1/R_1 + 1/R_2 + 1/R_3 + \ldots + 1/R_n$$

  • Resistance is low in smaller-diameter airways despite the fact that Poiseuille's equation states that resistance is inversely proportional to the fourth power of airway radius. This is because the branches of the small airways have a **total** cross-sectional area that is greater than that of the larger airways from which they branch. Additionally, flow in these small airways is laminar rather than turbulent, and it is very slow.

> **Pharmacology note:** Many classes of drugs affect large airway diameter by affecting bronchial smooth muscle tone. For example, **β2-adrenergic agonists** such as albuterol directly stimulate bronchodilation. Most other classes work by preventing bronchoconstriction or by inhibiting inflammation (which reduces airway diameter); these include **steroids, mast cell stabilizers, anticholinergics, leukotriene-receptor antagonists,** and **lipoxygenase inhibitors.**

2. **Compliance resistance (work)**
  • As the lungs inflate, work must be performed to overcome the intrinsic **elastic recoil of the lungs.**
  • This work, termed **compliance work,** normally accounts for the largest proportion (~75%) of the total work of breathing (Fig. 5-3).

> **Pathology note:** In **emphysema,** compliance work is **reduced** because of the destruction of lung tissue and the loss of elastin and collagen. In **pulmonary fibrosis,** compliance work is **increased,** because the fibrotic tissue requires more work to expand.

3. **Tissue resistance**
  • As the **pleural surfaces** slide over each other during the respiratory cycle, **friction** and therefore resistance is generated.
  • A small amount of **pleural fluid** in the pleural space acts to lubricate these surfaces, thereby minimizing the friction. Under normal conditions, tissue resistance accounts for a small portion (perhaps 5%) of the total work of breathing.

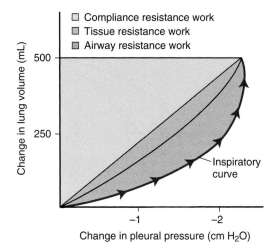

5-3: *Relative contributions of the three resistances to the total work of breathing.*

> **Pathology note:** In certain **pleuritic conditions,** inflammation or adhesions are formed between the two pleural surfaces, which increases tissue resistance substantially. An example is **empyema,** in which there is pus in the pleural space.

C. **Pulmonary compliance (C)**
  - This is a measure of **lung distensibility.** Compliant lungs are easy to distend, whereas less compliant lungs are more difficult to distend.
  - Defined as the change in volume (ΔV) required for a fractional change of pulmonary pressure (ΔP):

$$C = \frac{\Delta V}{\Delta P}$$

  - Highest in the midportion of the inspiratory curve (Fig. 5-4)

D. **Pulmonary elastance**
  - Elastance is the property of matter that makes it **resist deformation.** Highly elastic structures are difficult to deform, whereas inelastic structures are easy to deform.
  - Pulmonary elastance (E) is the pressure (P) required for a fractional change of lung volume (ΔV):

$$E = \frac{\Delta P}{\Delta V}$$

  - As elastance increases, increasingly greater pressure changes will be required to distend the lungs.

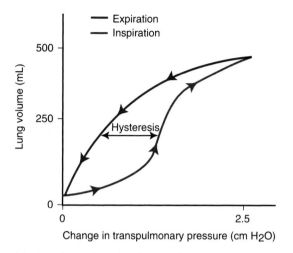

5-4: *Compliance curve of the lungs: lung volume plotted against changes in transpulmonary pressure (the difference between pleural and alveolar pressure). During inspiration, maximal compliance occurs in the midportion of the inspiratory curve. The difference between the inspiration curve and the expiration curve is referred to as hysteresis. Hysteresis is an intrinsic property of all elastic substances.*

Clinical note: In restrictive lung diseases such as **silicosis** and **asbestosis,** inspiration becomes increasingly difficult as the resistance to lung expansion increases due to **increased lung elastance,** resulting in reduced lung volumes.

In obstructive lung diseases such as emphysema, there is **reduced lung elastance** secondary to destruction of lung parenchyma and loss of proteins that contribute to the elastic recoil of the lungs (e.g., collagen, elastin). Expiration may therefore become an active process (rather than a passive one), even while at rest, because the easily collapsible airways "trap" air in the lungs. **"Pursed-lip breathing,"** an attempt to expire adequate amounts of air, is often seen: It creates an added pressure within the airways that keeps them open and allows for more effective expiration.

E. **Surface tension**
- The fluid lining the alveolar membrane is primarily water. The water molecules are attracted to each other via noncovalent hydrogen bonds and are repelled by the hydrophobic alveolar air. The **attractive forces between water molecules** generate **surface tension** (T), which in turn produces a **collapsing pressure,** which acts to collapse the alveoli.
- **Laplace's law** states that **collapsing pressure** (CP) is inversely proportional to the alveolar radius (R), such that smaller alveoli experience a larger collapsing pressure:

$$CP = \frac{2T}{R}$$

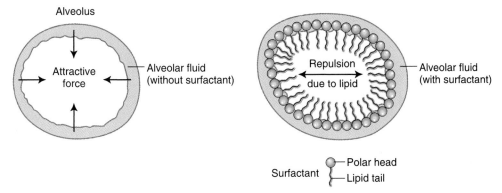

Surfactant
○─ Polar head
│─ Lipid tail

5-5: *Role of surfactant in reducing alveolar surface tension. Note the orientation of the hydrophilic "head" in the alveolar fluid and the hydrophobic "tail" in the alveolar air.*

> **Clinical note:** The collapse of many alveoli in the same region of lung parenchyma leads to **atelectasis.** Atelectatic lung may result from **external compression,** as may occur with pleural effusion or tumor; a prolonged period of **"shallow breaths,"** as may occur due to pain (e.g., rib fracture) or diaphragmatic paralysis; or **obstruction of bronchi** (e.g., tumor, pus, or mucus).

F. **Role of surfactant**
  - A moderate amount of surface tension is beneficial, because it generates a collapsing pressure that contributes to the elastic recoil of the lungs during expiration. Indeed, surface tension is typically responsible for about two thirds of the elastic recoil of the lungs. However, if collapsing pressure were to become pathologically elevated, lung inflation during inspiration would become impaired. So a balance needs to be reached, and this is mediated by surfactant.
  - **Surfactant** is a **complex phospholipid** secreted onto the alveolar membrane by **type II pneumocytes.** It minimizes the interaction between alveolar fluid and alveolar air (Fig. 5-5), which reduces surface tension. This increases lung compliance, which reduces the work of breathing.

> **Clinical note:** The collapsing pressure of alveoli in infants born before approximately 34 weeks of gestation may be pathologically elevated for two reasons: (1) the alveoli are small, which contributes to an elevated collapsing pressure, and (2) surface tension may be abnormally increased because **surfactant** is not normally produced until the **third trimester** of pregnancy. Therefore there is a high risk for respiratory failure and **neonatal respiratory distress syndrome.** Mothers in premature labor are frequently given corticosteroids to stimulate the infant to produce surfactant. After birth, **exogenous surfactant** or **artificial respiration** may also be required.

TABLE 5-3:
Comparison of Partial Gas Pressures (mm Hg)

Gas	Atmospheric	Alveolar	Arterial	Venous
O_2	160	100	100	40
CO_2	0.3	40	40	46
N_2	600	573	—	—
H_2O	0	47	—	—

IV. **Gas Exchange**
- Gas exchange across the pulmonary membrane occurs by **diffusion.**
- The **rate of diffusion** is dependent on the **partial pressure (tension)** of the gases on either side of the membrane and the **surface area** available for diffusion, among other factors.

A. **Partial pressure of gases**
- According to **Dalton's law,** the partial pressure exerted by a gas in a mixture of gases is proportional to the fractional concentration of that gas:

    Total pressure (mm Hg) × Concentration (%) = Partial pressure (mm Hg)

- The partial pressure of O_2 in the atmosphere, which is approximately 21% O_2, is calculated as follows:

    760 mm Hg × 21% = 160 mm Hg (at sea level)

- The importance of Dalton's law becomes evident when one considers the humidification of inspired air: The addition of H_2O vapor decreases the percent concentration of O_2 in alveolar air and hence decreases its partial pressure (Table 5-3).

    Pathology note: The "dilution" of partial pressures by H_2O (vapor) becomes extremely important at high altitudes, where atmospheric (i.e., alveolar) oxygen tension is already low.

B. **Diffusion**
- The **diffusion rate** of oxygen across the pulmonary membrane depends on
    (1) The **pressure gradient** (ΔP) between alveolar oxygen and oxygen within the pulmonary capillaries
    (2) The **surface area** (A) of the pulmonary membrane
    (3) The **diffusion distance** (T) across which O_2 must diffuse
- These variables are expressed in **Fick's law of diffusion,** where the solubility coefficient for oxygen (S) is an unchanging constant:

$$D = \frac{\Delta P \times A \times S}{T}$$

Clinical note: Oxygen diffusion is impaired by any process that decreases the O_2 pressure gradient (e.g., **high altitude**), decreases the surface area of the pulmonary membrane (e.g., **emphysema**), or increases the diffusion distance (e.g., **pulmonary fibrosis**).

C. **Diffusing capacity of the pulmonary membrane**
   - This is the **volume of gas** that can diffuse across the pulmonary membrane in 1 minute when the pressure difference across the membrane is 1 mm Hg. It is often measured using **carbon monoxide.**
   - The diffusing capacity of the lungs is normally so great that O_2 exchange is **perfusion limited;** that is, the amount of O_2 that enters the arterial circulation is limited only by the amount of blood flow to the lungs (cardiac output).
   - In various types of lung disease, the diffusing capacity may be reduced to such an extent that O_2 exchange becomes **diffusion limited.**

   Clinical note: A number pathophysiologic mechanisms **reduce diffusing capacity:** (1) increased thickness of the pulmonary membrane in restrictive diseases (the primary factor in **silicosis** and **idiopathic pulmonary fibrosis**); (2) collapse of alveoli and lung segments (atelectasis), which contributes to a decreased surface area available for gas exchange (e.g., with bed rest after surgery); (3) poor lung compliance, resulting in insufficient ventilation (e.g., silicosis); and (4) destruction of alveolar units, which also decreases surface area (e.g., **emphysema**).

V. **Pulmonary Blood Flow**
   - Although the lungs are well **perfused** (receiving the entire right ventricular output as well as contributions from the bronchial arteries), perfusion differs substantially in different sections of the lungs.
   - **Differential perfusion** becomes significant only in the upright position, when the effects of gravity are apparent, and essentially disappear in the supine position.
   - Pulmonary blood flow is often described as being divided into three different **zones** (Fig. 5-6).
A. **"Zones" of pulmonary blood flow**
   1. **Zone 1 blood flow**
      - Zone 1 has **no** blood flow during the cardiac cycle, a pathologic condition that *does not normally occur* in the healthy lung. The lack of perfusion that occurs with zone 1 pulmonary blood flow quickly leads to tissue necrosis and lung damage.
      - Zone 1 conditions occur when hydrostatic arterial and venous pressures are lower than alveolar pressures. This can occur in the lung apices, where arterial hydrostatic pressures are reduced relative to the pressures in arteries supplying the lower lung fields. Under these conditions, the blood vessel is completely collapsed and there is no blood flow during either systole or diastole.

      Clinical note: Zone 1 conditions can occur during severe hemorrhage and during positive pressure ventilation.

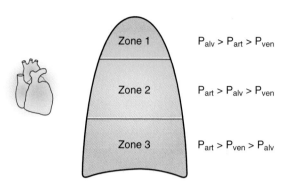

Zone 1 $P_{alv} > P_{art} > P_{ven}$

Zone 2 $P_{art} > P_{alv} > P_{ven}$

Zone 3 $P_{art} > P_{ven} > P_{alv}$

5-6: *Zones of pulmonary blood flow. Note the vertical position of the heart relative to the lung zones. P_{alv}, alveolar partial pressure; P_{art}, arterial partial pressure; P_{ven}, venous partial pressure.*

2. **Zone 2 blood flow**
   - Zone 2 has **intermittent** blood flow during the cardiac cycle, with no blood flow during diastole. This is typically exhibited by the **upper two thirds of the lungs.**
   - Alveolar pressures cause collapse of pulmonary capillaries during diastole, but pulmonary capillary pressures during systole exceed alveolar pressures, resulting in perfusion during systole.
3. **Zone 3 blood flow**
   - Zone 3 has **continuous blood flow** during the cardiac cycle. This pattern of blood flow is characteristic of the **lung bases,** which are situated below the heart.
   - Pulmonary capillary pressures are greater than alveolar pressures during systole and diastole, which means that the pulmonary capillaries remain patent throughout the cardiac cycle.

> **Clinical note:** Zone 3 conditions are exploited during hemodynamic monitoring with the use of a **Swan-Ganz** or **pulmonary artery catheter.** The catheter is inserted through a central vein and advanced into the pulmonary artery. An inflated balloon at the distal tip of the catheter allows it to "wedge" into a distal branch of the pulmonary artery. Under Zone 3 conditions, a static column of blood extends from the catheter, through the pulmonary capillary bed, to the left atrium and ultimately the left ventricle. When the balloon is inflated, the **pulmonary artery occlusion pressure** or **"wedge pressure"** is obtained. This is an indirect measurement of the **left ventricular end-diastolic pressure (LVEDP).** LVEDP is a surrogate measurement of **left ventricular end-diastolic volume,** which is an indicator of **cardiac performance** and **volume status.**

B. **Ventilation-perfusion (V/Q) matching** (Fig. 5-7)
   - For gas exchange to occur *efficiently* at the pulmonary membrane, pulmonary ventilation and perfusion should be well "**matched.**" Optimal matching

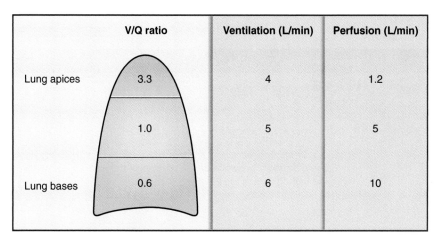

	V/Q ratio	Ventilation (L/min)	Perfusion (L/min)
Lung apices	3.3	4	1.2
	1.0	5	5
Lung bases	0.6	6	10

5-7: *Ventilation–perfusion (V/Q) matching in the different parts of the lungs (at rest). The value of V/Q at rest is approximately 0.8, with alveolar ventilation of about 4 L/min and cardiac output of 5 L/min. The lung apices at rest are underperfused and relatively overventilated (V/Q ratio ~3.3), but compared with the lung bases they do not receive as much ventilation. The high V/Q ratio indicates the discrepancy between the amount of blood flow and ventilation. Conversely, the lung bases at rest are relatively overperfused (V/Q ratio ~0.6).*

minimizes unnecessary ventilation of nonperfused regions and perfusion of nonventilated areas.

1. **Mechanisms of maintaining V/Q matching**
   - Optimal matching of pulmonary ventilation and perfusion is achieved by **hypoxia-induced vasoconstriction** and by changes in response to **exercise.**
   a. **Hypoxia-induced vasoconstriction**
      - In most capillary beds, hypoxia stimulates vasodilation (e.g., myogenic response of autoregulation; see Chapter 2). But in the pulmonary vasculature, hypoxia stimulates **vasoconstriction** of pulmonary arterioles, essentially preventing the perfusion of poorly ventilated lung segments (e.g., as might occur in pulmonary disease). This hypoxia-induced vasoconstriction allows the lungs to optimize V/Q matching for **more efficient gas exchange.**
      - Hypoxia-induced vasoconstriction is particularly well demonstrated in the **fetal lungs.** The resulting vasoconstriction of the pulmonary vessels shunts most of the blood from the pulmonary circulation to the rest of the body. After delivery, when ventilation is established, the pulmonary vascular resistance drops quickly and blood is pumped through the lungs for oxygenation.

> **Pathology note:** At **high altitudes,** where the alveolar partial pressure of O_2 is low, pulmonary vasoconstriction may become harmful, leading to a **global hypoxia-induced vasoconstriction.** This further inhibits gas exchange and increases pulmonary vascular resistance, contributing to the development of right-sided heart failure **(cor pulmonale).**

TABLE 5-4:
Types of Shunt

Type	Characteristics	Clinical Examples
Physiologic	Blood flow to unventilated portions of lungs	Pneumothorax, pneumonia
Anatomic	Blood flow bypasses lungs	Increased perfusion of bronchial arteries in chronic inflammatory lung disease
Left-to-right	Bypasses systemic circulation May cause pulmonary hypertension and eventual right-to-left shunt	Patent ductus arteriosus, ventricular septal defect
Right-to-left	Bypasses pulmonary circulation	Tetralogy of Fallot, truncus arteriosus, transposition of great vessels, atrial septal defect

   b. **Changes with exercise**
- **At rest,** only about one third of the pulmonary capillaries are open. Opening of additional pulmonary capillaries, particularly in the lung apices, occurs during exercise because of two factors:
  - (1) β_2-Mediated vasodilation (minor effect)
  - (2) Increased pulmonary artery blood pressure (major effect)
- **During exercise,** ventilation and perfusion (and hence gas exchange) occur more efficiently because
  - (1) With increased cardiac output, blood flow is increased to the relatively underperfused lung apices.
  - (2) Ventilation is increased to the relatively underventilated lung bases.

> **Clinical note:** At rest, a typical red blood cell (RBC) moves through a pulmonary capillary in approximately 1 sec. O_2 saturation takes only ~0.3 sec. The "safety cushion" of approximately 0.7 sec is essential for O_2 saturation of hemoglobin during **exercise,** when the velocity of pulmonary blood flow greatly increases and the RBC remains in the pulmonary capillary for much less time.

  C. **Shunts**
- A shunt refers to blood that **bypasses the lungs** or for another reason does not participate in gas exchange (Table 5-4).
  1. **Physiologic shunt**
     - This is the perfusion of nonventilated portions of the lungs.
     - The **bronchial arteries** are part of a physiologic shunt. The blood supplies the bronchial tissues but does not travel to the alveoli for gas exchange.
  2. **Anatomic shunt**
     - This is the **diversion of venous blood** from the lungs.
     - **Fetal blood flow** is the classic example. In the fetus, gas exchange occurs in the placenta, so most of the cardiac output is either shunted from the

pulmonary artery to the aorta through the ductus arteriosus or passes through the foramen ovale between the right and left atria.

3. **Cardiac defects causing shunting**
   • **Right-to-left shunts** result in the pumping of deoxygenated blood to the periphery, as occurs in a ventricular septal defect. Hypoxia always results and cannot be corrected with oxygen administration.
   • **Left-to-right shunts** do not cause hypoxia but can cause bilateral ventricular hypertrophy. Patent ductus arteriosus is an example.

VI. **Lung Volumes**
   • Total lung capacity comprises several individual **pulmonary volumes** and **capacities. Spirometry** is used to measure these (Fig. 5-8).
   • There are **four pulmonary volumes:** tidal volume, inspiratory reserve, expiratory reserve, and residual volume. All but residual volume can be measured directly with volume recorders.

> **Clinical note:** Lung volumes tend to decrease in restrictive lung diseases (e.g., **pulmonary fibrosis**) due to limitations of pulmonary expansion, and they tend to increase in obstructive lung diseases (e.g., **emphysema**) due to increased compliance. Note that in patients with **both** restrictive and obstructive disease, lung volumes may remain relatively normal.

A. **Tidal volume (V_T)**
   • The volume of air inspired or expired with each breath
   • Varies with such factors as age, activity level, and position
   • In a resting adult, the normal tidal volume is about **500 mL** (~10% of total lung capacity).

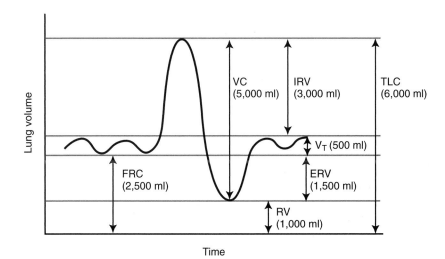

5-8: Spirogram showing changes in lung volume during normal and forceful breathing. Even after maximal expiration, the lungs cannot be completely emptied of air. ERV, expiratory reserve volume; FRC, functional residual capacity; IRV, inspiratory reserve volume; RV, residual volume; VC, vital capacity; V_T, tidal volume.

B. **Inspiratory reserve volume (IRV)**
- The maximum volume of air that can be inspired beyond a normal tidal inspiration
- Typically about **3000 mL** (~50% of total lung capacity)

C. **Expiratory reserve volume (ERV)**
- The maximum volume of air that can be exhaled after a normal tidal expiration
- Typically about **1100 mL** (~20% of total lung capacity)

D. **Residual volume (RV)**
- The amount of air remaining in the lungs after maximal forced expiration. The lungs cannot be completely emptied of air, because cartilage in the major airways prevent their total collapse; furthermore, not all alveolar units completely empty before the small conducting airways that feed them obstruct due to lack of cartilage support against elastic recoil pressures.
- Typically slightly more than **1000 mL** (~30% of total lung capacity)
- Because RV cannot be measured directly using spirometry, a helium dilution technique is used for **measurement of respiratory volume.** After maximal expiration, a 10% solution of helium gas (normal alveolar partial pressure of helium = 0) is inspired. The inspired helium is diluted by residual air in the lungs. After another maximal expiration, the air is again collected. The concentration of helium in this expired air is then measured, and the degree of dilution provides an indirect measurement of residual volume.

> **Clinical note:** Expiration is compromised in **obstructive airway diseases,** and residual volume may progressively increase because inspiratory volumes are always slightly greater than expiratory volumes. This explains the "barrel-chested" appearance of patients with **emphysema.** Dynamic air trapping during exercise is a major limitation to rigorous activity in patients with **chronic obstructive pulmonary disease (COPD).**

VII. **Lung Capacities**
- Lung capacities are the sums of two or more lung volumes.
- There are four lung capacities: functional residual, inspiratory capacity, vital capacity, and total lung capacity. Typical adult values for these are given in the calculations below.

A. **Functional residual capacity (FRC)**
- The amount of air remaining in the lungs after a normal tidal expiration.
- Can also be thought of as the equilibrium point at which the elastic recoil of the lungs is equal and opposite to the expansive forces of the chest wall.
- Calculated as follows:

$$FRC = RV + ERV$$
$$= 1200 \, mL + 1100 \, mL$$
$$= 2300 \, mL$$

- Mixing of small tidal volumes with this relatively large FRC prevents sudden fluctuations in alveolar oxygen tension with individual breaths. This explains why people do not immediately pass out after holding their breath for a short period.

> **Clinical note:** Because of the nature of their disease, patients with **COPD** "trap" air in their lungs, resulting in an **elevated FRC** at which tidal breaths occur. This increases the compliance work of breathing, because they are inspiring along a less efficient part of the curve (see Fig. 5-4).

B. **Inspiratory capacity (IC)**
   - The maximum volume of air that can be inhaled after a normal tidal expiration:

$$IC = V_T + IRV$$
$$= 500 \, mL + 3000 \, mL$$
$$= 3500 \, mL$$

   - Typically accounts for about 60% of the total lung capacity
C. **Vital capacity (VC)**
   - The maximum volume of air that can be expired after maximal inspiration; hence, it is sometimes called the **forced vital capacity (FVC):**

$$VC = IRV + V_T + ERV = IC + ERV$$
$$= 3000 \, mL + 500 \, mL + 1100 \, mL$$
$$= 4600 \, mL$$

   - Typically accounts for approximately 80% of total lung capacity

> **Clinical note:** VC may be decreased substantially in restrictive lung diseases (e.g., idiopathic pulmonary fibrosis) due to reduced pulmonary compliance.

D. **Forced expiratory volume (FEV_1) and FEV_1/FVC ratio**
   - FEV_1 is the maximum amount of air that can be exhaled in 1 second after a maximal inspiration.
   - In healthy individuals, the FEV_1 typically constitutes about 80% of FVC; this relationship is usually expressed as a ratio:

$$FEV_1/FVC = 0.8$$

   - The FEV_1/FVC ratio is clinically useful in helping to distinguish between restrictive and obstructive lung disease.

> **Clinical note:** Although FEV_1 and FVC are **both** reduced in lung disease, the degree of reduction depends on the nature of the disease:
> In **restrictive diseases,** inspiration is limited by noncompliance of the lungs, which limits expiratory volumes. However, because the elastic recoil of the lungs is largely preserved (if not increased), the FVC is typically reduced more than is the FEV_1, resulting in an **FEV_1/FVC ratio** that is **normal** or **increased.**

In **obstructive diseases,** expiratory volumes are reduced because of airway narrowing and sometimes a loss of elastic recoil in the lungs. Total expiratory volumes are largely preserved, but the ability to exhale rapidly is substantially reduced. Therefore, FEV_1 is reduced more than is FVC, and the **FEV_1/FVC ratio** is **reduced.**

E. **Total lung capacity (TLC)**
   - The maximum volume of air in the lungs after a maximal inspiration:

$$TLC = IRV + V_T + ERV + RV$$
$$= 3000\,mL + 500\,mL + 1100\,mL + 1200\,mL$$
$$= 5800\,mL$$

VIII. **Pulmonary Dead Space**
   - Refers to portions of the lung which are ventilated but in which no gas exchange occurs
   - There are **three types** of dead space: anatomic, alveolar, and physiologic.
   A. **Anatomic dead space**
      - Before inspired air reaches the terminal respiratory airways, where gas exchange occurs, it must first travel through the conducting airways. Anatomic dead space is the volume of those conducting airways that do not exchange oxygen with the pulmonary capillary blood.
      - It is estimated as approximately 1 mL per pound for thin adults, or about 150 mL in a 150-pound man.

      Clinical note: In patients who require **mechanical ventilation,** the amount of **anatomic dead space increases** considerably. This is because the volume of space occupied by the respiratory apparatus from the patient's mouth to the ventilator must be considered to be anatomic dead space. Therefore, alveolar ventilation (described later) is altered, and care must be taken to ensure adequate oxygenation.

   B. **Alveolar dead space**
      - If the terminal respiratory units are not ventilated for any reason (e.g., airway obstruction), or if they are ventilated but not supplied with blood (e.g., pulmonary embolism), the volume of these air spaces is referred to as alveolar dead space.
      - In healthy young adults, alveolar dead space is almost zero.
   C. **Physiologic dead space**
      - This is the total volume of lung space that does not participate in gas exchange. It is the sum of the anatomic dead space and the alveolar dead space.

      Clinical note: Alveolar dead space is typically of minimal significance. However, in **pulmonary airway** or **vascular disease,** it can become substantial, and it may contribute substantially to a pathologically **elevated physiologic dead space.**

D. **Alveolar ventilation**
- Because not all inspired air reaches the alveoli, pulmonary ventilation needs to be differentiated from alveolar ventilation.
- The **minute ventilation rate** (i.e., pulmonary ventilation per minute) is calculated as follows (typical values):

$$\text{Minute ventilation (V)} = \text{Respiratory rate} \times \text{Tidal volume}$$
$$= 12 \text{ breaths/minute} \times 500 \text{ mL}$$
$$= 6 \text{ L/minute}$$

- To calculate **alveolar ventilation,** the physiologic dead space must be taken into account. In a 150-pound healthy man with a physiologic dead space of 150 mL:

$$\text{Alveolar ventilation (V}_A) = \text{respiratory rate} \times$$
$$(\text{Tidal volume} - \text{Physiologic dead space})$$
$$= 12 \text{ breaths/minute} \times (500 \text{ mL/breath} - 150 \text{ mL})$$
$$= 4.2 \text{ L/minute}$$

- In the same man, if obstructive lung disease resulted in a substantial increase in physiologic dead space, from 150 to 350 mL, there would be a drastic reduction in alveolar ventilation:

$$V_A = 12 \text{ breaths/minute} \times (500 \text{ mL/breath} - 350 \text{ mL})$$
$$= 1.8 \text{ L/minute}$$

> **Clinical note:** If **alveolar ventilation falls** to a level too low to provide sufficient oxygen to the tissue, patients must compensate by increasing the rate of breathing **(tachypnea)** or by increasing the rate of ventilation **(hyperpnea),** or both.

IX. **Oxygen Transport**
- Oxygen is transported in the blood two forms, free dissolved oxygen and oxygen bound to the protein hemoglobin.
- Because O_2 is poorly soluble in plasma, it is transported in significant amounts only when bound to hemoglobin.

A. **Oxygen tension: free dissolved oxygen**
- Just as carbonated soft drinks are "pressurized" by dissolved carbon dioxide, so too is blood pressurized by dissolved O_2. The pressure this dissolved oxygen exerts in blood is termed the **oxygen tension** or **PaO_2,** which typically approximates **100 mm Hg** in arterial blood.
- The amount of dissolved O_2 that it takes to exert a pressure of 100 mm Hg is small, representing approximately **2% of the total volume of oxygen** in blood.

> **Clinical note: The alveolar-arterial (A-a) gradient** is helpful in detecting inadequate oxygenation of blood, in which case it is increased.

TABLE 5-5:
Conditions Associated with an Elevated Alveolar-Arterial Gradient

V/Q mismatch	Shunt	Diffusion Defect
Pulmonary embolism	Intracardiac (e.g., VSD)	Pulmonary fibrosis
Airway obstruction	Intrapulmonary (e.g., pulmonary AVM, pneumonia, CHF)	Emphysema
Interstitial lung disease	Atelectasis	Asbestosis

AVM, arteriovenous malformation; CHF, congestive heart failure; V/Q, ventilation-perfusion; VSD, ventricular septal defect.

It is the difference between the alveolar oxygen tension (PA_{O_2}) and the arterial oxygen tension (Pa_{O_2}):

$$\text{A-a gradient} = PA_{O_2} - Pa_{O_2}$$

The Pa_{O_2} is determined by an arterial blood gas (ABG) analysis, and the PA_{O_2} is calculated as follows:

$$PA_{O_2} \text{ (mm Hg)} = (FI_{O_2} \times [P_{atm} - P_{H_2O}]) - (Pa_{CO_2}/R)$$

where FI_{O_2} = fractional inspired oxygen concentration (0.21 mm Hg for room air), P_{atm} = atmospheric pressure (in mm Hg), P_{H_2O} = partial pressure of water (47 mm Hg at normal body temperature), Pa_{CO_2} = arterial CO_2 tension, and R = respiratory quotient (an indicator of the relative utilization of carbohydrates, proteins, and fats as "fuel"; although R varies depending on "fuel" utilization, a value of 0.8 is typically used).

Pa_{O_2} decreases and the normal A-a gradient increases with age and the A-a gradient ranges from 7 to 14 mm Hg when breathing room air. Conditions associated with an elevated A-a gradient are caused by V/Q mismatch, shunts, and diffusion defects. Examples are listed in Table 5-5.

B. **Oxygen-carrying capacity of the blood**
   • The amount of oxygen that can be transported in the blood **bound to hemoglobin.** Normally, about **98%** of the oxygen within blood is transported in this fashion.
   • Each gram of hemoglobin can bind between 1.34 and 1.39 mL of O_2. Therefore, a typical man with a hemoglobin concentration of 15 g/dL has an oxygen-carrying capacity of approximately **20 mL/dL,** or **20%.**

   Pathology note: Conditions associated with a reduced oxygen-carrying capacity include anemia and methemoglobinemia.

C. **Hemoglobin**
   1. **Types of hemoglobin**
      • **Adult hemoglobin (HbA)** is a tetrameric protein comprising **two α-** and **two β-subunits** which are held together by noncovalent bonds. Each

subunit can bind one molecule of O_2, so that one hemoglobin molecule can carry four O_2 molecules at a time.

- **Fetal hemoglobin (HbF)** comprises **two α- and two γ-subunits.** HbF has a **higher affinity for oxygen** than adult hemoglobin does. This causes increased release of oxygen to the fetal tissues, which is important for survival of the fetus in its relatively hypoxemic environment.

2. **O_2 binding to hemoglobin**
   - Each hemoglobin subunit contains a **heme group,** which is an iron-containing porphyrin moiety that contains iron in the ferrous state (Fe^{2+}).
   - This **heme group binds O_2** in a **cooperative** manner; that is, within a hemoglobin molecule, the binding of O_2 to one heme group enhances the binding of O_2 to another heme group, and so on.

> **Clinical note: Methemoglobin** is an altered form of hemoglobin in which the **ferrous (Fe^{2+}) irons** of **heme** are oxidized to the **ferric (Fe^{3+})** state. The ferric form of hemoglobin is unable to bind O_2, so patients with methemoglobinemia have functional anemia. Patients present with **cyanosis** despite having a normal PaO_2. The blood may appear a blue, dark red, or chocolate color and does not change with the addition of oxygen. Methemoglobinemia may be congenital, or it may occur secondary to certain drugs or exposures.

3. **Hemoglobin-O_2 dissociation curve**
   - The hemoglobin-O_2 dissociation curve (Fig. 5-9) has a sigmoidal shape, which represents the increasing affinity of hemoglobin for O_2 with increasing PaO_2 ("loading phase") and the decreasing affinity of hemoglobin for O_2 with decreasing PaO_2.

> **Clinical note:** Carbon monoxide (CO) is a colorless, odorless gas formed by hydrocarbon combustion that diffuses rapidly across the pulmonary capillary membrane. Hemoglobin has a very high affinity for CO (240 times its affinity for O_2). CO avidly binds to hemoglobin to form **carboxyhemoglobin,** which has greatly diminished ability to bind O_2. Nonsmokers may normally have up to 3% carboxyhemoglobin at baseline; this may increase to 10% to 15% in smokers.
>
> When CO binds to hemoglobin, the **conformation** of the hemoglobin molecule is changed in a way that greatly diminishes the ability of the other O_2-binding sites to offload oxygen to tissues. Blood PO_2 tends to remain normal, because PO_2 measurement usually reflects O_2 dissolved in blood, not that bound to hemoglobin. **Carbon monoxide poisoning** is treated with 100% oxygen and/or hyperbaric oxygen. When carboxyhemoglobin reaches a level of approximately 70% of total hemoglobin, death can occur from cerebral ischemia or cardiac failure. Autopsy shows bright red tissues due to the failure of CO to dissociate from hemoglobin. The blood appears bright red secondary to the inability of O_2 to dissociate from hemoglobin.

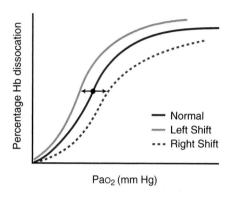

5-9: *The hemoglobin-O_2 dissociation curve. One cause of left shift is decreased temperature, explaining why people have rosy cheeks in cold weather.*

  a. **O_2 saturation (SaO_2)**
   - Each hemoglobin molecule contains four Fe^{2+}-containing groups to which oxygen can bind.
   - The percentage of the available heme groups that are bound to oxygen is termed the O_2 saturation, or the SaO_2 when referring to arterial blood.
   - In a healthy person, SaO_2 is approximately 98% at a typical O_2 tension (PaO_2) of 100 mm Hg.
   - O_2 saturation is measured in arterial, oxygenated blood, usually by using a sensor attached to a finger.
  b. **Increased O_2 delivery to the tissues**
   - **Right shift** of the O_2 dissociation curve (see Fig. 5-9) indicates a decrease in the affinity of hemoglobin for O_2 and a corresponding increased degree of oxygen unloading into the tissues. There is an increase in P_{50}, the pressure of oxygen (PO_2) at which hemoglobin is half saturated (i.e., two O_2 molecules are bound to each hemoglobin molecule), which facilitates the release of O_2 to the metabolically active tissues.
   - Factors that shift the curve to the right include **binding of 2,3-diphosphoglycerate (2,3-DPG), H^+ ions,** and **CO_2** to hemoglobin, as well as **increased body temperature.** The curve also shifts to the right during **exercise** due to the low pH secondary to lactic acidosis, increased CO_2, and increased temperature.
  c. **Decreased O_2 delivery to the tissues**
   - **Left shift** of the O_2 dissociation curve occurs when there is increased affinity of hemoglobin for O_2. The P_{50} decreases, and unloading of oxygen into the tissues is decreased.
   - Physiologic conditions that cause a leftward shift of the hemoglobin-O_2 dissociation curve include **raised pH** (to 7.6), **decreased PCO_2, decreased body temperature, decreased 2,3-DPG,** and the presence of large quantities of **fetal hemoglobin** blood.

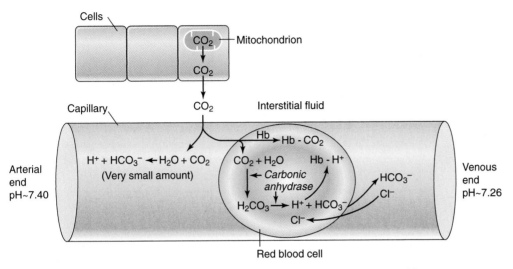

5-10: *Bicarbonate and the chloride shift. Hb, hemoglobin; Hb-CO₂, carbaminohemoglobin.*

X. **Carbon Dioxide Transport**
- CO_2 is a byproduct of cellular respiration. It diffuses across cell and capillary membranes into the bloodstream.
- Most (~70%) of the CO_2 then crosses the RBC membrane. Once inside the RBC, it is converted to bicarbonate ion (**HCO₃⁻**).
- The rest of the CO_2 travels in the blood as either **carbaminohemoglobin** (~20% of total CO_2), or **dissolved CO_2** (~10%).

> **Clinical note:** Whereas PaO_2 decreases and the A-a gradient widens with normal aging, the PCO_2 does **not** change with age.

A. **Bicarbonate ion**
- Approximately **70% of CO_2** is transported in the blood as HCO₃⁻ (Fig. 5-10).
- **Carbonic anhydrase,** present in abundance in RBCs, catalyzes the hydration of CO_2 to H_2CO_3. This dissociates to form HCO₃⁻ and H⁺. The HCO₃⁻ is exchanged for chloride ions (Cl⁻) across the RBC membrane to maintain a balance of charge. This **countertransport** is termed the **"chloride shift."** HCO₃⁻ then travels to the pulmonary capillaries via the venous blood.
- A **reverse chloride shift** and reversal of all of these reactions occurs in the RBCs in the pulmonary capillaries. This reverse reaction produces CO_2, which is expired.
- Low PACO_2 and a high solubility coefficient stimulate diffusion of CO_2 from pulmonary capillaries into the alveolar air. The consequent decrease in PCO_2 allows hemoglobin to bind oxygen more effectively (left shift; see Fig. 5-9).

B. **Carbaminohemoglobin**
- Approximately **20% of CO_2** is transported in the blood in a form that is chemically bound to the amino groups of hemoglobin.
- The binding of CO_2 to hemoglobin decreases the O_2 affinity of hemoglobin, causing a right shift of the hemoglobin-O_2 dissociation curve (**Bohr effect**).

This illustrates the dual roles of hemoglobin in unloading O_2 at the tissues and transporting CO_2 to the lungs.

   C. **Dissolved CO_2**

     • Approximately **10% of CO_2** is transported as dissolved CO_2 (compared to 0.3% of O_2), because of the high solubility constant of CO_2, which is approximately 20 times greater than that of O_2.

   D. **Buffering effect of deoxyhemoglobin**

     • For every HCO_3^- ion produced in the RBCs, one H^+ ion is also produced. Most of these ions are buffered by deoxyhemoglobin, which means that there is only a slight drop in plasma pH between arterial and venous blood.

     • Hydrogen binding to hemoglobin also increases O_2 unloading at the tissues, corresponding to a right shift of the dissociation curve.

  XI. **Control of Respiration**

    • Respiration is tightly controlled to maintain optimal Pa_{O_2} and Pa_{CO_2} in varying environmental and physiologic conditions. The act of breathing is under **central (brainstem) control** and is modulated by input from several types of **peripheral receptors,** including chemoreceptors and mechanoreceptors.

   A. **Central control**

     • **Basic control** of respiratory rhythm originates from two neuronal "groups" within the **medulla,** the dorsal and ventral respiratory groups.

     • **Fine control** of inspiration and expiration originates from the **pons** (pneumotaxic and apneustic groups) of the brainstem (Fig. 5-11).

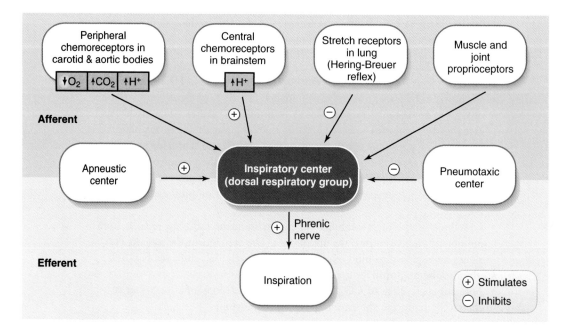

5-11: *Central (brainstem) control of respiration.*

- More complex regulation **(behavioral control)** by higher brain centers such as the **thalamus** and **cerebral cortex** is superimposed on these levels of control.

> **Clinical note:** Control by higher brain centers can override the basic controls of the brainstem, which makes it possible to induce one's own hyperventilation. For example, in some mental illnesses, patients may engage in voluntary suppression of breathing or hyperventilation.

1. **Dorsal respiratory group**
   - Located along the entire length of the **dorsal medulla**
   - **Controls the basic rhythm** of respiration. This is accomplished by neurons that spontaneously generate action potentials (similar to the sinoatrial node), which stimulate inspiratory muscles.
   - Input to the dorsal respiratory group from other respiratory centers and higher brain centers can have a significant effect on activity.

> **Clinical note: Ondine's curse,** a rare respiratory disorder, is a fascinating illustration of the dual control of respiration by **higher brain centers** (voluntary control) and **brainstem respiratory centers** (involuntary control). In this condition, the autonomic control of respiration may be impaired to such an extent that affected individuals must consciously remember to breathe. These patients may need mechanical ventilatory assistance while sleeping in order to prevent death.

2. **Ventral respiratory group**
   - Located on the ventral aspect of the medulla
   - **Stimulates expiratory muscles.** These muscles, which are inactive during normal quiet respiration because expiration is a passive process under normal conditions, become important only when ventilation is high (e.g., with exercise).
3. **Pneumotaxic center**
   - Located in the **superior pons;** its neurons project to the dorsal respiratory group.
   - **Inhibits inspiration,** limiting the size of tidal volume, and secondarily increasing the breathing rate.
4. **Apneustic center**
   - Located in the **inferior pons;** it projects to the dorsal respiratory group.
   - **Increases the duration of inspiratory signals,** increasing the duration of diaphragmatic contraction and resulting in more complete lung filling and a decreased breathing rate

B. **Chemoreceptors**
   - Groups of nerve terminals that are very sensitive to changes in pH, Pa_{O_2}, and Pa_{CO_2}, which lead to the firing of these afferent nerves to the brainstem respiratory centers.
   1. **Central chemoreceptors (chemosensitive areas)**
      - Located on the ventral surface of the medulla
      - Function to keep Pa_{CO_2} within normal limits, having an indirect response to the amount of CO_2 dissolved in cerebrospinal fluid (CSF) (Fig. 5-12):

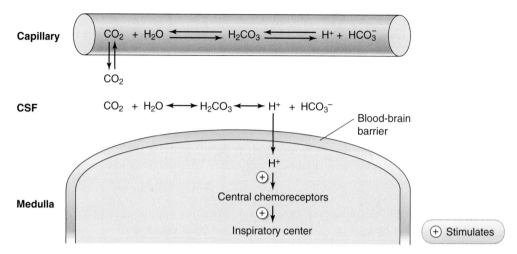

5-12: *Central chemoreceptors. CO_2 crosses the blood-brain barrier, diffusing from cerebral capillaries into the cerebrospinal fluid (CSF) bathing the medulla. At a steady but slow rate (slow because of the absence of carbonic anhydrase in the CSF), CO_2 reacts with H_2O to form HCO_3^- and H^+. Only the H^+ directly activates the central chemoreceptors, stimulating hyperventilation.*

    (1) Via the central chemoreceptors, high Pa_{CO_2} (hypercapnia) and the corresponding decrease in pH are powerful stimulants of **hyperventilation.**

    (2) These effects are **transient** due to desensitization of central chemoreceptors.

- Have a very slow response to increased plasma H^+, because H^+ **does not** cross the blood-brain and blood-CSF barriers.

> **Clinical note:** At **high altitudes,** hypoxia (decreased Pa_{O_2}) stimulates hyperventilation via **peripheral chemoreceptors,** leading rapidly to decreased Pa_{CO_2} and decreased $[H^+]$, both of which effectively antagonize hypoxia-induced hyperventilation. **Renal compensation,** which may take 1 to 2 days, increases excretion of HCO_3^{-P} and decreases secretion of H^+. After 1 to 2 days, the central chemoreceptors become sufficiently desensitized, and hypoxia is able to strongly stimulate hyperventilation. Climbers must ascend mountains slowly for this reason.

2. **Peripheral chemoreceptors**
   - Located in the **carotid** and **aortic bodies.** Afferent fibers travel from the carotid bodies along the glossopharyngeal nerve (cranial nerve [CN] IX), and from the aortic bodies along the vagus nerve (CN X), to the **dorsal respiratory group in the medulla.**
   - They respond primarily to pH and Pa_{CO_2} and are much less sensitive to Pa_{O_2}. When pH or Pa_{O_2} decreases or when Pa_{CO_2} increases, **breathing rate** is increased.

- They can also trigger **hyperventilation:** high Pa_{CO_2} **(hypercapnia)** or acidosis stimulates production of action potentials, which travel along afferents to the dorsal respiratory group, leading to hyperventilation.

> **Clinical note:** Hypoxia has a limited ability to stimulate hyperventilation, because hyperventilation rapidly decreases Pa_{CO_2} and $[H^+]$, thereby inhibiting the process. However, in conditions in which Pa_{CO_2} and $[H^+]$ do not decrease in response to hyperventilation (e.g., **emphysema, pneumonia**), hypoxia may remain a potent inducer of ventilation. Supplemental O_2 should be administered with great caution in these circumstances, because removal of the hypoxic stimulant to ventilation can inhibit ventilatory drive, leading to death from severe hypercapnia and acidosis.

C. **Mechanoreceptors and pulmonary reflexes**
  1. **Irritant receptors**
     - Located between the cells of **large-diameter airways,** primarily the trachea, bronchi, bronchioles
     - Respond to the presence of noxious gases, smoke, and dust, and **mediate reflexes** such as bronchoconstriction, coughing, and sneezing
  2. **Stretch receptors: the Hering-Breuer reflex**
     - Located in the muscular walls of the bronchi and bronchioles
     - Activated by distention of the airways in response to large tidal inspirations, they **inhibit further inspiration** and thereby play a protective role in preventing excessive filling of the lungs. The afferent nerve fibers travel via the glossopharyngeal (CN IX) and vagus (CN X) nerves to the dorsal respiratory group.
D. Effects of exercise
  - **Hyperventilation** in response to exercise is poorly understood but is thought to involve stimulation of respiratory centers by higher brain centers.
    (1) For example, the descending corticospinal fibers from the motor cortex, firing to induce motor functions, may have a stimulatory effect on brainstem respiratory centers as they pass through.
    (2) In the initial stages of exercise, hyperventilation occurs even *before* changes in blood gas levels are detectable, indicating that it is unlikely to be mediated via the actions of either the central or peripheral chemoreceptors.
  - **Body movements,** especially of the arms and legs, stimulate ventilation via excitatory signals from joint and muscle proprioceptors to the respiratory center.

XII. **Respiratory Responses to Stress**
  A. **Hypoxia and hypoxemia**
     - The distinction between these conditions is important:
       (1) **Hypoxemia** refers to insufficient O_2 in the **blood**
       (2) **Hypoxia** refers to insufficient O_2 in the **tissues.**
     - **Hypoxia** is caused either by a reduction in cardiac output or by hypoxemia (Table 5-6).

TABLE 5-6:
Types of Hypoxia

Type of Hypoxia	Pathophysiology	Example
Hypoxic	Decreased oxygenation of blood	Lung disease
Ischemic	Inadequate tissue perfusion	Myocardial infarction
Anemic	Decreased O_2-carrying capacity of blood secondary to low hemoglobin	Iron-deficiency anemia
Histotoxic	Inability of cells to use O_2 effectively	Cyanide poisoning

- **Hypoxemia** has many causes, including high altitude, anemia, carbon monoxide poisoning, hypoventilation, diffusion defects (fibrosis, pulmonary edema), V/Q defects, and shunts.
1. **Physiologic responses to hypoxia**
   - When PaO_2 drops, chemoreceptors increase their firing and the central breathing centers up-regulate the respiratory rate (tachypnea) and heart rate (tachycardia) and cause large tidal volume breaths (hyperpnea).

   > **Clinical note:** Treatment of hypoxia may vary depending on the type of hypoxia. For example, supplemental oxygen therapy may completely alleviate symptoms caused by **hypoxic hypoxia** (e.g., as with lung disease or high-altitude respiration), but it does little to improve symptoms associated with **histotoxic hypoxia** (e.g., cyanide poisoning).

2. **High-altitude respiration** (Fig. 5-13)
   - At high altitudes, atmospheric pressure and therefore PAO_2 is decreased
   - Several **physiologic responses** enable the body to acclimatize to this change, maintaining adequate oxygenation of tissues. The reduced PAO_2 triggers:
   (1) An increase in ventilation
   (2) An **increase in pulmonary vascular resistance,** as a result of hypoxia-induced vasoconstriction of the pulmonary vasculature
   (3) A **right shift** of the hemoglobin-O_2 dissociation curve
   - Hypoxia-induced **polycythemia,** an increase in number of RBCs, is responsible for longer-term acclimatization to high altitude: it increases the O_2-carrying capacity of the blood, compensating for the lower PAO_2. It is an additional cause of increased pulmonary vascular resistance, because it increases blood viscosity.

   > **Clinical note:** Hypoxia-induced polycythemia is a form of **secondary polycythemia** that occurs as a result of the increased renal secretion of erythropoietin in response to hypoxia; the erythropoietin stimulates RBC production in the bone marrow. In addition to high-altitude acclimatization, hypoxia-induced polycythemia can also be seen in smokers and in patients with lung and heart disease severe enough to cause hypoxia. Other types of secondary

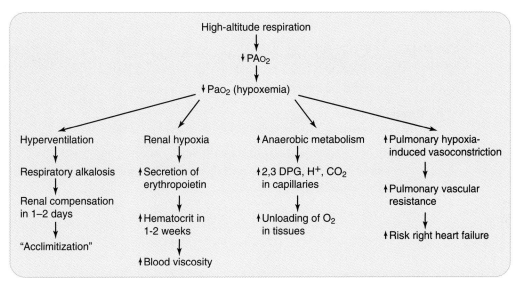

5-13: *Physiologic responses to high-altitude respiration. Note that relatively long-term exposure to high-altitude respiration can produce right-sided heart failure by increasing the work demand placed on the right ventricle in two ways: (1) increased blood viscosity and (2) increased pulmonary vasculature resistance. 2,3-DPG, 2,3-diphosphoglycerate.*

TABLE 5-7:
Altered Breathing Patterns and Their Causes

Type of Breathing	Description	Examples
Apnea	Temporary cessation of breathing	Sleep apnea
Dyspnea	"Air hunger" (sensation of difficulty breathing)	Congestive heart failure or lung disease
Eupnea	Normal breathing	—
Hyperpnea	Increased pulmonary ventilation in response to body's demand for O_2	Exercise
Biot's breathing	Several short breaths followed by period of apnea	Increased intracranial pressure
Cheyne-Stokes breathing	Periodic breathing; need higher P_{CO_2} to stimulate breathing	Head trauma
Hyperventilation	Pulmonary ventilation in excess of body's demand for O_2	Pulmonary, disease, asthma, metabolic acidosis, anxiety
Hypoventilation	Pulmonary ventilation that does not meet body's demand for O_2	Sedatives, anesthetics
Kussmaul's respirations	Rapid deep breathing associated with metabolic acidosis	Diabetic ketoacidosis
Ondine's curse	Impaired autonomic control of respiration	Patients need to be on respirator when sleeping

polycythemia occur in a hypoxia-independent manner (e.g., erythropoietin-secreting renal tumors). **Primary polycythemia** (often termed **"polycythemia vera"**) by contrast, occurs from an intrinsic proliferative abnormality within the bone marrow. Unlike in the secondary polycythemias, erythropoietin levels are low in this condition.

B. **Breathing disorders** (Table 5-7)
   • Altered breathing patterns often signify an underlying disease process.

   Clinical note: In **Kussmaul's respiration,** which is associated with metabolic acidosis (e.g., in diabetic ketoacidosis), patients may breathe rapidly (tachypnea) and deeply.

6

Renal Physiology

I. **Function of the Kidneys**
- The kidneys are an extraordinarily effective recycling facility into which the body's extracellular fluid compartment is cycled many times a day.
- Substances that are not needed (excess water and electrolytes and potentially toxic end-products of metabolism) are discarded into the urine.
- Substances that are needed (sodium, water, glucose, bicarbonate) are reclaimed and returned to the circulation. Thus, the kidneys have particularly strong control over **homeostasis** of water, sodium, potassium, calcium, phosphate, bicarbonate, and the nonvolatile acids.
- This allows them to regulate extracellular fluid volume, osmolality, and acid-base balance.

II. **Functional Anatomy of the Kidney** (Fig. 6-1)
- To achieve its recycling functions, the kidneys receive a substantial fraction (20% to 25%) of the **cardiac output.**
- This is supplied to the kidney by the **renal arteries.**
- In the **nephron,** the basic functional unit of the kidney, the blood is filtered.
- Fluid and compounds that are not recycled **(urine)** drain from the nephron into the **calyceal system.**
- This in turn drains into the **renal pelvis, ureter,** and **bladder.**

> **Clinical note:** Narrowing of the renal arteries (**renal artery stenosis**) most commonly occurs as a result of **atherosclerosis** or **fibromuscular dysplasia.** In unilateral renal artery stenosis, hypertension may occur because decreased perfusion of the affected kidney is incorrectly "interpreted" as intravascular volume depletion, which triggers a neurohormonal cascade response (the renin-angiotensin-aldosterone-antidiuretic hormone [ADH] system; see Chapter 3), causing fluid retention and vasoconstriction and resulting in hypertension. When both renal arteries are affected (*bilateral* renal artery stenosis), renal blood flow may become so compromised that the kidneys are unable to perform their normal recycling functions, resulting in the toxic accumulation of metabolic byproducts.

A. **Structure of the filtration unit: the nephron** (Fig. 6-2)
- There are approximately 1 million nephrons in each kidney.
- Filtration from the blood into the kidney takes place in the **glomerulus** (Fig. 6-3).
- Each **glomerulus** is an expansion of an afferent arteriole into a diffuse capillary bed, the glomerular capillaries, which have an extensive surface area for

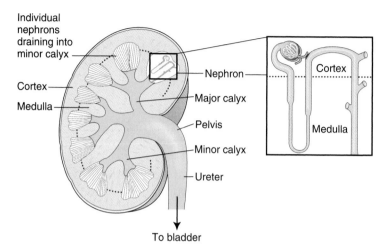

6-1: *Structure of the kidney. The inset shows the location of the nephron depicted in Figure 6-2.*

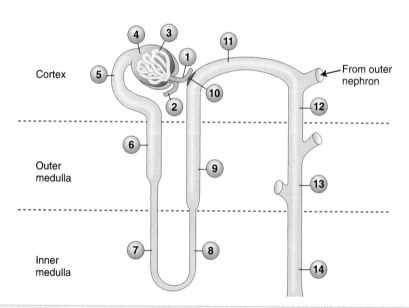

1. Afferent arteriole	**6.** Proximal straight tubule	**11.** Distal convoluted tubule
2. Efferent arteriole	**7.** Thin descending limb	**12.** Cortical collecting duct
3. Glomerular capillaries	**8.** Thin ascending limb	**13.** Outer medullary collecting duct
4. Bowman's space	**9.** Thick ascending limb	**14.** Inner medullary collecting duct
5. Proximal convoluted tubule	**10.** Macula densa	

6-2: *Anatomy of the nephron. (The shape of the proximal convoluted tubule has been simplified; see Fig. 6-8 for detail.)*

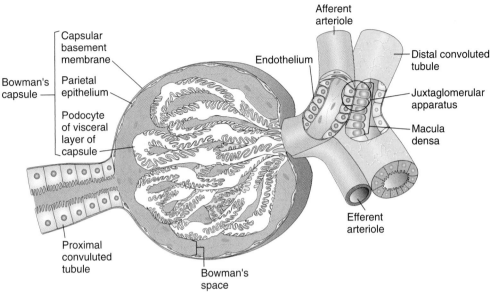

6-3: *Anatomy of the glomerulus.*

filtration; these capillaries are surrounded by an expansion of the renal tubular system.

- The **ultrafiltrate** of plasma created in the glomerulus flows into the **tubular system,** where selective reabsorption and secretion of solutes and water occurs along the various segments of the nephron.
- The terminal segments of the nephron empty into the **calyceal system.**

B. **The glomerular filtration barrier**

1. **Function of the filtration barrier**
   - For substances in the lumen of the glomerular capillaries to be filtered into the renal tubular system, they must traverse the three component layers of the **glomerular filtration barrier.**
   - Each of these layers is highly specialized for filtration.
   - They effectively prevent the passage of cells and larger-molecular-weight proteins into the glomerular ultrafiltrate, thereby preventing their loss into the urine.

2. **Layers of the filtration barrier** (Fig. 6-4)
   - **Endothelial cells** of the glomerular capillaries are **fenestrated** (have many holes), which markedly increases capillary permeability and so permits the production of large volumes of filtrate.
   - The **glomerular basement membrane** is negatively charged, which helps prevent filtration (and subsequent loss in the urine) of negatively charged plasma proteins.
   - The overlying **visceral epithelial cells** or **podocytes,** project foot-processes that overlie the glomerular basement membrane. These podocytes, and their

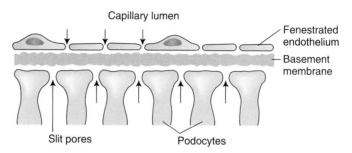

Capillary lumen

Fenestrated
endothelium

Basement
membrane

Slit pores

Podocytes

6-4: Layers of the glomerular filtration barrier.

adjoining **slit pores,** which are closed by a **slit diaphragm,** form a final **negatively charged barrier** for filterable molecules to traverse before they enter **Bowman's space.**

> **Pathology note:** In a condition known as **minimal change disease,** the negative charges on the glomerular filtration barrier are lost for unknown reasons. Certain proteins are then able to pass through the basement membrane, resulting in proteinuria. This disease is the most common cause of the **nephrotic syndrome** (loss of >3.5 g of protein per day into the urine) in children, and is usually responsive to treatment with corticosteroids. Of note, the positively charged immunoglobulin light chains, which are overproduced in **multiple myeloma,** are small enough to pass through the glomerular filtration barrier (and therefore into the urine) without any pathologic changes in the glomerulus.

III. **Regulation of Glomerular Function**
   A. **Filtration forces at the glomerulus** (Fig. 6-5)
   - The forces that drive fluid across the glomerular membrane and into Bowman's space are the same as the **Starling forces** that cause fluid movements in systemic capillaries.
   - Forces that promote filtration are the **hydrostatic pressure** in the **glomerular capillaries** (P_{GC}) and the **oncotic pressure in Bowman's space** (Π_{BS}); however, because most proteins are not readily filtered into Bowman's space, the latter is typically negligible.
   - The forces that oppose fluid movement across the glomerular membrane are the **hydrostatic pressure in Bowman's space** (P_{BS}) and the **oncotic pressure in the glomerular capillaries** (Π_{GC})
   - Summation of these forces gives the **net filtration pressure (NFP)**, the pressure gradient driving filtration across the glomerulus. For a typical adult:

$$\mathbf{NFP} = (\mathbf{P_{GC}} + \mathbf{\Pi_{BS}}) - (\mathbf{P_{BS}} + \mathbf{\Pi_{GC}})$$
$$= (60 + 0) - (18 + 32)$$
$$= 10\,\text{mm Hg}$$

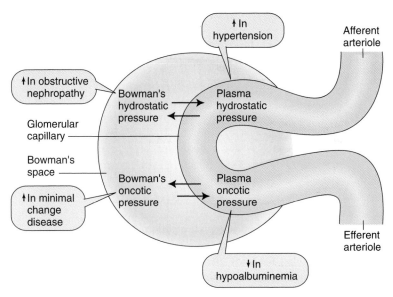

6-5: Filtration forces at the glomerulus. Note how individual forces can be affected in pathologic states.

> **Clinical note:** In the presence of a damaged basement membrane (e.g., membranous nephropathy), where protein can be filtered across the glomerular membrane, the resulting increase in oncotic pressure in Bowman's space can result in an elevated NFP and increased filtrate production.

B. **Glomerular filtration rate (GFR)**
  - This describes the volume of plasma filtered by all the renal glomeruli each minute (milliliters per minute).
  - GFR is dependent on the **filtration forces** acting at the glomerulus and the **unit permeability** (Lp) and available **surface area** (S) of the glomerular capillaries. In the healthy kidney, LpS is equal to approximately 12.5 mL/minute per mm Hg filtration pressure, whereas the NFP is equal to approximately 10 mm Hg. GFR can therefore be calculated as follows:

$$GFR = LpS \times NFP$$
$$= 125 \text{ mL/minute}$$

  - A typical value for GFR in a healthy adult is approximately 90 mL/minute in women and 120 mL/minute in men.
  - This rate of filtration exceeds that seen in muscle capillaries by more than 1000-fold. This is due to the high Lp of glomeruli (50–100 times greater than that of muscle capillaries) and their higher hydrostatic pressure (approximately 60 versus 30 mm Hg).
  - The **filtration fraction** is the percentage of renal plasma flow (RPF) that is filtered across the renal glomeruli. It is normally about 20%.

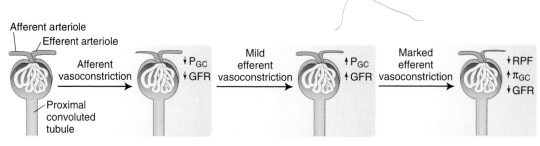

6-6: *Effects of afferent and efferent vasoconstriction on glomerular forces and glomerular filtration rate (GFR). P_{GC}, hydrostatic pressure in glomerular capillary; Π_{GC}, oncotic pressure in glomerular capillary; RPF, renal plasma flow.*

C. **GFR regulation by glomerular hydrostatic pressure**
- Although alteration of any of the determinants of NFP at the glomerulus can substantially alter the GFR, the primary physiologic mechanism through which GFR is normally regulated is the **glomerular hydrostatic pressure.**
- This pressure depends on the systemic arterial pressure and afferent and efferent arteriolar resistance.
- The **sympathetic nervous system** and hormones such as **angiotensin II** primarily regulate GFR by varying the degree of afferent and efferent arteriolar resistance. This is discussed later in the context of overall plasma volume regulation.
1. **Systemic arterial pressure**
   - As systemic arterial pressure increases, the increased renal perfusion tends to increase glomerular hydrostatic pressure and GFR, and the reverse (decrease) is also true.
   - However, the changes in glomerular hydrostatic pressure are relatively small compared with the often substantial fluctuations in systemic arterial pressure. This attenuation is due to intrinsic **autoregulatory mechanisms** in the kidneys, which maintain a relatively constant renal perfusion despite fluctuations in systemic arterial pressure (see later discussion and Fig. 6-7).
   - Consequently, the contribution of systemic arterial pressure is minor, and the primary determinants of glomerular hydrostatic pressure are afferent and efferent arteriolar resistance.
2. **Afferent arteriolar resistance** (Fig. 6-6)
   - Dilation of the afferent arteriole increases renal blood flow, glomerular hydrostatic pressure, and, hence, GFR.
   - Vasoconstriction has the opposite effect.
3. **Efferent arteriolar resistance** (see Fig. 6-6)
   - **Mild to moderate vasoconstriction** of the efferent arteriole (i.e., increased resistance) increases glomerular hydrostatic pressure, resulting in increased filtration across the glomerulus.
   - However, this increased resistance comes at the expense of reducing overall renal blood flow to some degree and increasing the filtration fraction at the glomerulus because of that reduced flow, which in turn increases the glomerular oncotic pressure that opposes filtration.

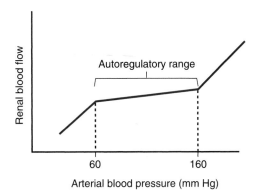

6-7: *Autoregulation of renal blood flow. At extremes of blood pressure, systemic arterial pressure and renal blood flow are in direct proportion.*

- Therefore, with **marked vasoconstriction** of the efferent arteriole, the GFR typically decreases, because the reduced renal blood flow and increased glomerular oncotic pressure overcome the effects of the increased glomerular hydrostatic pressure on GFR.

D. **Autoregulation of renal blood flow**
- Autoregulation by intrinsic mechanisms ensures that renal blood flow, and therefore the filtration forces at the glomerulus and the GFR, remain relatively constant even while systemic arterial pressures fluctuate across a relatively broad range between 80 and 160 mm Hg.
- Outside this range, the autoregulatory mechanisms fail, and renal blood flow parallels changes in systemic arterial pressure (Fig. 6-7).
- The autoregulatory mechanisms are called the **myogenic response** and **tubuloglomerular feedback;** both function largely by regulating renal vascular resistance, and in the absence of any neural or hormonal input.

1. **Myogenic response**
   a. **Response to increased arteriolar pressure**
      - As in other arterioles, an increase in pressure in the afferent arteriole stimulates reflexive vasoconstriction by stimulating smooth muscle cell contraction.
      - This is important in minimizing the increase in glomerular hydrostatic pressure that would otherwise occur in response to increased systemic arterial pressure.
      - It also prevents damage to the glomerular capillaries, which already function at hydrostatic pressures that are much greater than those in the systemic capillaries.
   b. **Response to decreased arteriolar pressure**
      - If the pressure in the afferent arteriole decreases significantly, this triggers reflexive vasodilation, which increases blood flow and filtration pressure in the glomerulus.
      - This helps to ensure adequate filtration for removal of wastes when systemic arterial pressures drop.

2. **Tubuloglomerular feedback**
   - In this mechanism, the rate of NaCl delivery to the distal nephron significantly influences the glomerular blood flow and therefore the GFR. (The rate of NaCl delivery to the distal tubule is dependent on the tubular concentration of NaCl as well as the tubular flow rate.)
   - This mechanism is dependent on the presence of a specialized structure termed the **macula densa,** which is located at the end of the thick ascending limb and abuts the glomerulus adjacent to the afferent arteriole (see Figs. 6-2, 6-3, and 6-8).
   - The macula densa, along with specialized cells within the glomerulus and the walls of the afferent arteriole, are referred to as the **juxtaglomerular apparatus.**
   - The mechanism has three components:
     (1) A **signal** (NaCl delivery to the distal tubule)
     (2) A **sensor** (macula densa)
     (3) An **effector** (vascular smooth muscle cells within the wall of the afferent arteriole)
   - When filtration increases, the increased NaCl delivery to the macula densa triggers vasoconstriction of the afferent arteriole (Fig. 6-8). The result is reduced renal blood flow (RPF) and therefore decreased GFR, which reduces delivery of NaCl to the macula densa.
   - When filtration decreases, decreased NaCl delivery to the macula densa triggers vasodilation of the afferent arteriole, which increases GFR and increases delivery of NaCl to the macula densa.

   Pharmacology note: The juxtaglomerular apparatus is informed of NaCl in the tubular lumen by virtue of its transport into the cells of the macula densa by the same Na^+-K^+-$2Cl^-$ cotransporter that is inhibited by **loop diuretics.** One reason for the potency of loop diuretics is their ability to **blunt tubuloglomerular feedback** and thereby maintain GFR despite increased NaCl traffic past the macula densa.

   Clinical note: Acute tubular necrosis (ATN) is a common cause of **acute renal failure,** which results when hypotension or tubular toxins damage renal tubular epithelial cells. In ATN, sodium and water reabsorption in the proximal tubule, where the majority of NaCl and fluid reabsorption normally occurs, is impaired. Large amounts of NaCl and water are therefore presented to the macula densa. Through tubuloglomerular feedback, this decreases renal blood flow and GFR by stimulating vasoconstriction of the afferent arteriole. The subsequent decrease in GFR may play a role in limiting potentially life-threatening losses of sodium and water that might otherwise occur.

IV. **Measuring Renal Function**
   - The kidney performs many functions such as removal of toxins and regulation of the acid-base balance.

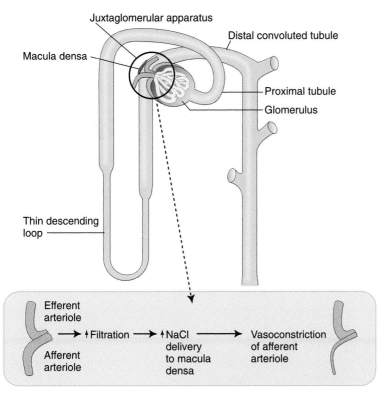

Juxtaglomerular apparatus

Distal convoluted tubule

Macula densa

Proximal tubule

Glomerulus

Thin descending loop

Efferent arteriole

Afferent arteriole

→ ↑Filtration → ↑NaCl delivery to macula densa → Vasoconstriction of afferent arteriole

6-8: *Tubuloglomerular feedback. Because of the hairpin loop structure of each nephron, the macula densa is located adjacent to its originating glomerulus and is positioned adjacent to the afferent and efferent arterioles that supply that glomerulus.*

- However, the term **renal function** is used to refer to the rate at which the kidney removes **toxins** from the circulation.

A. **Clearance**
- The main mechanism of toxin removal is filtration of toxin-laden plasma through the glomerulus, leaving the toxins behind in the tubule and reabsorbing 99% of the filtrate.
- Plasma that has undergone this process has been **"cleared."**
- **Clearance,** actually more a conceptual than a physiologic reality, is the volume of plasma from which a substance has been completely cleared by the kidneys per unit of time.
- If a substance is freely filtered across the glomerulus and then neither reabsorbed nor secreted into the tubule, its rate of its clearance from blood is equivalent to the GFR. Therefore, measures of renal function involve use of the concept of clearance to directly measure or estimate GFR.

B. **Calculating clearance**
- If a substance is present in the blood at a concentration of 1 mg per 100 mL, then the clearance of the substance from 100 mL of blood per minute will result in 1 mg of this substance being excreted into the urine each minute.

- If the amount of the substance excreted in the urine is divided by its plasma concentration (Px, in milligrams per milliliter), the quotient reflects the volume of plasma that has been cleared of that substance in 1 minute, called its **clearance** (Cx):

$$\text{Clearance} = \frac{\text{Amount excreted in urine in 1 minute}}{\text{Plasma concentration}}$$

- This can be expressed in terms of urinary flow rate (V, in milliliters per minute) and urinary concentration (Ux, in milligrams per milliliter):

$$Cx = \frac{V \times Ux}{Px} \quad \frac{\frac{ml}{min} \cdot \frac{mg}{ml}}{mg/ml}$$

- For example, a typical excretion rate of urea into the urine is 15 mg/min, and typical plasma concentration of urea is 0.2 mg/mL. Therefore, the clearance of urea (C_{urea}) is typically

$$C_{urea} = \frac{15}{0.2} = 75 \, \text{mL/min}$$

- Note that the C_{urea} is less than the typical GFR, which is approximately 90 to 120 mL/minute. This is consistent with **net reabsorption** of urea along the nephron.
- A clearance value that is greater than GFR indicates **net secretion** of the substance along the nephron.

> **Clinical note:** In clinical settings, clearance is calculated from the serum concentration of a substance and the substance's concentration in a timed urine sample (typically a 24-hour sample).

C. **Measuring the GFR**
  1. **Creatinine clearance**
     - Creatinine is formed continually as a breakdown product in **skeletal muscle** and is released into the bloodstream.
     - Circulating creatinine is useful for measuring **renal function** because it is freely filtered across the glomeruli: It is not reabsorbed, secreted, or metabolized to any significant extent in the kidney (see later discussion), and therefore the amount that enters the urine is approximately equal to the amount that is filtered across the glomeruli.
     - The amount of creatinine that enters the urine in 1 minute is equal to the product of the urinary flow rate and the urinary creatinine concentration (creatinine = $V \times U_{cr}$),
     - The amount of creatinine that filters across the glomeruli is equal to the product of the plasma creatine concentration and the GFR (creatinine = $P_{cr} \times$ GFR).
     - Because these two expressions define the same quantity, they can be equated and solved for the **GFR,** as follows:

$$V \times U_{cr} = P_{cr} \times \text{GFR}$$

so that

$$GFR = \frac{V \times U_{cr}}{P_{cr}}$$

- This is the same equation as the equation for creatinine clearance ($C_{cr} = V \times U_{cr}/P_{cr}$). Therefore, the creatinine clearance is approximately the **same as the GFR.**
- Creatinine clearance is used clinically as an estimate of GFR; however, because there is in fact a mild degree of tubular secretion of creatinine, it is actually a slight overestimate of GFR.
- Note that if GFR decreases, plasma creatinine will increase until a new steady state is reached, at which point urinary excretion of creatinine will again match daily creatinine production.

> **Clinical note:** Because measuring renal clearance involves collecting urine and is a nuisance for patients, **plasma creatinine** levels are usually measured as a surrogate marker of renal function. However, because the plasma creatinine concentration is dependent on both muscle mass and renal function, this method may significantly overestimate renal function in patients with reduced muscle mass and, hence, lower creatinine production. Similarly, renal function may be underestimated in very muscular individuals and in situations, such as crush injury, where extensive muscle damage leads to increased creatinine release into the circulation.

(handwritten margin note: low muscle mass, overestimated — High muscle mass, underestimate)

2. **Inulin clearance**
   - Inulin is a nonmetabolized polysaccharide that is freely filtered at the glomerulus.
   - Unlike creatinine, it is neither reabsorbed nor secreted along the tubule, so inulin clearance is a more **accurate measurement of the GFR.**

> **Clinical note:** Unlike creatinine, inulin must be administered intravenously and is therefore almost never used clinically except in clinical research where precise assessments of GFR are required.

D. **Clearance and reabsorption/secretion**
   - After filtration at the glomerulus, substances can be either reabsorbed or filtered (Fig. 6-9).
   - The **clearance value** for a given substance provides useful information about renal handling of that substance (i.e., filtration, reabsorption, secretion) (Fig. 6-10).
     (1) Renal clearance for a given substance approximates to GFR if that substance is **freely filtered** and does not undergo net reabsorption or secretion along the nephron (e.g., **inulin**).
     (2) If a substance undergoes net **reabsorption** along the nephron, its clearance is less than GFR because some of it is returned to the plasma from which it was initially cleared (e.g., **urea**).

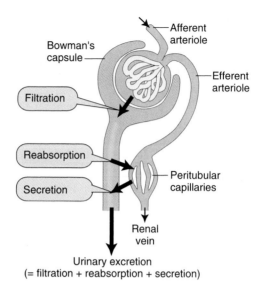

6-9: *Filtration, reabsorption, and secretion along the nephron.*

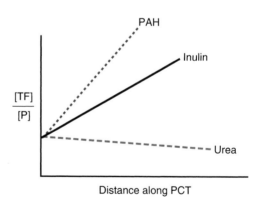

Distance along PCT

6-10: *Due to the reabsorption of water, the tubular fluid concentration of inulin increases roughly threefold compared to plasma concentration along the proximal convoluted tubule (PCT). Because inulin is neither secreted nor reabsorbed, substances that become concentrated more than inulin (e.g., PAH) must therefore be secreted and substances that becomes less concentrated than inulin (e.g., urea) must be reabsorbed. PAH, para-aminohippuric acid. [P], plasma concentration; [TF], tubular fluid concentration.*

(3) If a substance undergoes net **secretion** along the nephron (e.g., para-aminohippuric acid [**PAH**]), its clearance is greater than GFR because it is removed both from the filtered plasma at the glomerulus and from the unfiltered plasma in the peritubular capillaries.

• Notice that the clearances of substances that are freely filtered but then actively reabsorbed (e.g., sodium, glucose, amino acids) are quite low (Table 6-1).

TABLE 6-1:
Summary of Important Clearance Values

Substance	Approximate Clearance Rate (% of GFR)
Urea	50 → nt reabsorpt
Inulin	100
Creatinine	100
PAH	>>100 → net secretion
Sodium	1
Potassium	10
Glucose	0
Amino acids	0

GFR, glomecular filtration rate; PAH, para-aminohippuric acid.

E. **Using clearance values to estimate effective renal plasma flow**
   • If a substance were filtered and secreted so efficiently that it was completely eliminated from plasma by the time blood leaves the kidney (i.e., concentration in renal vein = 0), its clearance would give a very good approximation of RPF, because the amount of plasma cleared of the substance would represent all the plasma that initially entered the kidney, including the filtered fraction at the glomerulus and the unfiltered fraction in the peritubular capillaries.
   • An example of such a substance is **para-aminohippuric acid (PAH)**; if this nonmetabolized organic acid is administered, it is freely filtered and very efficiently secreted but not reabsorbed.
   • If PAH is present in relatively low amounts in the plasma, approximately 90% of the amount entering the kidney is removed in its first pass. Therefore, the rate at which PAH is excreted in the urine ($U_{pah} \times V$) approximately equals the rate at which PAH is delivered to the kidneys ($P_{pah} \times RPF$). In other words, PAH clearance approximates RPF:

$$U_{pah} \times V \approx P_{pah} \times RPF$$

since

$$C_{pah} = U_{pah} \times V/P_{pah}$$

this becomes

$$RPF \approx C_{pah}$$

   • Estimating RPF from this calculation really yields the **effective RPF** rather than the **true RPF**, because a small amount of blood leaving the efferent arterioles (~10%) perfuses the **vasa recta** in the **medulla** rather than the peritubular capillaries. This PAH, therefore, cannot be secreted into the nephron. More precision can be achieved by correcting for this factor:

$$\text{True RPF} = C_{pah}/0.90$$

   • Even more precision can be achieved by inserting a catheter in the renal vein and measuring the concentration of PAH in the renal venous plasma.

- Note that most clinicians speak in terms of **renal blood flow** (RBF) rather than renal plasma flow (RPF). Although RBF is not normally measured clinically, it can be calculated from the hematocrit:

$$RBF = \frac{RPF}{1 - Hematocrit}$$

> **Clinical note:** Renal blood flow is not normally measured in routine clinical practice because it involves the intravenous administration of PAH and catheterization of the renal vein in order to determine the concentration of PAH in the renal venous plasma. However, this is more commonly performed in clinical research investigations, for example, when evaluating a new drug to see whether it effects renal hemodynamics.

V. **Renal Transport Mechanisms**
- Impaired transport along the various nephron segments result in numerous conditions, as shown in Table 6-2.
- A huge amount of glomerular filtrate is delivered into the tubules each day. Potentially life-threatening fluid and electrolyte disturbances would rapidly occur if the tubules did not reclaim the majority of this filtrate.
- Therefore, the tubules of the nephron undertake a complex array of activities to excrete unneeded substances (excess electrolytes, toxins, hydrogen ions) while reclaiming the rest.

TABLE 6-2:
Function of Nephron Segments

Nephron Segment	Primary Functions	Hormonal Regulation	Associated Disorders
Proximal convoluted tubule	Reabsorption and secretion	Ang II, PTH	Fanconi syndrome, renal diabetes, carbonic anhydrase deficiency
Loop of Henle	Concentration followed by dilution of tubular fluid	ADH	Nephrogenic diabetes insipidus, volume derangements
Thin ascending Limb	Permeable to water	—	—
Thick ascending limb	Impermeable to water, dilution of tubular fluid via activity of Na-K-2Cl channel	Aldosterone and ADH	Diuretic-induced volume depletion, Bartter syndrome (chronic metabolic alkalosis)
Distal tubule	Site of macula densa, tubuloglomerular feedback	ADH, aldosterone, PTH	Gitelman's syndrome
Cortical collecting tubules	Baseline permeability to urea		Hyperkalemia secondary to potassium-sparing diuretics
Medullary collecting tubules	Variable permeability to urea	ADH	Liddle's syndrome, pseudohypoaldosteronism

Ang II, angiotensin II; ADH, antidiuretic hormone; PTH, parathyroid hormone.

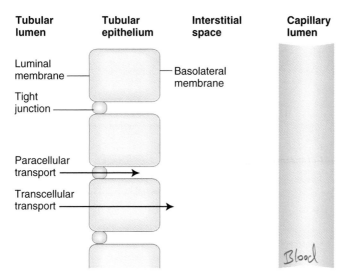

| Tubular lumen | Tubular epithelium | Interstitial space | Capillary lumen |

6-11: *Paracellular and transcellular transport from the tubular lumen into the interstitial space and circulation. Substances traversing the transcellular route pass through two distinct portions of the tubular cell membrane, which are separated by the tight junctions: the luminal membrane, which is in contact with the tubular lumen, and the basolateral membrane, which contacts the interstitial space.*

A. **General tubular function**
- As a consequence of **selective reabsorption** and **secretion,** the solute composition of tubular fluid, which is initially plasma-like, changes dramatically along the course of the nephron.
- There are two basic routes of transport across the **tubular epithelium** into the **interstitial space** (Fig. 6-11):
    (1) The **paracellular route:** transport across **tight junctions** between tubular epithelial cells
    (2) The **transcellular route:** transport across tubular epithelial cells by way of **channels, pumps,** or **transporters;** this includes transport from the tubular lumen across the luminal aspect of the tubular epithelial cell membrane (the **luminal membrane**) and from within the tubular epithelial cell across the basolateral aspect of the cell membrane (the **basolateral membrane**).
- The reabsorption and secretion of fluids and solutes from the tubular fluid is accomplished by a variety of tubular epithelial cell types, which have distinctly different transport capabilities and are located in different segments of the nephron.
- One example of these variations is the "tightness" of the tight junctions: these are relatively leaky in the proximal tubule and quite tight in the **collecting tubules** (tubes, ducts).
    (1) The leakiness in the **proximal tubule** facilitates the reabsorption of large amounts of fluid and solute via the **paracellular route.**

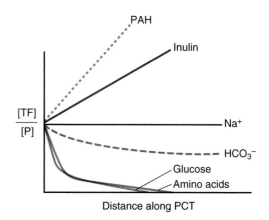

6-12: *Relative changes in concentration of substances in the tubular fluid ([TF]) with respect to their concentration in plasma ([P]) along the proximal convoluted tubule (PCT). Note that the concentration of sodium remains constant along the length of the PCT because water is simultaneously reabsorbed. Filtered substances that are neither reabsorbed nor secreted (e.g., inulin) increase in concentration along the PCT, but not as much as do substances that are secreted but not reabsorbed (e.g., PAH). This graph also reflects the fact that the majority of glucose and amino acids are reabsorbed in the early segments of the PCT.*

      (2) In contrast, paracellular transport in the collecting tubules is much more limited; steep concentration gradients can be maintained across the very tight junctions that separate tubular and interstitial fluids.

  B. **Reabsorption of salt and water**

    1. **Reabsorption from the proximal tubule**

- Approximately two-thirds of the glomerular filtrate is reabsorbed from the proximal tubule.
- However, reclamation of components in the filtered load is not uniform (Fig. 6-12). For example, reabsorption of glucose and amino acids in the proximal tubule is almost complete, whereas only about 65% of filtered sodium is reabsorbed at this site.
- The primary driving force behind **transcellular proximal tubular reabsorption** is the active transport of sodium out of the tubular epithelial cells and into the interstitium, via the sodium-potassium adenosine triphosphatase pump (**Na$^+$,K$^+$-ATPase pump**) located on the **basolateral membrane** of the tubular epithelial cell. This pump creates a favorable electrochemical gradient that facilitates further sodium entry into the cell from the tubular lumen via the **luminal membrane** by maintaining
  - (1) A low intracellular sodium concentration
  - (2) A negatively charged intracellular environment, because the pump moves three sodium molecules into the interstitium in exchange for only two potassium molecules
- Despite this favorable electrochemical gradient, because it is a charged ion sodium cannot simply pass out of and into tubular epithelial cells through the lipid bilayer. Instead, it moves through the luminal membrane by way of **cotransporters** (e.g., Na$^+$-glucose, Na$^+$-amino acid, Na$^+$-phosphate) and **countertransporters** (Na$^+$-H$^+$) (Fig. 6-13).

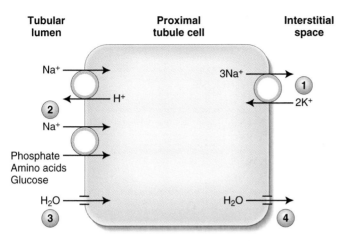

6-13: *Steps in proximal tubular solute and water reabsorption: (1) the Na⁺,K⁺-ATPase pump creates a favorable intracellular electrochemical gradient for further entry of Na⁺; (2) luminal sodium cotransporters and countertransporters move solute into the cell, which increases intracellular osmolality; (3) water enters the cell via luminal water channels in response to the increased intracellular osmotic gradient; (4) basolaterally located cotransporters and water channels transport water and solute into the interstitial space.*

- This solute movement into the tubular epithelial cells increases the intracellular osmolality relative to tubular fluid osmolality, which then causes water to move from the lumen into the cells via water channels in the luminal membrane of the tubular epithelial cells.
- **Cotransporters** and **water channels** located in the **basolateral membrane** then move solute and water into the **interstitial space** (see Fig. 6-13).
- Although osmotic forces are involved in reabsorbing water and sodium from the proximal tubule, the net changes are such that the osmolarity of the tubular fluid does not change along the proximal tubule. This is referred to as **isosmotic reabsorption.**
- Although the bulk of reabsorption in the proximal tubule is via the transcellular route, paracellular transport is also important, particularly for the electrolytes potassium and calcium.

> **Pathology note:** Excessive urinary loss of neutral and cationic (basic) amino acids (aminoaciduria) occurs in **Hartnup disease** and **cystinuria,** respectively, due to impaired reabsorption in the proximal tubule. Both are inherited as autosomal recessive disorders.

2. **Reabsorption into the peritubular capillaries**
   - The **Starling forces** (see section III, A, on filtration forces at the glomerulus) are responsible for reabsorption of fluid from the renal interstitium into the peritubular capillaries.
   - Because a significant amount of protein-free plasma is filtered across the glomerulus, the plasma that remains in the efferent arteriole, and therefore the plasma in the peritubular capillaries, is relatively high in protein, creating a strong capillary oncotic pressure that draws fluid into these

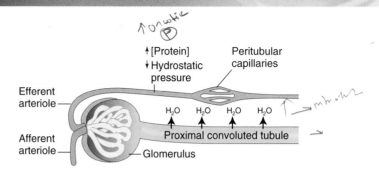

6-14: *Increased plasma oncotic pressure and reduced hydrostatic pressure in the peritubular capillaries drive salt and water reabsorption from the proximal tubule.*

capillaries. This may also be responsible for glomerulotubular balance (discussed later).

- Additionally, the hydrostatic pressure in the peritubular capillaries is relatively low, because the blood has already passed through the resistance beds of the afferent arteriole, glomerular capillaries, and efferent arteriole. This low hydrostatic pressure also favors reabsorption from the interstitium (Fig. 6-14).
- The peritubular capillaries emerge from the efferent arteriole of the glomerulus and drain into the renal veins

3. **Glomerulotubular balance: coupling of reabsorption to GFR**
   - Despite a GFR that may spontaneously vary, when total body sodium balance is normal a relatively constant *fraction* of the filtrate is reabsorbed from the proximal tubule.
   - The mechanism is unclear, but it may involve the increased oncotic pressure within the efferent arteriole and peritubular capillaries that is present after glomerular filtration, which promotes reabsorption from the proximal tubule.
   - This phenomenon—termed **"glomerulotubular balance"**—tends to minimize the effects of a fluctuating GFR on sodium and water excretion, which promotes a constant plasma volume, as follows:
     (1) In a state of expanded plasma volume in which renal blood flow (and therefore GFR) is increased, if a constant fraction of the filtrate produced is reabsorbed, then a much larger absolute amount of urine is produced. This diuresis returns the plasma volume back to normal.
     (2) In a volume-contracted state in which renal blood flow (and therefore GFR) is decreased, if a constant fraction of the filtrate produced is reabsorbed, then a much smaller absolute amount of urine is produced. This antidiuresis facilitates volume expansion.

> **Clinical note: Glomerulotubular balance** and **tubuloglomerular feedback** are easy to confuse. In glomerulotubular balance, the tubules try to strike a proper *balance* between reabsorption and glomerular filtration, whereas in tubuloglomerular feedback, the tubules provide *feedback* to the glomerulus and "tell" it whether filtration needs to be increased or decreased.

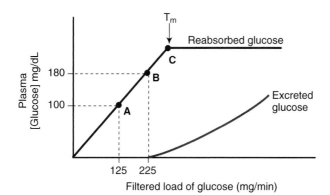

6-15: *A typical concentration of plasma glucose of 100 mg/dL corresponds to a glucose load of 125 mg/minute (point A), which is well below the transport maximum (Tm) for glucose of 320 mg/minute. As plasma glucose levels become pathologically elevated (e.g., in diabetes), a threshold value (point B) is reached, at which point glucose begins to appear in the urine. At still higher plasma levels of glucose (point C), the transport maximum is reached. At this point, all transporter proteins are saturated, and excess glucose is lost in the urine.*

C. **Transport maximum (Tm)**
- This is the maximum rate at which a substance can be reabsorbed from the tubular fluid. It exists for certain substances because their reabsorption is dependent on membrane receptor proteins that have a finite transport capacity (i.e., they are saturable).
- The importance of the Tm is its relationship to **renal (filtered) load,** which describes the amount of any substance delivered to the renal tubular system. The renal load can be calculated, as shown here for glucose (where $[P_{glucose}]$ is the plasma glucose concentration in milligrams per deciliter and GFR is in milliliters per minute):

$$Renal\ load\ for\ glucose = [P_{glucose}] \times GFR$$
$$= 100 \times 125$$
$$= 125\ mg/minute$$

- If the **renal load exceeds the Tm,** as might occur with an abnormal increase in the plasma concentration of a substance, that substance will begin to **accumulate** in the urine, as shown for glucose in Figure 6-15.

Clinical note: The threshold value for plasma glucose (i.e., the level at which glucose begins to appear in the urine) is 180 mg/dL, which corresponds to a glucose load of 225 mg/minute (assuming a GFR of 125 mL/minute). Given that 225 mg/minute is still well below the Tm for glucose (320 mg/minute), it may seem strange that glucose begins to appear in the urine at 180 mg/dL. This is believed to reflect the fact that there is variation in the transport capacity of different nephrons. Consequently, the glucose reabsorptive capacity of some nephrons may become saturated sooner than others, spilling the remainder into the urine, while other nephrons may still be able to increase reabsorption until their higher Tm is reached.

D. **Tubular secretion**
  - A number of substances are **secreted** rather than filtered into the tubular lumen.
  - The proximal tubule plays a significant role in the transport of organic cations and anions into the tubular lumen, the opposite of the route of reabsorbed solutes discussed earlier.
  - The substances being secreted enter the interstitial space from the peritubular capillaries and are transported by organic cation or organic anion **transporters** in the basolateral membrane into the tubular epithelial cell, after which luminal membrane **transporters** facilitate movement into the tubular lumen.
  - The transporters move endogenous substances, typically toxic end products of metabolism such as **bile salts, uric acid,** and **ketoacids.**
  - The relative lack of specificity of these transporters allows them to serve as an important route of elimination of a number of different **drugs** and **exogenous chemicals.**

    > **Clinical note:** With the exception of spironolactone, an aldosterone receptor antagonist, **diuretics** must gain access to the tubular lumen to reach their site of action. Because they are highly protein bound, they are not filtered through the glomerulus. Instead, they are transported into the tubular lumen via the organic ion transporters located in the basolateral membrane of the proximal tubular epithelial cells. Diuretics become less effective in individuals with **renal failure.** This diminished efficacy occurs in part because other organic ions accumulate in renal failure and compete with diuretics for transport into the tubular lumen. Large doses of diuretics, particularly loop diuretics, are given in renal failure to overcome this competition for tubular secretion.

  - The transporters are **saturable** (i.e., they have a Tm) and demonstrate **competitive inhibition.**

    > **Pharmacology note:** Probenecid and penicillin utilize organic anion transporters for elimination into the urine. Probenecid can be used clinically to reduce elimination of penicillin because it competes for the anion transporter, thereby increasing plasma penicillin levels.

VI. **Concentration and Dilution of Urine**
  - The kidney is the body's major route of excretion of solute and water.
  - It has the ability to excrete urine that either has a **high solute load** or is **very dilute.**
  - If this were not the case and reabsorption of fluid and electrolytes along the nephron occurred in an isosmotic fashion (as it does in the proximal tubule), urine would have an osmolality equivalent to that of plasma. Consequently, maintenance of plasma osmolality in the tight range that is physiologically required would fall largely to regulation of dietary intake, which would not be feasible.

A. **Obligatory urine output**
  - This is the minimum amount of urine that must be produced each day in order to excrete the waste products of daily metabolism.

- It is determined by the kidney's concentrating capacity and solute production and is approximately 500 mL, reflecting a normal maximum concentrating capacity of 1200 milliosmoles per liter (mOsm/L) and typical daily solute production of 600 mOsm.

B. **The interstitial osmotic gradient from cortex to medulla**
   - In order to regulate total body sodium and water balance, the kidney must be able to excrete urine across a high range of concentrations.
   - To remove **excess water,** the kidney must be able to excrete a dilute urine. The nephron does this by reabsorbing solute and retaining water in the tubular lumen (because the water channels across the tubular epithelial cells are closed). Excretion of this dilute urine eliminates the excess water.
   - To remove **excess solute,** the kidney must be able to excrete a concentrated urine. This is achieved by the nephron passing through a hyperosmolar region of the kidney, with open water channels across the tubular epithelial cells. Water moves out of the tubule into the interstitial space, and then the remaining solute-rich urine can be excreted. Excretion of this concentrated urine eliminates the excess solute.
   - The ability of the kidney to produce a concentrated urine hinges on the creation and maintenance of a region of **high interstitial osmolality.**

   1. **The countercurrent mechanism**
      - The kidney's ability to establish an osmotic gradient rests primarily in the structure of the **loop of Henle,** which folds back on itself to form a physiologic **countercurrent system** (Fig. 6-16).
      - Other factors, such as the active transport of NaCl from the ascending limb of the loop of Henle and urea trapping within the medullary interstitium, are also important.

   2. **The loop of Henle as a countercurrent system**
      - The loop of Henle functions as a countercurrent system in which the flows in the individual limbs interact with one another (Fig. 6-17).
      - As in the example in Figure 6-16B, where the heat from the ascending tube was used to heat the cold water in the descending tube, the salts removed from the ascending limb are used to concentrate the fluid within the descending limb, by creating a hyperosmolar interstitium.
        (1) In the **descending limb,** which is permeable to water but not to salts, water is removed and solute remains, increasing the concentration and causing an increase in tubular fluid osmolality.
        (2) In the **thick ascending limb** (see Fig. 6-2), which is permeable to salts but not water, the removal of solute dilutes the tubular fluid and helps generate and maintain the interstitial osmotic gradient.
      - Note that the loop of Henle functions as an imperfect countercurrent system, because the fluid emerging from the ascending limb is more dilute than the fluid entering. This is partly because the hyperosmotic tubular fluid in the **thin ascending limb** (see Fig. 6-2) draws in water from the medullary interstitium (which also helps maintain the hyperosmolar interstitium of the medulla).

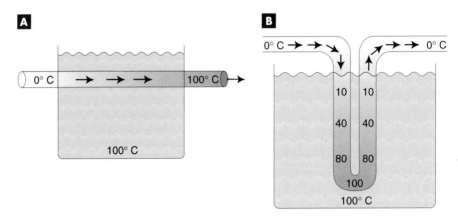

6-16: *Flow-through and countercurrent systems.* **A,** *In a flow-through system, initially the water in the tube is at 0°C; as it passes through the beaker, it draws heat from the fluid such that it emerges from the tube in a changed state at 100°C. This arrangement represents a flow-through system. The capillaries in the renal cortex (as in most tissues) can be thought of as flow-through capillaries that rapidly equilibrate with the surrounding interstitial fluid.* **B,** *In a countercurrent system with a hairpin bend (such as the loop of Henle), the fluid emerges from the tube unchanged from its initial temperature of 0°C. Thus, countercurrent systems isolate environments despite intimate contact. For the countercurrent mechanism to work efficiently, two requirements must be met: The fluid must be moving slowly, and the two vertical "limbs" of the "U" must be contiguous.*

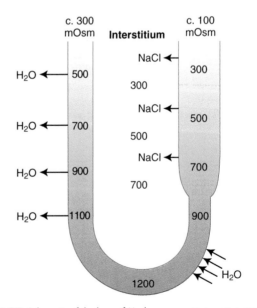

6-17: *Schematic of the loop of Henle as a countercurrent system.*

Pharmacology note: Recall that a slow flow rate is required for a countercurrent system to work effectively. If the tubular flow rate increases substantially within the loop of Henle, its ability to function as a countercurrent system and maintain a hyperosmolar interstitium will become compromised. Dilute urine will then be produced in large amounts. This is one mechanism by which loop diuretics function in promoting diuresis—by increasing the tubular flow rate and compromising the ability of the loop of Henle to function as a countercurrent system.

3. **Antidiuretic hormone and control of urine concentration**
   - The distal nephron delivers a very dilute tubular fluid to the **collecting tubules.**
   - If fluid intake has been high, then all this dilute urine is excreted through the collecting tubules. However, if solute load is such that fluid retention is needed, then mechanisms must be in place to allow the needed water to be reclaimed.
   a. **Plasma osmolality**
      - Plasma osmolality is determined by the ratio of solute to plasma water. The major plasma solute is **sodium** and its accompanying anions, so plasma osmolality is typically equal to slightly more than 2 times the plasma sodium concentration.
      - Plasma osmolality is tightly regulated and normally is 275 to 290 mOsm/L.
      - The addition of water (or the removal of solute) decreases the osmolality of plasma (Fig. 6-18).
   b. **Renal responses to changes in plasma osmolality** (see Fig. 6-18)
      - The permeability of the collecting tubules to water is determined by secretion of **ADH,** which is controlled by the response of **hypothalamic osmoreceptors** to **plasma osmolality.**
      - When ADH is secreted, it travels to the kidney, where it stimulates insertion of water channels (**aquaporins**) into the membranes of the tubular epithelial cells of the collecting tubules, allowing water to move by osmosis into the hypertonic interstitium.
      - In response to **decreased plasma osmolality** (addition of water or loss of solute), osmoreceptors trigger cessation of the release of ADH, and so the collecting tubules remain relatively impermeable to water. Because of this, the excess water is excreted into the urine. The loss of this excess water returns plasma osmolality to normal.
      - In response to **raised plasma osmolality** (addition of solute or loss of water), the osmoreceptors stimulate ADH secretion. As a result, the collecting tubules become permeable to water, allowing water to move by osmosis into the hypertonic interstitium, and so less water is excreted and plasma osmolality returns to normal.
      - Note that the osmoreceptors that regulate ADH secretion may also stimulate thirst, leading to increased water intake. The combination of

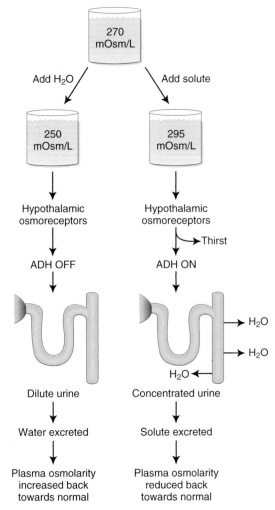

6-18: *Renal response to water and solute loads. The addition of water decreases plasma osmolality, which triggers the hypothalamic osmoreceptors to turn off production of antidiuretic hormone (ADH), which results in the excretion of the excess water as dilute urine. The addition of solute increases plasma osmolality. This triggers ADH release, which stimulates thirst and the reabsorption of water by the kidney.*

water retention, solute excretion, and increased water intake serves to lower the plasma osmolality toward normal.

4. **Urea trapping**
   - Approximately one half of the solute that contributes to the medullary concentrating gradient is urea.
   - Urea is freely filtered through the glomerulus and only partially reabsorbed in the proximal tubule.
   - The cortical and outer medullary portions of the collecting tubules are impermeable to urea, whereas the inner medullary collecting tubules are variably permeable to urea.

- In the presence of **ADH,** urea concentration in the collecting tubules becomes quite high, because water is removed via open water channels. ADH further increases the permeability of the inner medullary collecting tubules to urea, allowing more urea to diffuse into the medullary interstitium. This creates a more hypertonic medulla, which enables further concentration of the urine.

5. **Vasa recta**
   - This is the capillary network that supplies the nephron.
   - The vascular supply to the loop of Henle and collecting tubules could easily wash away the medullary concentrating gradient if the vessels traveled past the nephron in a manner similar to the flow-through model depicted in Figure 6-16A. However, the vasa recta also have a **hairpin configuration** that prevents these vessels from dissipating the concentrating gradient. The ascending portions of the vasa recta remove water reabsorbed from the collecting tubules, which helps maintain the medullary hypertonicity.
   - These vessels also supply the **oxygen** and **nutrients** required by the tubular epithelial cells. Because of their hairpin configuration, oxygen can diffuse from the descending vessels into the ascending vessels, leaving the tubular epithelial cells at the innermost part of the loop of Henle in a relatively **oxygen-poor** environment.

> **Clinical note:** The poor oxygenation of tubular epithelial cells makes them susceptible to hypoxia or hypotension. A hypotensive insult that leaves the heart, liver, and brain unscathed can cause **acute renal failure** because of **hypoxic injury** to tubular epithelial cells. This leads to one of the most common causes of acute renal failure, **acute tubular necrosis.**

VII. **Renal Control of Extracellular Fluid Volume**
   - **Extracellular fluid** (ECF) consists of multiple fluid compartments in the body (see later discussion), and its primary constituents are total body sodium and salts
   - **ECF volume** is a major determinant of **plasma volume.**
     (1) It is determined by the total amount of sodium and water in the extracellular compartment.
     (2) It is mainly controlled by the kidneys, primarily by their regulation of the excretion of sodium and other salts (Fig. 6-19).
   - Under normal conditions, the kidneys maintain a constant ECF volume by matching salt intake with salt excretion:
     (1) If salt intake exceeds excretion, ECF volume increases as a result of neurohormonal compensatory mechanisms that increase water intake and decrease water excretion.
     (2) If salt intake is less than excretion, ECF volume decreases.

> **Clinical note:** Appropriate **plasma volume** is critical for adequate tissue **perfusion;** a reduced volume may impair tissue perfusion, whereas an elevated plasma volume may result in **hypertension, edema,** and **heart failure.**

	Volume depleted	Euvolemic	Volume overloaded
	Na140 mOsm/L	Na140 mOsm/L	Na140 mOsm/L
Sodium concentration (mEq/L)	140	140	140
Total sodium content (mEq)	70	140	210
Total volume (mL)	500	1000	1500

6-19: *Osmolality and total fluid volume. The sodium concentration is 140 mEq/L in each hypothetical example (volume depletion, euvolemia, and volume overload). However, the total sodium content and total fluid volume are very different in each example.*

A. **Distribution of body fluids**
   1. **Fluid compartments**
      - Approximately 50% to 60% of total body weight consists of water (50% in women because of higher fat content, and 60% in lean men).
      - Of that, roughly two thirds is located in the intracellular space (i.e., **intracellular fluid**), with the remaining fluid in the extracellular space (i.e., ECF).
      - This **ECF** is divided into the **interstitial fluid** (~75% of ECF) and **plasma volume** (~25% of ECF), and a relatively small fraction consisting of **transcellular fluids.**
      - **Transcellular fluids** include many small fluid compartments (such as the peritoneal, pleural, synovial, pericardial, and cerebrospinal fluids and the aqueous humor of the intraocular compartment).
      - In a 70-kg man there are approximately 28 L of **intracellular fluid,** 10 L of **interstitial fluid,** and 3.5 L of **plasma.**
   2. **Composition of fluid compartments**
      - **Intracellular fluid,** relative to the ECF, has large amounts of protein, potassium, and phosphate and low levels of sodium and chloride.
      - **Interstitial fluid** is separated from the plasma compartment by a plasma membrane that is freely permeable to water and many electrolytes but not to most proteins. It is therefore very similar in content to plasma, except that it contains much less protein. **Plasma** is the fluid component of the blood that remains after blood cells are removed.

> **Clinical note:** To measure the volume of one of the fluid compartments, an **indicator** substance can be used that is diffusion-restricted to that particular fluid compartment. For example, **deuterium** and **tritiated water** can be used to measure total body water, **inulin** and **mannitol** to measure ECF volume, and radiolabeled **albumin** (^{125}I-albumin) to measure plasma volume. These measurements are not used in clinical practice.

B. **Effective circulating volume**
   - This is not a separate fluid compartment; it is that portion of the ECF that is in the vascular space and is effectively perfusing tissue.
   - It varies directly with the **ECF volume** and with **total body sodium.**
   - The ECF volume is directly proportional to total body **sodium** content because sodium, as the primary extracellular solute, acts to hold fluid within the extracellular space.
   - The kidney regulates the size of the ECF space (i.e., the volume of ECF) by regulating **sodium retention** or **excretion.**
   - The body perceives the effective circulating volume in relation to the pressure that is perfusing the arterial **stretch receptors** in the carotid sinus, the aortic arch, and the glomerular afferent artery.
   - When **stretch receptors** are activated by reduced blood flow, they send signals to the brainstem to increase sympathetic outflow, which stimulates vasoconstriction and plasma volume expansion (through activation of the remaining renin-angiotensin-aldosterone system) in an attempt to restore an effective circulating volume.

> **Clinical note:** The effective circulating volume is not directly proportional to extracellular volume in certain conditions such as **congestive heart failure** and **cirrhosis with ascites.** In the former, the impaired cardiac output is unable to stretch the baroreceptors; this leads to the perception of inadequate circulating volume, which triggers further fluid retention. In cirrhosis, fluid sequestration in ascitic fluid and in the dilated splanchnic bed results in a markedly expanded extracellular volume. However, this expanded volume is effectively invisible to the detectors of effective circulating volume, which trigger further fluid retention and consequent exacerbation of the ECF excess.

C. **Response to changes in effective circulating volume**
   1. **Changes in sympathetic tone**
      a. **In response to decreased effective circulating volume**
         - There is an increase in sympathetic tone, which alters the circulatory system in several ways:
            (1) Increased cardiac contractility and heart rate
            (2) **Constriction** of the venous system, which moves blood into the arterial circulation. (Approximately 70% of blood is usually in the venous system, and a shift of some of this volume to the arterial circulation increases the effective circulating volume.)
            (3) **Arteriolar constriction,** which raises systemic blood pressure

- An increase in sympathetic tone also results in
  (1) Production of **renin** (in the kidneys)
  (2) Production of **angiotensin II** (primarily in the pulmonary vasculature)
  (3) Direct stimulation of **renal sodium retention**
- The sympathetic nervous system also regulates plasma volume (and therefore blood pressure) by regulating volume loss by the kidneys. It does this primarily by regulating renal perfusion, which directly affects the GFR. If blood pressure falls, sympathetic stimulation causes preferential constriction of the afferent arteriole relative to the efferent arteriole. This reduces renal perfusion (and therefore GFR) but also avoids increasing the glomerular hydrostatic pressure, which could otherwise increase filtration.

b. **In response to increased effective circulating volume**
- All of the changes in the previous section are reversed.
- The increased cardiac output causes stretching of baroreceptors, which triggers cessation of sympathetic outflow from the brainstem.
- This has multiple effects, including vasodilation, reduced cardiac contractility, and decreased renal fluid retention, which lower cardiac output and blood pressure, thereby reducing baroreceptor stretch.

2. **Changes in renal sodium retention** (Fig. 6-20)
- In individuals with normal renal function, the glomeruli filter approximately 20,000 mEq of sodium each day. In **euvolemic states** (normal fluid status), the kidney reabsorbs all but the 100 to 300 mEq of excess ingested sodium in order to maintain sodium homeostasis.
- When there is a decrease in circulating volume, the kidney retains sodium so that plasma volume increases accordingly.
- With a decrease in effective circulating volume, the kidney can retain sodium so effectively that only 1 mEq is excreted per liter of urine. This is achieved by the renal responses to an increase in sympathetic tone described earlier and as follows:
  (1) Increased sympathetic tone directly stimulates renal **sodium reabsorption** in the proximal tubule.
  (2) Renal hypoperfusion and increased sympathetic tone stimulate increased **renin production** by the juxtaglomerular cells in the afferent arteriole.
  (3) Renin stimulates the production of **angiotensin II** and, consequently, **aldosterone.**
  (4) **Angiotensin II,** in addition to its ability to induce systemic vasoconstriction, directly stimulates sodium **reabsorption** by the proximal tubule.
  (5) **Aldosterone** stimulates sodium **reabsorption** in the collecting tubule by increasing the number of open Na^+ (and K^+) channels.
  (6) **ADH** is produced in response to hypovolemia. ADH stimulates sodium retention in the thick ascending limb and increases water retention in the collecting tubule (see earlier discussion).
  (7) Volume depletion turns off the production of **atrial natriuretic peptide,** which further decreases renal sodium excretion.

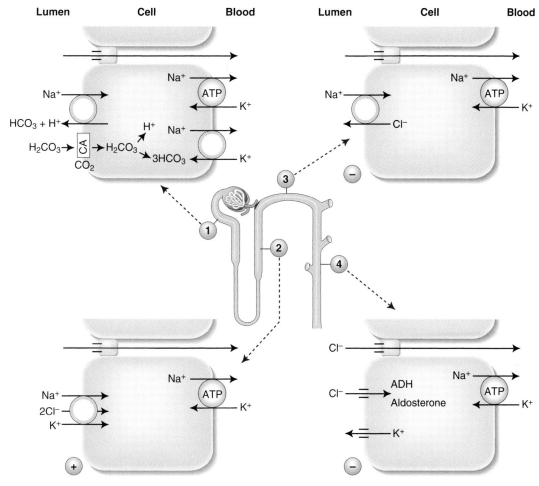

6-20: *Major sites of sodium reabsorption along the nephron. The mechanism for sodium transport through the luminal membrane differs at different sites along the nephron. ADH, antidiuretic hormone; ATP, adenosine triphosphate; CA, carbonic anhydrase. In the proximal tuble (1) sodium reabsorption is coupled to hydrogen ion secretion; in the thick ascending limb of the loop of Henle (2) sodium is actively reabsorbed along with chloride and potassium; in the distal convoluting tubule (3) sodium reabsorption is coupled to chloride secretion; chloride reabsorption and potassium secretion, respectively, are also illustrated in the distal collecting tubules (4) of this diagram.*

- In states of volume expansion, these sympathetic nervous system and renal responses are reversed, so that the kidney excretes the excess sodium and water.

VIII. Renal Control of Acid-Base Homeostasis
- The kidney has a major role in the control of acid-base homeostasis.
- It does this by returning filtered bicarbonate to the plasma, using buffers to facilitate acid excretion, and by generating bicarbonate *de novo.*
A. Maintenance of plasma pH
- The plasma pH is kept within a narrow range by means of **plasma buffers,** the **lungs,** and the **kidneys.**

1. **Buffers**
   - In a reaction of the form, HA → H⁺ + A⁻, the **Henderson-Hasselbach equation** reveals that the higher the concentration of a conjugate base (A⁻) relative to its acid (HA), the higher the pH:

$$pH = pKa + \log A^-/HA$$

   - The pKa equals the pH at which the acid is half dissociated (i.e., the point at which $[A^-] = [HA]$).
   - In the **plasma,** the most important buffer is the **bicarbonate system,** and consequently the most important conjugate base is bicarbonate, from the reaction

$$H_2CO_3 \rightarrow H^+ + HCO_3^-$$

   - Raising the plasma bicarbonate level (without adding protons) raises the plasma pH, and lowering the plasma bicarbonate lowers the plasma pH.
2. **The lungs**
   - Daily metabolism of fats, carbohydrates, and proteins generates tremendous quantities of **carbon dioxide.** When carbon dioxide dissolves in water, the following reaction occurs:

$$CO_2 + H_2O \rightarrow H_2CO_3 \rightarrow H+ + HCO_3^-$$

   - The hydrogen ions thus generated lower the plasma pH.
   - However, in the **lungs,** the reverse reaction takes place: hydrogen ions are consumed, and **CO₂** is **blown off.** This ability of the lungs to blow off CO_2 prevents the development of an overwhelming acidosis.
3. **The kidneys**
   - Daily metabolism, primarily the metabolism of proteins, generates a number of **nonvolatile acids** that cannot be eliminated by the lungs. These acids consume bicarbonate, the major plasma buffer, via the following reaction:

$$HA + HCO_3^- \rightarrow A^- + H_2CO_3 \rightarrow A^- + H_2O + CO_2$$

   - The resulting CO_2 is blown off. The attendant decrease in plasma bicarbonate **decreases plasma pH.** The kidney compensates for this by generating bicarbonate *de novo* (see later discussion), in an amount equivalent to that consumed by these nonvolatile acids. The kidneys also excrete the conjugate base of the nonvolatile acids to prevent their accumulation.
B. **Bicarbonate reclamation and synthesis in the kidney**
   - The kidneys reclaim most of the 3500 mEq of bicarbonate that is filtered through the glomeruli into the tubular lumens each day.
   - They also synthesize bicarbonate *de novo* to offset nonvolatile acid production.
   - Urinary acidification is the result of bicarbonate reclamation and *de novo* bicarbonate synthesis in the kidney, so acidification will be discussed here as well.
1. **Bicarbonate reclamation**
   - More than 99.9% of filtered plasma bicarbonate is reabsorbed in the kidney—approximately 80% in the proximal tubule, 10% in the thick ascending limb, and 10% in the distal nephron.

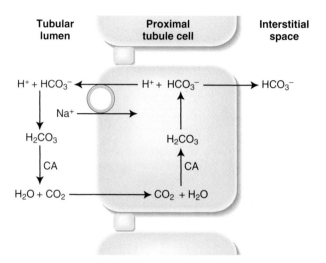

Tubular   Proximal   Interstitial
lumen   tubule cell   space

6-21: Reclamation of filtered bicarbonate. Filtered bicarbonate combines with secreted H^+ to form carbonic acid, which, under the influence of carbonic anhydrase (CA), dissociates to H_2O and CO_2. The CO_2 diffuses into the tubular epithelial cell, where it combines with H_2O to form carbonic acid. The intracellular carbonic acid dissociates to form HCO_3^-, which is returned to the circulation, and H^+, which is secreted into the tubular lumen to be used in absorbing more filtered bicarbonate.

- A single mechanism operates at all sites in the nephron (Fig. 6-21).
- **Hydrogen ions** are secreted into the tubular lumen, where they react with bicarbonate to form **carbonic acid,** which the enzyme **carbonic anhydrase** dissociates into **CO_2** and **water.**
- The CO_2 and water diffuse across the tubular cell membrane, and inside the cell the reverse reaction takes place: the **CO_2** and water react to form **carbonic acid,** which then dissociates into **H^+ ions** and **bicarbonate.**
- The resulting **bicarbonate** is pumped out of the basolateral surface of the cell and returned to the **plasma.**
- Notice that there is no net acid secretion or generation because the hydrogen ions are continually recycled in this reclamation process.

> **Pharmacology note:** Because sodium reabsorption in the proximal tubule is indirectly compled to bicarbonate reabsorption, carbonic anhydrase inhibitors such as acetazolamide exert a diuretic effect by blunting sodium reabsorption. However, this **diuretic** action is weak because of the capacity of more distal sites, particularly the Na^+-K^+-$2Cl^-$-cotransporter in the loop of Henle, to increase sodium reabsorption. They also interfere with reclamation of bicarbonate in the proximal tubule, the site at which 80% of filtered bicarbonate is reclaimed (the distal sites do not have a capacity to greatly increase their bicarbonate absorption). The loss of bicarbonate can cause **acidosis** when carbonic anhydrase inhibitors are used as diuretics. In fact, clinically,

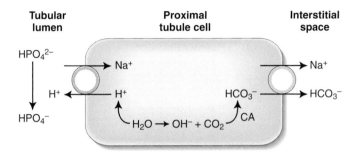

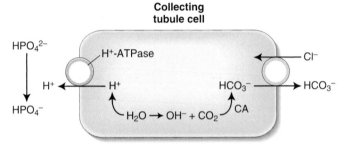

6-22: *Titratable acidity. The secretion of each H⁺ ion into the tubular lumen for buffering with titratable acids in the proximal tubule, and further down the nephron in the collecting tubule, is associated with the generation of a molecule of HCO_3^-, which is returned to the interstitial space for absorption into the circulation. In the proximal tubule the bicarbonate is transported into the interstitium along with sodium, whereas in the collecting tubule the bicarbonate is exchanged for chloride. ATPase, adenosine triphosphatase; CA, carbonic anhydrase.*

the carbonic anhydrase inhibitors are used much more often for their ability to increase bicarbonate excretion and thus treat a **metabolic alkalosis** than they are used as a diuretic.

2. ***De novo* bicarbonate synthesis**
   - The removal of a hydrogen ion is the biochemical equivalent of bicarbonate generation, so the kidney needs to excrete hydrogen ions to generate bicarbonate and to prevent acidosis.
   - If H⁺ were excreted as free ions in the urine, this would lower urine pH to physiologically intolerable levels. In fact, negligible amounts of free H⁺ ions are excreted, because the kidney uses **urinary buffers** to facilitate H⁺ excretion.
   - The **buffers** used are filtered **weak acids** that make up what is called **titratable acidity** and **ammonium.** (Using bicarbonate as a buffer would accomplish nothing, because the effect of losing H⁺ would be offset by the simultaneous loss of HCO_3^-.)
   a. **Titratable acidity**
      - Filtered phosphate (**HPO_4^{2-}**) is the major contributor to titratable acidity (Fig. 6-22). Less abundant acids with less favorable pKa values (e.g. **creatinine** and **uric acid**) also contribute.

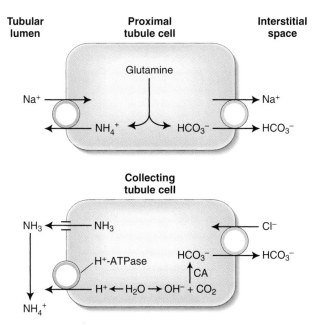

6-23: *Formation of urinary ammonium. Metabolism of glutamine in the proximal tubule generates ammonium (NH₄⁺) and bicarbonate (HCO₃⁻) ions. Ammonium is transported into the tubular lumen, and bicarbonate is transported to the interstitial space, where it is absorbed into the peritubular capillaries. In the collecting tubule, secreted hydrogen ions combine with ammonia (NH₃) that has diffused into the tubular lumen. Bicarbonate is also generated and supplied to the interstitial space as part of this process. ATPase, adenosine triphosphatase; CA, carbonic anhydrase.*

- The amount of titratable acidity present in the urine can be determined by determining the amount of OH^- required to titrate the urine pH back to 7.4 (hence, the name). Normally, about 10 to 40 mEq of H^+ that has been secreted into the tubular lumen is buffered in this manner each day.

b. **Ammonium production**
  - The deamination of the amino acid **glutamine** in the **proximal tubule** cells yields two **ammonium** (NH_4^+) molecules and two **bicarbonate** molecules (Fig. 6-23). The bicarbonate molecules are transported across the basolateral membrane and absorbed into the plasma. The NH_4^+ is transported across the luminal membrane by substitution of NH_4^+ on the **Na⁺-H⁺ countertransporter.**
  - In the **collecting tubule,** lipid-soluble **ammonia (NH_3)** diffuses across the luminal membrane, where it combines with secreted H^+ ions to form the polar, nondiffusible, NH_4^+, which is then trapped in the tubular lumen.
  - **Note:** The model of nondiffusible NH_4^+ being trapped in the tubular lumen is an oversimplification of renal NH_4^+ handling. In fact, NH_4^+ is produced, partially reabsorbed, then dissociated to NH_3 that is recycled in the renal medulla, where its high concentration prompts diffusion

back into the tubular lumen; there, it combines again with secreted H^+ to form NH_4^+. The net result is that NH_4^+ ends up back in the tubular lumen.

> **Clinical note:** In **renal failure,** in which the GFR is substantially reduced, less H^+ may be secreted into the tubular fluid because of a reduced number of functioning nephrons. The result is an accumulation of acid in the plasma, leading to the **acidosis** that is characteristic of advanced renal failure.

c. **Regulation of *de novo* bicarbonate synthesis**
  - Under normal physiologic circumstances, all of the filtered bicarbonate is reabsorbed, and the additional amount of bicarbonate required to offset the 40 to 80 mEq of H^+ produced daily is generated in the kidney by excretion of titratable acids and ammonium.
  - Renal acid excretion, and hence bicarbonate synthesis, varies to adapt to different physiologic circumstances:
    (1) The amount of H^+ excreted varies inversely with extracellular pH. As systemic pH falls, the activities of the kidney's Na^+-H^+ **countertransporter** H^+-ATPase cotransporter and Na^+-HCO_3 cotransporter increase.
    (2) The capacity of titratable acidity to increase is fairly limited, so the required increase in renal buffering capacity is derived from increased production of NH_4^+.
  - Systemic alkalosis results in a reversal of these H^+ secreting processes and a decrease in bicarbonate reabsorption.
  - These processes are so efficient that enormous amounts of bicarbonate can be ingested without generating a significant increase in bicarbonate concentration.

> **Clinical note: Acidosis** can develop because of bicarbonate depletion (**metabolic acidosis**) or carbon dioxide accumulation (**respiratory acidosis**) or both. In either situation, the kidneys attempt to compensate by increasing H^+ excretion. Similarly, **alkalosis** can occur because of an increase in bicarbonate or a decrease in CO_2. In this situation, the kidneys decrease H^+ excretion in an effort to normalize systemic pH.

IX. **Renal Control of Plasma Potassium**
  - Most potassium is **intracellular** (140 mEq/L), and only ~2% is extracellular (~4.5 mEq/L). Therefore, a shift of only a small fraction of intracellular potassium to or from the plasma can have a significant impact on the plasma potassium concentration.
  - The distribution of **sodium** and **potassium** between the **intracellular** and **extracellular** compartments is maintained by the activity of the **Na^+,K^+-ATPase pump,** which moves sodium out and potassium into cells.
  - The kidneys play a major role in regulating potassium excretion.

Clinical note: Regulation of the extracellular potassium pool is extremely important, because modest changes in plasma levels can precipitate neuromuscular symptoms and lethal cardiac arrhythmias. These occur because the resting membrane potentials of nerves and muscle are directly related to the ratio of intracellular and extracellular potassium concentrations.

A. **Potassium distribution**
- The activity of the Na^+,K^+-ATPase pump is regulated by insulin, catecholamines, and K^+ concentration.
- Regulation by **K^+ concentration** is particularly advantageous after ingestion of a potassium-containing meal. The meal-induced increase in insulin activates Na^+,K^+-ATPase, which moves the absorbed potassium into the intracellular compartment; this circumvents the large increase in extracellular potassium that would otherwise occur.
- **Catecholamines** also stimulate intracellular movement of potassium. Activation of β_2-adrenergic receptors promotes entry of potassium into cells; α-receptors impair this movement.

Clinical note: The role of extracellular K^+ concentration in regulating potassium distribution is demonstrated in patients with **insulin deficiency (type 1 diabetes)** and **pharmacologically induced β-adrenergic blockade.** In these situations, the shift in potassium into the intracellular compartment is impaired but not absent. The increase in plasma K^+ concentration is thought to prompt K^+ movement into the intracellular compartment.

- **Extracellular pH** can also prompt shifts in the distribution of potassium, especially in certain types of **metabolic acidosis** in which large amounts of the H^+ excess are buffered intracellularly. In order to maintain mandatory electroneutrality, K^+ shifts to the extracellular location to offset an increase in positive charges caused by intracellular movement of H^+. The result is an increase in plasma K^+ concentration of 0.2 to 1.7 mEq/L for every 0.1-unit fall in extracellular pH. H^+ shifts are much less prominent with **metabolic alkalosis,** and K^+ levels typically exhibit only small decreases.

Pharmacology note: Several drugs can affect potassium distribution. **Digitalis** is a drug commonly used in the treatment of congestive heart failure; overdose impairs the activity of Na^+,K^+-ATPase and can cause severe **hyperkalemia** because of the inability of potassium to be moved intracellularly. Other drugs that affect potassium distribution are **insulin** and **albuterol** (a β_2-receptor agonist). Because of their ability to shift potassium to the intracellular location, these drugs are used to treat severe hyperkalemia.

B. **Control of potassium homeostasis**
- Ultimately, control of potassium balance requires the **excretion** of excess potassium by the **kidneys.**
- Under normal circumstances, the kidneys maintain potassium homeostasis simply by matching potassium excretion with potassium intake.

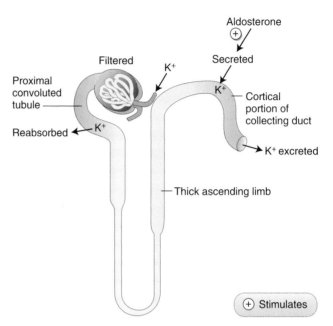

6-24: *Renal handling of potassium. Because the absorption of K^+ is so complete, most urinary potassium is derived primarily from secreted rather than filtered potassium. This diagram depicts the typical situation of dietary potassium excess. In potassium-depleted states, net reabsorption of potassium might occur in the distal nephron.*

- The **colon** also plays a minor role in potassium excretion.
1. **Renal handling of potassium**
   - Most potassium (~90%) is **reabsorbed** in the **proximal nephron** (primarily the **proximal convoluted tubule** and the **thick ascending limb**). The result is a fairly limited delivery of potassium to the distal nephron (late distal tubule and cortical collecting tubules) (Fig. 6-24).
   - The **distal nephron** has the ability to either **reabsorb** or **secrete potassium** and therefore is the site that ultimately determines renal potassium handling.
   - Under normal conditions, the distal nephron favors potassium secretion over potassium reabsorption, because this is normally what is required to maintain potassium balance. This secretory ability is so powerful that if there is high dietary intake of potassium, the amount of urinary potassium actually exceeds the filtered potassium load.
   a. **Mechanism of potassium secretion by distal nephron**
      - In the distal nephron, **Na^+,K^+-ATPase pumps** on the basolateral membrane of tubular cells pump sodium out and potassium into the cells (Fig. 6-25). The potassium that accumulates in the cells then passively diffuses into the tubular lumen via luminal potassium channels. Therefore, anything that affects the electrochemical gradient for passive potassium diffusion from cell to tubular lumen affects potassium secretion in the distal nephron.

| Tubular | Principal | Interstitial |
| lumen | cell | space |

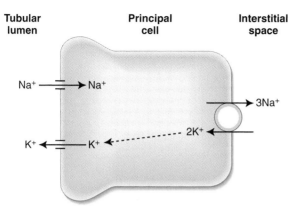

6-25: *Potassium secretion by the principal cells in the cortical collecting tubule of the distal nephron. Potassium that has entered the tubular cells via the basolateral Na^+,K^+-ATPase diffuses into the tubular lumen via luminal K^+ channels.*

- If the **tubular flow rate** is increased, less potassium accumulates in the tubular lumen, and this maintains a larger electrochemical gradient for potassium diffusion into the tubules, increasing potassium secretion.
- If the **Na^+,K^+-ATPase** is more active, this increases intracellular potassium levels in the tubular cells and causes increased potassium diffusion into the tubules.
- The **transcellular electrical potential** affects potassium secretion: more **negative** luminal potentials increase the diffusion of the positively charged potassium ions. Such an increase in transcellular potential occurs with increased **sodium** movement from the tubular lumen into the cells via the luminal sodium channels (see Fig. 6-25).

> **Clinical note:** In **renal failure,** the GFR is reduced. This reduces the rate of flow through the renal tubules, limiting the amount of potassium that can be excreted. Therefore, **hyperkalemia** is a common complication of severe renal failure.

b. **Regulation of renal potassium secretion and reabsorption**
  - **Aldosterone** and **plasma K^+ concentration** are the major regulators of K^+ secretion by the kidney. Small increases (0.1 mEq/L) in plasma potassium concentration promote significant increases in aldosterone secretion by the **adrenal glands.**
  - **Aldosterone** has two effects on the potassium-secreting cells in the kidney. It increases the activity of the **Na^+,K^+-ATPase pump** in the basolateral membrane, and it causes a marked increase in the number of open **Na^+ and K^+ channels** in the luminal membrane. These factors favor potassium secretion into the urine as outlined in the previous section, and hence excretion of potassium from the body.
  - **Plasma potassium** levels themselves can regulate renal potassium excretion:

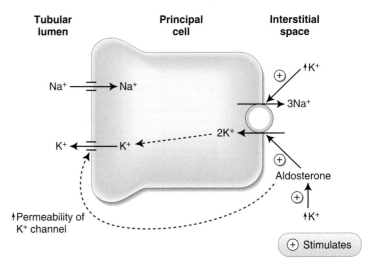

Tubular   Principal   Interstitial
lumen   cell   space

6-26: *Effect of aldosterone and hyperkalemia on potassium excretion. Aldosterone or elevated interstitial K^+ concentrations generate changes in the principal cell that favor potassium excretion. The activity of Na^+,K^+-ATPase is increased, and the number of open sodium and potassium channels on the luminal membrane is increased.*

   (1) An **increase in plasma K^+ concentration,** and thus interstitial K^+ concentration, replicates all the activities of aldosterone (Fig. 6-26).

   (2) The response to **potassium depletion** is a decrease in the release of aldosterone and a fall in intracellular potassium concentration in the distal portions of the nephron. This effectively shuts down potassium secretion into the tubular lumen by the principal cells; however, reabsorption must be employed to reclaim potassium that is still present in the tubular lumen.

• A second cell type, the **intercalated cell,** plays an active role in distal potassium **reabsorption.** These cells have a luminal H^+,K^+-ATPase pump that reabsorbs K^+ and secretes H^+. The activity of this pump increases with K^+ depletion and promotes reabsorption of potassium.

> **Pharmacology note:** The volume depletion triggered by **carbonic anhydrase inhibitors, loop diuretics,** and **thiazide diuretics** stimulates **aldosterone** secretion. Because this increases the number of open sodium and potassium channels in the collecting tubule, the high distal flow rates and sodium retention at this site set the stage perfectly for high levels of potassium secretion into the tubule. **Hypokalemia** commonly results. This potassium-wasting property of diuretics is so consistently observed that the one class of diuretics that does not prompt hypokalemia is distinguished by being known as the "potassium-sparing" diuretics (see later discussion). The **potassium-sparing diuretics** are those that act in the collecting tubule to decrease the number of open sodium channels in principal cells; examples include amiloride, triamterene, and spironolactone.

Tubular | Proximal | Interstitial
lumen | tubule cell | space

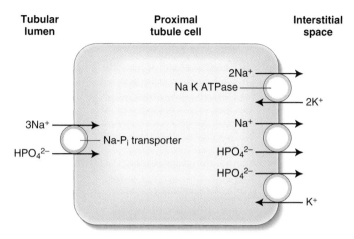

6-27: *Phosphate transport in the proximal tubule. An increase in PTH levels decreases the number of Na⁺-Pi cotransporters located in the luminal membrane, thus increasing renal phosphate excretion. Energy for phosphate transport is derived from the basolateral Na⁺,K⁺-ATPase. Phosphate is transported into the interstitum for absorption into the circulation.*

X. Renal Contribution to Control of Phosphate and Calcium

- The contribution of the kidney to phosphate homeostasis involves a more complex regulatory system than does its contribution to acid-base, bicarbonate, and potassium homeostasis, which all involve near-complete absorption of electrolytes from the gut together with a matching of daily intake with urinary losses.
- Regulation of plasma **phosphate** levels is tightly linked to regulation of plasma **calcium** and is influenced by the same compounds, **parathyroid hormone (PTH)** and **vitamin D.**
- Gut absorption of phosphate and calcium is highly variable and is controlled by PTH and vitamin D, as is the distribution of high concentrations of calcium and phosphate in the bone in the form of hydroxyapatite.
- Renal excretion of phosphate is controlled by PTH.

A. Parathyroid hormone

- PTH is secreted by the **parathyroid gland,** the primary role of which is the precise regulation of **serum calcium levels.**
- A decrease in serum calcium increases circulating **PTH;** this triggers increased **gut absorption** of **calcium** and **phosphate,** increased **mobilization** of calcium and phosphate from stores in bone, and decreased renal calcium excretion. These factors raise plasma calcium back to normal.
- However, in the absence of renal control, this would also have the unwanted effect of increasing serum phosphate. This does not occur because **PTH** also increases **renal phosphate excretion.** It does this by causing a marked decrease in the number of **sodium phosphate (Na⁺-Pi) cotransporters** present on the luminal membrane of epithelial cells of the proximal convoluted tubule, the major site of phosphate reabsorption (Fig. 6-27).
- **Hyperphosphatemia** also stimulates an increase in PTH, which increases renal phosphate losses by decreasing the number of Na⁺-Pi cotransporters.

B. **Vitamin D**
  - **Calcitriol (1,25-dihydroxyvitamin D),** the most active form of vitamin D, is the primary hormone that responds to changes in **phosphate balance.**
  - **Vitamin D (cholecalciferol)** is obtained from the diet and also is synthesized in skin exposed to ultraviolet light. In the liver, a hydroxyl group is added in the 25 position to yield **calcidiol,** which then travels via the circulation to the kidney.
  - In the kidney, calcidiol is hydroxylated at the 1 position to yield **calcitriol,** which is returned to plasma by the kidney. Phosphate depletion raises renal calcitriol production, and phosphate loading decreases renal calcitriol production.
  - Changes in plasma calcitriol concentration normalize phosphate balance by regulating the absorption of **dietary phosphate** and **phosphate mobilization** from bone: increased calcitriol increases bone formation/mineralization and decreases bone resorption/mobilization (see Chapter 3).
  - Calcitriol also modulates **PTH production:** a low calcitriol level stimulates PTH production, and a high calcitriol level decreases PTH production.
C. **Hypophosphatemia and hyperphosphatemia**
  - Physiologic responses to **hypophosphatemia** include the following:
    (1) Increased number of Na^+-Pi cotransporters, which serves to increase proximal phosphate reabsorption
    (2) Increased calcitriol synthesis, which increases phosphate availability from the gut and bone
    (3) Suppression of PTH secretion, which further increases the activity of the proximal Na^+-Pi cotransporters and lowers urinary phosphate losses
  - The reverse happens in response to **hyperphosphatemia,** which is commonly seen in individuals with **moderate renal failure:**
    (1) A reduction in proximal tubular phosphate reabsorption occurs because of reduced production of the Na^+-Pi cotransporter.
    (2) Calcitriol levels fall.
    (3) Increased PTH secretion further lowers Na^+-Pi cotransporter activity.
    (4) The net result is a decrease in serum phosphorus levels toward normal.

Clinical note: In **primary hyperparathyroidism,** the primary problem is overproduction of PTH by the parathyroid glands. The typical laboratory findings in this disease are **hypercalcemia** and **hypophosphatemia.**

Secondary hyperparathyroidism is commonly seen secondary to **chronic kidney disease.** Impaired 1,25-dihydroxyvitamin D production by the diseased kidney, hyperphosphatemia due to impaired renal phosphate excretion, and mild hypocalcemia combine to increase PTH production. The hyperparathyroidism tends to normalize calcium levels and increase renal phosphorus excretion. The result is that both calcium and phosphorus levels may be normal. The price for this normalcy is sustained elevation of PTH, which can induce **bone disease** because of the continued stimulatory effects of PTH in mobilizing bone stores of calcium and phosphate.

TABLE 6-3:
Classes of Diuretics

Class of Diuretic (Example)	Site of Action	Mechanism	Potency	Clinical Use	Side Effects
Carbonic anhydrase inhibitors (acetazolamide)	Proximal convoluted tubule	Promote metabolic acidosis by inhibiting bicarbonate reclamation (i.e., increase bicarbonate excretion), weak diuretic effect by inhibiting Na reabsorption	Weak diuretic effect because of the capacity of more distal sites, particularly the Na^+-K^+-Cl^- cotransporter in the loop of Henle, to increase sodium reabsorption	High-altitude sickness, glaucoma	Metabolic acidosis
Thiazide diuretics (HCl-thiazide)	Distal convoluted tubule	Inhibit the activity of the Na^+-Cl^- cotransporter	Relatively weak because act at sites where smaller amounts of sodium (5–10%) are reabsorbed	Hypertension	Hyponatremia, hypercalcemia
Potassium-sparing diuretics	Collecting tubule	Decrease number of open Na^+ channels in principal cells of the tubule	Relatively weak because act at sites where smaller amounts of sodium (3–5%) are reabsorbed	—	Hyperkalemia (rarely), gynecomastia (spironolactone)
Loop diuretics (furosemide)	Loop of Henle	Inhibit Na^+-K^+-$2Cl^-$ carrier in thick ascending limb of loop of Henle	More potent because act at a site responsible for reabsorption of approximately 25% of filtered sodium	Pulmonary edema associated with congestive heart failure	Hyponatremia, hearing loss
Osmotic diuretics (mannitol)	—	Osmotic diuresis	—	Cerebral edema	—

XI. **Diuretics**
- Diuretics primarily reduce extracellular volume by preventing reabsorption of **sodium** and **water** from the tubular lumen.
- **Sodium,** the most abundant plasma electrolyte, is freely filtered through the glomerulus and then almost completely reabsorbed via transporters located at several different sites along the nephron.
- The basolaterally located **Na^+,K^+-ATPase** is important at each of these sites; however, the mechanism of sodium entry through the luminal membrane differs (see Fig. 6-20).
- Different classes of diuretics act at different **nephron sites,** because each class of diuretics interacts with one type of luminal sodium transporter (Table 6-3).
- The ability of diuretics to increase sodium excretion is dependent on the amount of sodium absorbed at the site of diuretic action and the ability of more distal sites in the nephron to increase their sodium reabsorption.

Gastrointestinal Physiology

I. **Structure and Function of the Gastrointestinal Tract**

  A. **Functional anatomy**

- The gastrointestinal (GI) tract is essentially a **hollow digestive tube** that extends from the mouth to the anus. Secretions from accessory digestive structures such as the salivary glands, pancreas, and liver empty into this tube and are essential for efficient digestion and absorption.
- The digestive tract can be subdivided into three sections based on embryologic origin and vascular supply (Fig. 7-1). The **foregut** extends from the esophagus to the second part of the duodenum and is supplied by the **celiac artery.** The **midgut** extends from the second part of the duodenum to the splenic flexure of the colon and is supplied by the **superior mesenteric artery.** The **hindgut** extends from the splenic flexure of the colon to the anus and is supplied by the **inferior mesenteric artery.**
- Venous return of all three arterial beds is through the **portal vein** into the liver.

> **Pathology note:** The portal vein normally carries nutrient-rich blood from the intestines to the liver, after which the blood is shunted to the inferior vena cava via the hepatic vein. In **cirrhosis,** a variety of pathophysiologic changes result in elevated portal vein pressures, termed **"portal hypertension."** Because the portal vein has multiple **anastomoses with systemic veins,** pressures likewise increase in these vessels. These systemic veins may then become abnormally dilated and are at increased risk of rupture. In the anterior abdominal wall, venous dilatation can result in **caput medusae,** a rather harmless clinical examination finding that nonetheless indicates severe liver disease. In the esophagus, venous dilatation can result in **esophageal varices.** Rupture of esophageal varices can be rapidly fatal.

    1. **Layers of the gut wall**

- Throughout most of the GI tract, the gut wall is composed of four layers; from inside to outside, these are the mucosa, submucosa, muscularis propria, and serosa (Fig. 7-2).

      a. **Mucosa**

- The mucosa is composed of three distinct layers: the **mucosal epithelium,** the **lamina propria,** and the **muscularis mucosae.**
- The structure of the **mucosal epithelium** varies depending on its location in the GI tract. **Stratified squamous** mucosal epithelium is present in the esophagus. In contrast, **columnar** mucosal epithelium is

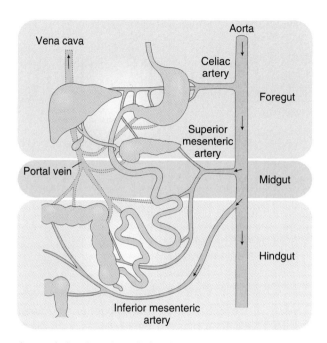

7-1: *Splanchnic circulation, which is derived entirely from the celiac artery, the superior mesenteric artery, and the inferior mesenteric artery.*

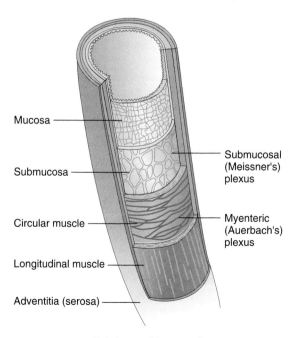

7-2: *Layers of the gut wall.*

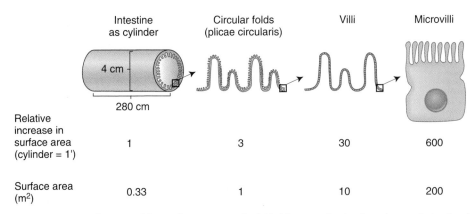

	Intestine as cylinder	Circular folds (plicae circularis)	Villi	Microvilli
Relative increase in surface area (cylinder = 1')	1	3	30	600
Surface area (m²)	0.33	1	10	200

7-3: Arrangement of mucosa of the small intestine. Circular folds (plicae circularis), villi, and microvilli significantly increase the surface area of the mucosa. Surface areas are shown in square meters.

present in the rest of the GI tract (except for the rectum, where it changes back to squamous at the dentate line). In the stomach, the mucosa is folded into **rugae.** In the small intestine, there are folds of cells in the mucosa (**villi**) and projections on individual cells (**microvilli**), which increase the surface area for absorption (Fig. 7-3). In the large intestine, there are **crypts** but no villi.

> **Pathology note:** In **gastroesophageal reflux disease** (GERD), the mucosal epithelium of the esophagus takes on the appearance of the gastric mucosal epithelium: It differentiates from a **stratified squamous epithelium** into a **columnar epithelium.** This process, whereby one cell type transforms into another, is termed **"metaplasia."** Columnar metaplasia in the lower esophagus is called **Barrett's esophagus,** which can be detected by endoscopy and substantially increases the risk for development of **esophageal adenocarcinoma.**

- The **lamina propria** is a thin sheet of connective tissue just outside the mucosa.
- The **muscularis mucosa** is a thin sheet of smooth muscle just outside the lamina propria.

b. **Submucosa**
  - The submucosa is a single layer of loose connective tissue.
  - It is located between the mucosa (inside) and the muscularis propria (outside).

c. **Muscularis propria (externa)**
  - The muscularis propria is a thick muscular layer that plays an important role in **intestinal motility** (e.g., peristalsis).
  - It is composed of **two muscle layers,** an inner circular layer and an outer longitudinal layer, that extend the entire length of the GI tract.

> **Anatomy note:** In the colon, the outer longitudinal muscle layer is discontinuous and clustered into three distinct strips called the **taeniae coli.**

  d. **Serosa (adventitia)**
  - This outermost layer is essentially a fibrous covering that is continuous with the peritoneal lining.
  - The serosa is not present in much of the esophagus, because the esophagus is extraperitoneal.

> **Clinical note:** Absence of the serosa from much of the esophagus may contribute to the tendency for esophageal cancers to spread locally before they are detected.

2. **Neural regulation of the gastrointestinal tract**
  a. **Enteric nervous system**
  - The enteric nervous system is contained entirely within the gut wall.
  - It is composed of the **submucosal plexus** and the **myenteric plexus.** These plexuses regulate entirely different aspects of intestinal activity, and they receive sensory information from the GI tract.
    (1) **Submucosal (Meissner's) plexus:** This is located between the muscularis mucosa and the muscularis propria. It gives rise to efferent fibers that synapse directly on mucosal epithelial cells. Therefore, it is involved mainly in coordinating activity of the mucosal layer. Stimulation of the submucosal plexus promotes digestion in part by stimulating secretions from the mucosal epithelium.

> **Clinical note:** In **Hirschsprung's disease** (aganglionic megacolon), the neural crest cells that form the myenteric plexus **fail to migrate** to the colon. Newborns with this condition are likely to be severely **constipated,** and imaging studies may reveal a massively **dilated colon.**

    (2) **Myenteric (Auerbach's) plexus:** This is situated between the inner circular and the outer longitudinal muscle layer of the muscularis propria. It is involved mainly in coordinating intestinal motility. Stimulation of the myenteric plexus increases intestinal motility mainly by stimulating peristalsis and also by inhibiting contraction of sphincter muscles throughout the intestinal tract.
  b. **Extrinsic regulation: autonomic nervous system** (Fig. 7-4)
  - The **parasympathetic nervous system** generally **promotes digestion and absorption** by stimulating GI secretions and peristalsis while inhibiting sphincter muscle contraction. In contrast, the **sympathetic nervous system** generally **inhibits digestion and absorption,** stimulates sphincter muscle contraction, and causes vasoconstriction in the splanchnic circulation (Table 7-1).

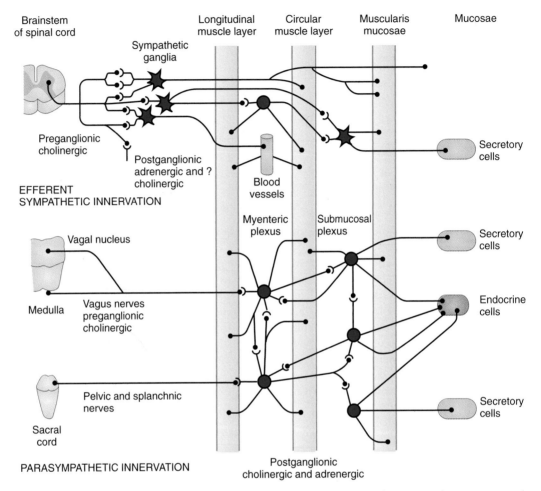

7-4: *Innervation of the gastrointestinal tract by the autonomic nervous system. The myenteric plexus synapses mainly on the inner circular and outer longitudinal muscles, whereas the submucosal plexus synapses mainly on the muscularis mucosae and epithelial cells of the mucosa.*

TABLE 7-1:
Effect of the Autonomic Nervous System on the Gastrointestinal Tract

Effect	Parasympathetic	Sympathetic
Motility	+	−
Sphincter tone	−	+
Secretion	+	−
Vasoconstriction	No effect	+

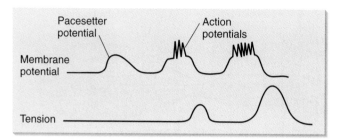

7-5: *Slow waves of the enteric nervous system. The tension occurs slightly after the action (spike) potentials, and the magnitude of the tension depends on the frequency of the spike potentials.*

> **Clinical note:** The parasympathetic nervous system stimulates intestinal motility by releasing acetylcholine onto neurons of the myenteric plexus. Therefore, cholinergic drugs should never be given to a patient if an intestinal obstruction is suspected. The resulting increase in pressure could rupture a viscus.

    c. **Anatomy of reflex loops**
- Local reflexes, such as the **gastrocolic reflex,** involve afferent and efferent arcs that are contained entirely within the enteric nervous system.
- **Vagovagal reflexes,** such as **receptive relaxation** of the stomach as it fills with food, involve afferent fibers from the gut that travel via the vagus nerve to the brainstem and then back to the gut.
- **Afferent fibers** from the gut may travel to the spinal cord (or sympathetic ganglia) and then back to the gut. Some of the afferent fibers that travel to the spinal cord synapse, directly or indirectly, on lower-order neurons of the anterolateral system and send pain signals to the brain. These afferent fibers that sense pain typically travel to the spinal cord together with the nerves of the sympathetic nervous system.

B. **Gastrointestinal functions**
  1. **Motility**
    a. **Electrical basis for intestinal motility: slow waves**
- Similar to cardiac nodal cells, intestinal smooth cells have a continually **changing resting membrane potential.** Rather than constantly generating action potentials, intestinal smooth muscle cells are subject to undulating oscillations in resting membrane potential. These **slow waves** have a resting membrane potential that varies between approximately -60 and -30 mV (Fig. 7-5).
- In the absence of spike potentials, the slow waves are **unable to elicit smooth muscle contractions,** except in the stomach. However, if the peak of the slow wave reaches the threshold potential, an action (**spike**) potential may be initiated, which then stimulates smooth muscle contraction. This **rhythmic contraction** results in the intermittent propulsion of intestinal contents toward the anus.

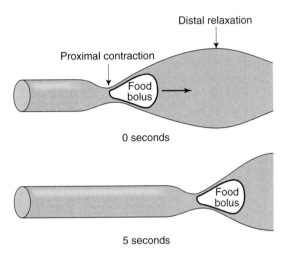

7-6: Peristalsis.

Clinical note: Patients with a long history of poorly controlled diabetes mellitus can sometimes develop severe gastric motility dysfunction, termed **"gastroparesis."** In diabetes, gastroparesis can occur as a result of **damage to the autonomic nerves supplying the stomach.** These patients may suffer from intractable **nausea** and **vomiting** because of the failure of the stomach to empty after a meal. In such patients, promotility agents such as **metoclopramide** can provide substantial symptomatic relief. A more aggressive option is to surgically implant a **gastric pacemaker,** although this is rarely done.

  b. **Types of contractions**
   • **Peristalsis:** Distention of the gut wall by a food bolus triggers reflexive contractions of smooth muscle (mainly the inner circular and outer longitudinal muscle layers) that **push the food bolus forward along the intestinal tract.** This forward propulsion requires smooth muscle contraction just proximal to the food bolus and simultaneous relaxation just distal to the food bolus (Fig. 7-6). The **myenteric plexus** is almost entirely responsible for **coordination of peristalsis.** In its absence, peristaltic contractions may be severely impaired or even absent.

   Pathology note: In a condition called **achalasia,** esophageal peristalsis is severely compromised because of damage to the myenteric plexus (see later discussion).

   • **Segmentation:** The primary function of segmentation is to assist digestion by promoting mixing of the intestinal contents (e.g., food, digestive enzymes, bile salts). This is achieved by simultaneous

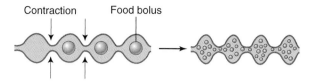

7-7: Segmentation.

TABLE 7-2:
Composition and Function of Saliva

Component	Primary Function
Potassium bicarbonate	Neutralizes bacterial acid, preventing digestion of tooth enamel and dentine (prevents cavities)
Lingual lipase	Initiates lipid digestion
Salivary amylase	Initiates carbohydrate digestion
Mucins	Lubrication of food bolus, primary determinant of viscosity
Lysozyme	Bacterial lysis
Immunoglobulins (IgA)	Immune protection

contractions both proximal and distal to the food bolus (Fig. 7-7). In contrast to peristalsis, segmentation does not result in forward propulsion of the food bolus.

- **Tonic contractions:** The tonic contractions of sphincter muscles throughout the intestinal tract separates different segments of the tract and **prevents premature passage of intestinal contents into the next segment.**

2. **Digestion**
   - Digestion entails the enzymatic hydrolysis of macromolecules (fats, carbohydrates, and proteins) into smaller compounds.
   - These can then be absorbed across the intestinal epithelial barrier.

3. **Absorption**
   - Absorption involves the transport of luminal substances across the mucosal barrier.
   - Absorption is facilitated by the large surface area of the mucosal epithelium, particularly in the small intestine.

II. **Salivation and Mastication**
   A. **Salivation**
      1. **Composition and functions of saliva**
         - Salivation plays several important roles in facilitating digestion in addition to its vital role in maintaining oral health (Table 7-2).

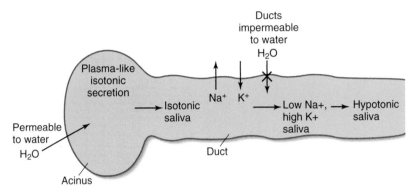

7-8: Saliva production.

Clinical note: Sjögren's syndrome is an autoimmune disorder characterized by lymphocytic infiltration of exocrine glands, mainly affecting the salivary and lacrimal glands. It is relatively common in the elderly (3% to 5% of people >60 years of age) and is characterized by dry mouth (**xerostomia**) and dry eyes (**keratoconjunctivitis sicca**). Low levels of saliva may cause dysphagia and increased dental caries; a deficiency in tear production may cause corneal ulceration and scarring. Pilocarpine, a muscarinic receptor agonist, is effective in increasing salivary production, and **artificial tears** can be used for treating dry eyes.

2. **Mechanism of saliva production**
   - Secretions from the salivary acinus are very similar in tonicity to plasma (i.e., they are isotonic).
   - However, as these secretions move along the salivary duct, **they are constantly modified.** The salivary ducts are relatively impermeable to water, and sodium is continually reabsorbed. Therefore, saliva is usually **hypotonic relative to plasma** by the time it is secreted (Fig. 7-8).
3. **Types of salivary glands**
   - There are two types of salivary glands: serous and mixed.
   - **Serous glands** (e.g., **parotid**), which are primarily composed of serous cells, secrete a nonviscous saliva containing water, electrolytes, and enzymes.
   - **Mixed glands (submandibular, sublingual),** which are composed of serous and mucous cells (Fig. 7-9), secrete a viscous saliva rich in mucin glycoproteins.
4. **Regulation of salivation**
   - Salivation is mainly controlled by the **autonomic nervous system.**
   - Both branches of the autonomic nervous system stimulate salivation, but the parasympathetic nervous system does so much more strongly than the sympathetic nervous system.

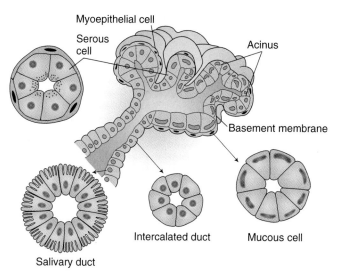

7-9: *Structure of a mixed salivary gland, showing both serous and mucous cells as well as contractile myoepithelial cells.*

Pharmacology note: The muscarinic acetylcholine receptor mediates the effects of the parasympathetic nervous system on the salivary glands. Blockade of this receptor can substantially decrease salivary secretions. This effect is associated with several classes of drugs, most notably **antimuscarinic drugs** (e.g., atropine, ipratropium), but also with drugs that have anticholinergic side effects, especially the antipsychotics and tricyclic antidepressants.

B. **Mastication**
- Mastication (chewing) is the first step in the breakdown of complex foodstuffs. It serves several important functions. Not only does it break large food pieces into smaller pieces, which increases the surface area available for digestion, but it also lubricates food with saliva, which makes the food more conducive to swallowing.
- The **muscles of mastication** are the **masseter, temporalis,** and **medial** and **lateral pterygoids.** They are all innervated by the mandibular division of the trigeminal nerve (cranial nerve V$_3$).

III. **Esophagus**
A. **Functional anatomy**
- The sphincter muscles, the upper and lower esophageal sphincters, are located at the top and bottom of the esophagus, respectively.
- Alternating contraction and relaxation of these sphincter muscles help coordinate movement of the food bolus from the pharynx to the stomach.

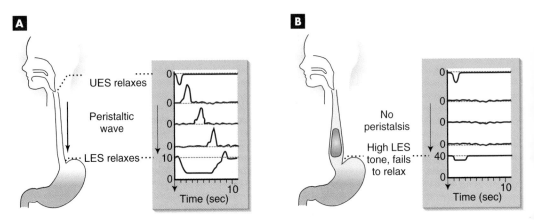

7-10: Pressure changes in the esophagus during swallowing. **A,** Normal pressure changes during peristalsis. There is decreased pressure in the lower esophagus because of relaxation of the lower esophageal sphincter (LES) (receptive relaxation). **B,** Abnormal pressure changes that occur in achalasia. UES, upper esophageal sphincter.

B. **Esophageal motility**
- Esophageal motility is under both voluntary and involuntary control. This reflects the differential distribution of striated and smooth muscle fiber throughout the esophagus.
- The upper third of the esophagus is composed of **striated muscle fibers,**
- The lower third is composed mainly of **smooth muscle fibers** that are controlled by nerve fibers from the myenteric (Auerbach's) plexus.
- The middle third is composed of a **mixture of striated and smooth muscle fibers.**
1. **Opening of the upper esophageal sphincter**
   - Relaxation of the upper esophageal sphincter **allows food to enter the esophagus** from the pharynx.
   - The sphincter then closes immediately after the food bolus passes to prevent reflux into the pharynx.
2. **Peristalsis: coordinated muscular contraction**
   - Swallowing or distention of the esophagus by a food bolus triggers a series of local reflexes, which result in coordinated esophageal contractions that move the food bolus toward the stomach.
   - **Primary peristalsis** is triggered by swallowing, whereas **secondary peristalsis** is triggered by esophageal distention.
3. **Opening of the lower esophageal sphincter**
   - When not eating, the lower esophageal sphincter (LES) is normally **tonically constricted,** in part because of the additional sphincteric pressure provided by the diaphragm. This helps prevent reflux of gastric contents into the esophagus.
   - When eating, the LES relaxes in response to **deglutition** (swallowing) and distention of the esophagus. This relaxation is mediated both by vagal stimulation and by some intrinsic properties of the LES (Fig. 7-10).

Pathology note: In a **sliding hiatal hernia,** the esophagogastric junction herniates upward through the **esophageal hiatus** in the diaphragm. This removes the contribution to LES tone provided by the diaphragm and **predisposes to reflux. In a rolling (paraesophageal) hiatal hernia,** the esophagogastric junction remains fixed in place and LES tone remains largely preserved. These patients therefore are less likely to suffer from reflux.

Clinical note: In **achalasia,** destruction of the myenteric plexus of the enteric nervous system causes dysregulation of esophageal smooth muscle activity. Pressure-recording studies (esophageal manometry) show decreased or **absent peristaltic activity** in the distal esophagus, **impaired LES relaxation,** and **increased LES pressure.** The result is that food cannot pass easily into the stomach. There may be difficulty swallowing (dysphagia), chest pain from esophageal distention, and frequent bouts of pneumonia from aspiration of esophageal contents. Achalasia is most commonly idiopathic, but it can also be seen in **Chagas' disease,** which is caused by infection with the protozoan parasite, *Trypanosoma cruzi* (found in South America). In Chagas' disease, the myenteric plexus of the colon may also be destroyed, causing **toxic megacolon.**

IV. **Stomach** (Fig. 7-11)
  - The stomach functions mainly as a "holding area" for food waiting to be digested in the small intestine.
  - It also prepares food for digestion in the small intestine by converting the food into chyme and then regulating the release of this chyme into the duodenum.
  A. **Gastric response to a meal: phases of digestion**
    - Multiple cues can **trigger** the stomach to prepare for the process of digestion.
    - In the **cephalic phase,** the sight or even the mere thought of food can stimulate gastric secretions.
    - In the **gastric** phase, after eating has begun, the presence of food in the stomach and the distention it causes can also stimulate gastric secretions.
    - In the **enteric** or **intestinal phase,** the entry of gastric contents into the small intestine stimulates the release of multiple factors, which then inhibit gastric activity.
  B. **"Receptive" relaxation of the stomach**
    - As the food bolus travels through the lower esophagus, the stomach reflexively begins to relax. This anticipatory relaxation is referred to as **receptive relaxation.**
    - This phenomenon allows the stomach to accept large amounts of food with only a minimal increase in gastric pressure; it also minimizes esophageal reflux.
    - **Note:** The stomach relaxes in response to **distention** of the stomach itself, which also allows the stomach to accept and to store larger quantities of food. This process is termed **"gastric accommodation."**

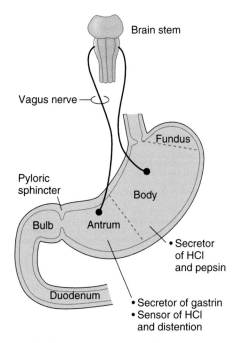

7-11: Functional anatomy of the stomach.

C. **Gastric cell types and their secretions**
  1. **Parietal cells** (Table 7-3)
     • Parietal cells secrete hydrogen ions, which creates a low gastric pH. This low pH serves many functions: it **denatures proteins, activates protein-digesting enzymes** such as pepsinogen, and creates a **harsh environment for bacterial growth.** Parietal cell activity is promoted by vagal stimulation (via acetylcholine) and by the hormones histamine and gastrin.
     • Parietal cells secrete intrinsic factor, which binds vitamin B_{12} in protein-rich foods such as meats to prevent its degradation in the small intestine and to allow absorption in the terminal ileum.

     > **Clinical note:** In **pernicious anemia,** autoimmune destruction of parietal cells results in the deficient secretion of **intrinsic factor** by parietal cells, causing impaired absorption of vitamin B_{12} (cobalamin). This produces a **macrocytic anemia,** because vitamin B_{12} is required for **DNA synthesis** in erythrocyte progenitor cells within the bone marrow.

     • Figure 7-12 shows how certain drugs regulate parietal cell activity.
     • Figure 7-13 shows the mechanism by which hydrogen ions are generated and secreted from parietal cells into the gastric lumen.
  2. **G cells**
     • G cells secrete the hormone **gastrin,** which promotes parietal cell activity.

TABLE 7-3:
Gastric Secretions

Secretion	Cell of Origin	Stimulus	Actions	Pathophysiology
Hydrochloric acid	Parietal	Parasympathetic innervation, histamine, gastrin	Converts pepsinogen to pepsin, denatures proteins, kills most bacteria	Excessive secretion due to gastrin-secreting tumor (Zollinger-Ellison syndrome) may lead to peptic ulcer disease Hypochlorhydria from atrophic gastritis → G cell hyperplasia; ↑ gastrin → ↑ risk of gastrinoma
Intrinsic factor	Parietal	Parasympathetic innervation, histamine, gastrin	Prevents vitamin B_{12} from degrading in small intestines (i.e., necessary for vitamin B_{12} absorption)	Destruction of parietal cells in pernicious anemia (atrophic gastritis) → vitamin B_{12} deficiency → macrocytic anemia
Mucus and HCO_3^-	Mucous	Prostaglandins	Protects gastric mucosa from low pH	NSAIDs → ↓ prostaglandins → ↓ activity of mucous cells → peptic ulcer disease
Pepsinogen	Chief	Ingestion of food	Digests proteins to peptides (major) and amino acids (minor)	
Gastrin	G cell	Food in stomach, particularly protein	Stimulates parietal cell activity, resulting in secretion of hydrochloric acid and intrinsic factor	May be elevated in Zollinger-Ellison syndrome or with prolonged administration of proton pump inhibitors such as omeprazole

NSAID, nonsteroidal anti-inflammatory drug.

- Gastrin release is stimulated mainly by the presence of **protein** in the stomach, and its secretion is controlled mainly by H^+ via feedback inhibition.

> **Clinical note:** In **atrophic gastritis,** many of the glands containing acid-secreting cells (parietal cells) are destroyed, thereby limiting the extent of gastric acidification (**achlorhydria**). This lack of acid production causes a loss of feedback inhibition of gastrin secretion. As a result, **hypergastrinemia often develops.**

3. **Chief cells**
   - Protein digestion (i.e., hydrolysis of proteins to peptides and amino acids) begins in the stomach because of the activity of chief cells (see Table 7-3).
   - These cells secrete the inactive precursor protein, pepsinogen, which is activated to the proteolytic enzyme, pepsin, in the presence of acid and/or small amounts of active **pepsin.** Pepsin functions optimally at a pH of approximately 2.

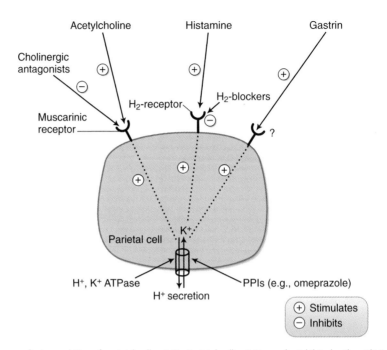

7-12: *Pharmacologic regulation of parietal cell activity. Parietal cell activity can be inhibited with antihistamines (H$_2$-blockers such as ranitidine) and anticholinergics (e.g., atropine). Proton pump inhibitors (PPIs such as omeprazole) inhibit the final common pathway of acid secretion in parietal cells (H$^+$,K$^+$-ATPase pump on the apical surface) and are the most potent agents for reducing gastric acid secretion. H$^+$,K$^+$-ATPase, hydrogen-potassium-adenosine triphosphatase pump.*

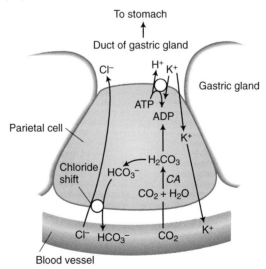

7-13: *Mechanism of secretion by parietal cells. Plasma CO$_2$ is generated within the parietal cells or diffuses into parietal cells, where it reacts with water to form HCO$_3^-$ and H$^+$ ions. H$^+$ ions are then secreted into the gastric lumen in exchange for K$^+$ ions, and HCO$_3^-$ diffuses from parietal cells into the plasma in exchange for chloride. This results in a brief "alkaline tide" after a meal. The reason that large meals do not precipitate a metabolic alkalosis is because these secretions are counteracted by the secretion of HCO$_3^-$ into the gut lumen by organs such as the pancreas. ADP, adenosine diphosphate; ATP, adenosine triphosphate; CA, carbonic anhydrase.*

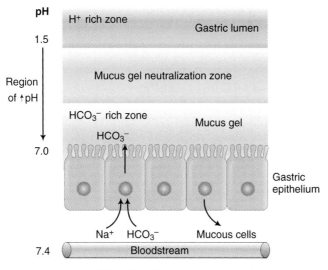

7-14: *Mucus-bicarbonate layer.*

4. **Mucous cells** (see Table 7-3)
   - If it were not for the protective activity of mucous cells, which secrete mucus and HCO_3^-, the low gastric pH would continually damage the gastric mucosa and predispose to ulcers.
   - The mucous layer protects the gastric mucosa by preventing "back-diffusion" of H^+ ions into the gastric mucosa (Fig. 7-14). Beneath this mucous layer, a layer rich in HCO_3^- neutralizes H^+ as it passes through the mucous barrier. In addition, the alkaline HCO_3^- layer prevents activation of any pepsinogen that "escapes" through the mucous layer.

   > **Clinical note:** Mucosal blood flow is highly dependent on the local production of prostaglandins. **Nonsteroidal anti-inflammatory drugs** (NSAIDs), such as aspirin, can impair mucosal blood flow by **inhibiting prostaglandin synthesis.** This compromises the protective abilities of the mucosa (mucus and HCO_3^- secretion) and can cause irritation of the mucosa (gastritis) or even ulceration (peptic ulcer disease).

D. **Gastric motility: regulation of gastric emptying**
   - Depending on the composition of the meal, food typically stays in the stomach for 3 to 6 hours. When the pyloric sphincter relaxes, chyme enters the duodenum.
   - Gastric motility and pyloric sphincter tone are primarily regulated by hormones produced in the small intestine. The production of these hormones is in turn somewhat dependent on the volume and composition of chyme entering the small intestine (e.g., high versus low fat content) (Table 7-4).

TABLE 7-4:
Hormones Produced in the Duodenum

Hormone	Structure of Origin	Primary Stimuli	Actions
Secretin	S cells	Acidic chyme entering duodenum	↓ Gastric emptying ↑ HCO_3^--rich secretion from ductal cells of pancreas to buffer acidic chyme
Cholecystokinin	I cells	Fatty acids	↑ Enzyme-rich secretion by pancreatic acinar cells ↑ Gallbladder contraction ↓ Tone of sphincter of Oddi ↓ Gastric emptying
Gastric inhibitory peptide	Mucosa	Carbohydrates, proteins, and fatty acids entering duodenum	↓ Gastric activity
Somatostatin	Mucosa (also δ cells of pancreas)	↓ pH of duodenum ↑ Levels of various gastrointestinal hormones	Various inhibitory actions

Clinical note: A normally functioning pyloric sphincter is tonically contracted and relaxes only periodically to allow small volumes of chyme to enter the duodenum. If the pyloric sphincter is incompetent, as is often caused by **gastric surgery,** large volumes of **hypertonic chyme** may enter the duodenum, resulting in massive loss of water from the circulation and the extracellular fluid. The ensuing **hypovolemia** may result in dizziness, tachycardia, sweating, flushing, and vasomotor collapse; this is called **dumping syndrome.** Symptoms occur shortly after eating. Treatment consists primarily of eating very small meals to limit the hyperosmolar load to the duodenum.

1. **Secretin**
   - The entry of acidic chyme into the small intestine stimulates the release of the hormone secretin from specialized S cells in the duodenum.
   - Secretin then stimulates the release of a **HCO_3^--rich secretion** from the ductal cells of the pancreas to neutralize the acidic chyme and to allow pancreatic digestive enzymes to function close to their pH optima. Secretin also stimulates the secretion of HCO_3^- by the duodenum and inhibits further gastric emptying.
2. **Cholecystokinin**
   - The entry of chyme that is abundant in fatty acids into the small intestine stimulates the release of the hormone cholecystokinin (CCK).
   - CCK then powerfully **inhibits relaxation** of the **pyloric sphincter** to prevent further gastric emptying. This occurs because fats require more time to digest than proteins or carbohydrates.

3. **Other hormones**
   - The hormone **gastric inhibitory peptide** is released in response to a variety of substances, particularly carbohydrates. It interferes with numerous aspects of gastric activity.
   - Likewise, the hormone **somatostatin,** which is released from the duodenal mucosa and pancreatic δ cells, globally inhibits gastric activity.

V. Pancreas

A. **Functional anatomy** (Fig. 7-15)
   - The pancreas is a retroperitoneal organ located behind the stomach.
   - Although the pancreas serves critical endocrine functions (e.g., regulation of plasma glucose), most of this organ is devoted to exocrine functions that are critical for the efficient digestion of macromolecules.

> **Anatomy note:** During embryologic development of the pancreas, the ventral and dorsal pancreatic buds may become abnormally **fused** as they rotate around the second part of the duodenum. If this occurs, it can cause **duodenal obstruction** and is termed **"annular pancreas."** Newborns with annular pancreas may present with **projectile vomiting** in the first few days of life. It is also a very rare cause of chronic pancreatitis in adults.

B. **Pancreatic secretions**
   - The exocrine secretions of the pancreas that ultimately drain into the small bowel are derived from two distinct cells, **ductal cells** and **acinar cells.**
   - Acinar secretions are enzyme-rich secretions that provide the enzymes necessary for digestion.
   - Ductal secretions are HCO_3^--rich and neutralize acidic chyme (Fig. 7-16).

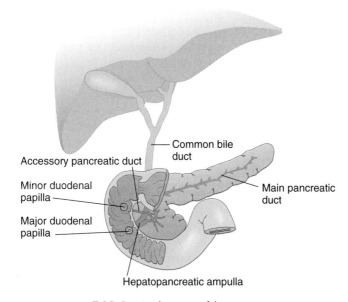

Accessory pancreatic duct

Common bile duct

Minor duodenal papilla

Major duodenal papilla

Main pancreatic duct

Hepatopancreatic ampulla

7-15: *Functional anatomy of the pancreas.*

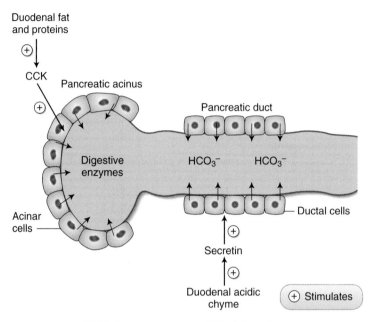

7-16: *Pancreatic secretions. CCK, cholecystokinin.*

C. **Pathophysiology**
  • With loss of pancreatic exocrine function, as may occur in **pancreatitis** or **pancreatic insufficiency,** fewer digestive enzymes are secreted, which impairs nutrient digestion and absorption.
  • The most common causes of pancreatitis are **alcohol abuse** and **gallstones.** Other well established but less common causes include **hypercalcemia, hypertriglyceridemia,** and various **drugs** such as azathioprine.

> **Pathology note:** In the genetic disease **cystic fibrosis,** thick secretions into the pancreatic duct may obstruct the duct and cause pancreatic insufficiency. Usually fat digestion is affected to the greatest extent, resulting in a fatty diarrhea (**steatorrhea**). These patients are often treated with supplementary pancreatic enzymes.

VI. **Liver and Biliary Tree**
  A. **Functional anatomy**
    • The functional anatomy of the liver and biliary tree is shown in Figure 7-17.
  B. **Gallbladder**
    • The gallbladder is involved in the digestion and absorption of dietary fats and the removal of waste products such as bilirubin and excess cholesterol.
    • The bile within the gallbladder serves several functions. Bile acids and bile salts, as well as lecithin, are important in the solubilization of cholesterol. An imbalance of these substances can produce cholesterol stones. In addition, bile

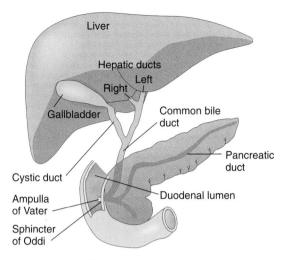

7-17: *Anatomy of the biliary tree.*

TABLE 7-5:
Composition and Function of Bile

Component	Function
Bile acids/bile salts	Emulsify fats to facilitate digestion by lipases Form micelles to deliver fatty acids to mucosal surface for absorption Solubilize cholesterol Cholesterol degradation product for elimination
Lecithin	Solubilizes cholesterol
Bilirubin	Forms waste product from metabolism of heme
Cholesterol	Effects waste elimination

acids and bile salts play a role in the formation of the lipid micelles, which enable fatty acid absorption across the intestinal mucosa (Table 7-5).

> **Clinical note:** When fatty acids enter the duodenum, they stimulate the release of CCK, which stimulates the gallbladder to contract and excrete bile into the small intestine and to inhibit gastric emptying. In **biliary dyskinesia,** the gallbladder does not contract effectively in response to CCK. Often, the symptoms of biliary dyskinesia and biliary obstruction by gallstones are similar.

C. **Enterohepatic circulation**
- The term "enterohepatic circulation" describes the **cycling** of substances **between the liver and intestinal tract;** it does not refer to a distinct anatomic circulation.

- For example, **bile salts** are synthesized by the liver and secreted into the duodenum. Most bile acids (>90%) are then reabsorbed in the terminal ileum and returned to the liver. The small percentage of bile acids that are not reabsorbed in the distal ileum are eliminated in the feces. This is the primary mechanism of excretion of excess **cholesterol.**

> **Clinical note: Bile-sequestering agents,** such as **cholestyramine,** act by preventing reabsorption of bile in the distal ileum, thereby depleting hepatic stores of bile acids. Because bile acids are synthesized from cholesterol, a compensatory hepatic synthesis of new bile acids necessitates increased uptake of plasma low-density lipoprotein (LDL) cholesterol by the liver, resulting in **decreased plasma LDL.** Unfortunately, inhibiting the actions of bile in the small intestines also leads to a reduced ability to digest fats, potentially resulting in **steatorrhea** and a **deficiency of fat-soluble vitamins.**

VII. **Small Intestine**
   A. **Functional anatomy**
      - The small intestine extends from the pylorus to the ileocecal valve and is composed of the duodenum, jejunum, and ileum.
      - Most absorption occurs in the duodenum and proximal jejunum, although important fat-soluble vitamins, bile acids, and vitamin B_{12} are absorbed in the distal ileum.
   B. **Digestion and absorption**
      1. **Carbohydrates** (Table 7-6)
         - Complex carbohydrates are long-chain polymers of simple sugars such as glucose. Complete degradation to the monosaccharides glucose, galactose, and fructose is necessary for absorption across the intestinal mucosa (Fig. 7-18).

TABLE 7-6:
Digestion and Absorption of the Major Fuels

Fuel	Enzymes Used in Digestion	Structural Form Absorbed	Comments
Proteins	Pepsin in stomach Protease in pancreas	Amino acids and small peptides	Small peptides broken down into amino acids in enterocytes
Carbohydrates	Amylase in saliva Amylase in pancreas Disaccharidases in intestinal mucosa	Monosaccharides	
Fats	Lipase in saliva and stomach Lipase/colipase in pancreas	Free fatty acids	Bile acids/salts emulsify for digestion and form micelles to facilitate absorption Resynthesized to triglycerides and packed into chylomicrons by enterocytes

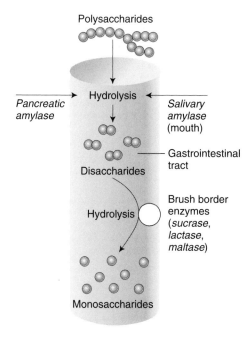

Polysaccharides

Pancreatic amylase

Hydrolysis

Salivary amylase (mouth)

Gastrointestinal tract

Disaccharides

Hydrolysis

Brush border enzymes (*sucrase*, *lactase*, *maltase*)

Monosaccharides

7-18: *Carbohydrate digestion.*

- Although this degradation begins in the mouth in the presence of salivary amylase, most carbohydrate digestion occurs in the small intestine via **pancreatic amylase.** Pancreatic amylase mainly breaks down carbohydrates to disaccharides, which are then further hydrolyzed to monosaccharides by intestinal brush border enzymes (**disaccharidases**) such as sucrase, lactase, and maltase.

  Clinical note: In disaccharidase-deficient states, such as **lactase deficiency,** the osmotically active disaccharide lactose is delivered to the colon, where it is **fermented by colonic bacteria** to produce gases such as hydrogen and carbon dioxide. Symptoms include flatulence, bloating, cramping, and diarrhea.

  Pharmacology note: Carbohydrate digestion can be intentionally impaired in patients with diabetes mellitus by α-**glucosidase inhibitors** such as **acarbose.** These drugs competitively inhibit intestinal enzymes such as sucrase, maltase, and amylase, thus impairing carbohydrate digestion and therefore intestinal glucose absorption. Reduced intestinal absorption of glucose facilitates **glucose control** in diabetes. However, because carbohydrates remain in the gut, these drugs typically cause adverse effects such as **flatulence, nausea,** and **diarrhea.**

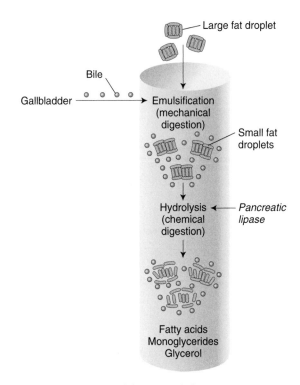

7-19: *Lipid digestion and absorption.*

2. **Proteins** (see Table 7-6)
   - Protein digestion begins in the stomach because of the acidic pH and the presence of the enzyme pepsin, but most protein digestion occurs in the small intestine. By neutralizing the acidic chyme, the HCO_3^--rich ductal secretions allow the pancreatic proteases to function optimally in degrading proteins and large peptides into small peptides and amino acids.
   - Products of protein digestion are absorbed as small peptides (major) and free amino acids (minor) via cotransport with Na^+ into enterocytes. In the cytoplasm of enterocytes, the peptides are degraded to amino acids, which then enter the portal blood destined for the liver.
   - **Note:** The gastric contribution to protein digestion is so minor that even patients with **achlorhydria** (such as in patients with pernicious anemia or in those taking protein pump inhibitors such as omeprazole) have no observable impairment of protein assimilation.
3. **Lipids** (Fig. 7-19; see Table 7-6)
   - In most people, with the possible exception of vegetarians, intake of fats (lipids) is in the form of **triglycerides.**
   - Most triglyceride digestion occurs in the small intestine, although a small amount (no more than 10%) occurs in the mouth (due to **lingual lipase**) and stomach (due to **gastric lipase**).

a. **Digestion**
  - In the presence of bile and the phospholipid lecithin, mechanical mixing in the stomach and small intestine converts large lipid droplets to much smaller lipid globules by the process of **emulsification.** This process markedly increases the surface area for water-soluble digestive enzymes such as pancreatic lipase.
  - Pancreatic lipase (and colipase) then hydrolyzes triglycerides into free fatty acids and monoglycerides. Micelles formed by bile salts then efficiently absorb these free fatty acids. This is a critical step in fat digestion, because the free fatty acids and monoglycerides would otherwise rapidly recombine to form triglycerides, which are unable to diffuse across the intestinal mucosa.
b. **Absorption**
  - Once lipids in the form of fatty acids and monoglycerides are absorbed across the intestinal mucosa, they are reesterified to produce triglycerides.
  - The triglycerides are then packaged as **chylomicrons** and transported through the intestinal **lymphatics** to the **thoracic duct,** not the portal vein.

> **Pathology note:** In **celiac sprue** (celiac disease), massive **loss of intestinal surface area** occurs because of a hypersensitivity reaction to the **gliadin** component of the protein gluten, found in grains such as wheat. This hypersensitivity reaction results in **autoimmune destruction** of intestinal villi, which causes **malabsorption** of numerous nutrients and predisposition to a variety of nutrient deficiency diseases. Patients with celiac sprue may respond dramatically to elimination of gluten from the diet.

4. **Absorption of other substances**
  a. **Sodium**
    - The intestinal lumen–intracellular sodium gradient can be used to drive absorption of numerous substances, including glucose, amino acids, dipeptides, and water-soluble vitamins (Fig. 7-20).
  b. **Vitamin B_{12} (cobalamin)**
    - Vitamin B_{12} complexes with R protein in the mouth and with intrinsic factor in the stomach. It is then absorbed in the distal ileum of the small intestine.
    - **Note:** Patients with disease of the distal ileum (e.g., **Crohn's disease**) are likely to have impaired intestinal absorption of vitamin B_{12}.

> **Clinical note:** Disease involvement of the distal ileum can also impair reabsorption of bile salts, resulting in fat malabsorption (**steatorrhea**) as well as impaired absorption of the **fat-soluble vitamins** (vitamins A, D, E, and K).

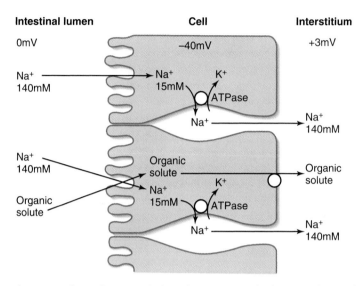

Intestinal lumen	Cell	Interstitium

7-20: *Sodium absorption in the small intestine. The luminal concentration of sodium is much larger than the intracellular concentration because of the continual activity of the basolateral Na^+,K^+-ATPase pumps. Sodium entry can therefore be coupled to entry of a wide variety of organic solutes, including glucose, hexoses, dipeptides, amino acids, and water-soluble vitamins.*

   c. **Iron**
- Dietary iron is released in relatively large amounts after the digestion of proteins such as myoglobin and hemoglobin, which are particularly **abundant in meats.** It is absorbed primarily in the duodenum and proximal jejunum.
- After absorption, iron is transported in plasma bound to **transferrin** and stored within cells as **ferritin.**

> **Clinical note:** Iron is essential for the production of red blood cells within the bone marrow (erythropoiesis). A **deficiency of iron** may therefore result in **impaired erythropoiesis** and a **microcytic anemia.** The term "microcytic" refers to the small size of the red blood cells, which results from a lack of hemoglobin within the cytoplasm. Patients susceptible to iron deficiency anemia include **premenopausal women** with heavy menstrual bleeding, **vegetarians** with limited dietary intake, and patients with **chronic blood loss** (e.g., intestinal bleeding from an ulcer or colon cancer).

C. **Motility: migrating myoelectric complex**
- During the **interdigestive period,** a pattern of motor activity functions to clear food debris from the intestinal tract, including the stomach, small intestine, and large intestine. Bursts of peristalsis occur at 90-minute intervals during fasting. The hormone **motilin,** secreted by duodenal mucosa, is thought to play an important role in this process.

- The migrating myoelectric complex is characterized by three phases:
  (1) **Phase I:** long period in which peristalsis is absent
  (2) **Phase II:** sporadic contractions
  (3) **Phase III:** short period of intense peristalsis to clear the lumen of debris

> **Pharmacology note:** The antibiotic **erythromycin,** sometimes known as "erythroterrible," has frequent side effects (e.g., nausea, diarrhea) associated with the GI system. Indeed, it is sometimes used specifically because of these side effects; for example, as a laxative in adults. It is believed to produce these effects by stimulating the motilin receptor. Erythromycin is also implicated as a cause of **hypertrophic pyloric stenosis.** Infants who are given the drug orally have about a 10-fold increased risk of developing hypertrophic pyloric stenosis.

D. **Reflexes**
  - Gastric and/or duodenal distention after a meal stimulates various reflexes. These reflexes are controlled entirely by the **enteric nervous system,** as shown by their continuation after **autonomic denervation.**
  - Perhaps the best known is the **gastrocolic reflex,** which results from distention of the stomach, causing mass movements after meals.
  - The **gastroileal** (gastroenteric) **reflex** promotes passage of intestinal contents from the small intestine into the colon by stimulating intestinal peristalsis and relaxation (opening) of the ileocecal valve.
  - The **enterogastric reflex,** which is triggered by the entry of acidic chyme into the duodenum, inhibits further gastric emptying.

VIII. **Large Intestine**
  A. **Functional anatomy** (Fig. 7-21)

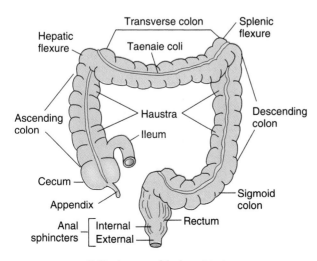

7-21: Anatomy of the large intestine.

TABLE 7-7:
Structural Comparison of Small and Large Intestines

Characteristic	Small Intestine	Large Intestine
Plicae circularis	+	–
Villi	+	–
Microvilli	+	Fewer in number
Glycocalyx	+	+
Peyer's patches	+ (Ileum)	–
Brunner's glands	+ (Duodenum)	–
Outer longitudinal muscle	Continuous sheet	Arranged as taeniae coli

- The large intestine has much less mucosal surface area available for absorption than does the small intestine, reflecting the absence of villi and fewer microvilli on epithelial cells (Table 7-7).
- The main functions of the colon are **absorption of salt and water** and **storage** and **elimination of feces.** Initially, the fecal contents in the right colon are fairly liquid; they gradually become more solid as they move through the large intestine.

B. **Electrolyte movements**
  1. **Sodium**
     - Absorption of sodium by the large intestine is very efficient.
     - **Aldosterone** and high doses of **glucocorticoids** increase sodium absorption and potassium secretion.
  2. **Bicarbonate and potassium**
     - The colon actively secretes bicarbonate. Therefore, a patient with diarrhea may lose large amounts of **bicarbonate** and have a **metabolic acidosis.**
     - The colon also secretes potassium, so large volumes of diarrhea can also precipitate **hypokalemia.**

C. **Defecation reflex**
   - When the rectum becomes distended with feces, it initiates a spinal reflex that causes relaxation of the internal and external anal sphincters.
   - Fortunately, we can consciously override the relaxation of the external anal sphincter when we wish to.

Common Laboratory Values

Test	Conventional Units	SI Units
Blood, Plasma, Serum		
Alanine aminotransferase (ALT, GPT at 30°C)	8–20 U/L	8–20 U/L
Amylase, serum	25–125 U/L	25–125 U/L
Aspartate aminotransferase (AST, GOT at 30°C)	8–20 U/L	8–20 U/L
Bilirubin, serum (adult): total; direct	0.1–1.0 mg/dL; 0.0–0.3 mg/dL	2–17 μmol/L; 0–5 μmol/L
Calcium, serum (Ca^{2+})	8.4–10.2 mg/dL	2.1–2.8 mmol/L
Cholesterol, serum	Rec: <200 mg/dL	<5.2 mmol/L
Cortisol, serum	8:00 AM: 6–23 μg/dL; 4:00 PM: 3–15 μg/dL	170–630 nmol/L; 80–410 nmol/L
	8:00 PM: ≤50% of 8:00 AM	Fraction of 8:00 AM: ≤0.50
Creatine kinase, serum	Male: 25–90 U/L	25–90 U/L
	Female: 10–70 U/L	10–70 U/L
Creatinine, serum	0.6–1.2 mg/dL	53–106 μmol/L
Electrolytes, serum		
Sodium (Na^+)	136–145 mEq/L	135–145 mmol/L
Chloride (Cl^-)	95–105 mEq/L	95–105 mmol/L
Potassium (K^+)	3.5–5.0 mEq/L	3.5–5.0 mmol/L
Bicarbonate (HCO_3^-)	22–28 mEq/L	22–28 mmol/L
Magnesium (Mg^{2+})	1.5–2.0 mEq/L	1.5–2.0 mmol/L
Estriol, total, serum (in pregnancy)		
24–28 wk; 32–36 wk	30–170 ng/mL; 60–280 ng/mL	104–590 nmol/L; 208–970 nmol/L
28–32 wk; 36–40 wk	40–220 ng/mL; 80–350 ng/mL	140–760 nmol/L; 280–1210 nmol/L
Ferritin, serum	Male: 15–200 ng/mL	15–200 μg/L
	Female: 12–150 ng/mL	12–150 μg/L
Follicle-stimulating hormone, serum/plasma (FSH)	Male: 4–25 mIU/mL	4–25 U/L
	Female:	
	Premenopause, 4–30 mIU/mL	4–30 U/L
	Midcycle peak, 10–90 mIU/mL	10–90 U/L
	Postmenopause, 40–250 mIU/mL	40–250 U/L
Gases, arterial blood (room air)		
pH	7.35–7.45	[H^+] 36–44 nmol/L
PCO_2	33–45 mm Hg	4.4–5.9 kPa
PO_2	75–105 mm Hg	10.0–14.0 kPa
Glucose, serum	Fasting: 70–110 mg/dL	3.8–6.1 mmol/L
	2 hr postprandial: <120 mg/dL	<6.6 mmol/L
Growth hormone–arginine stimulation	Fasting: <5 ng/mL	<5 μg/L
	Provocative stimuli: >7 ng/mL	>7 μg/L

Test	Conventional Units	SI Units
Blood, Plasma, Serum—cont'd		
Immunoglobulins, serum		
IgA	76–390 mg/dL	0.76–3.90 g/L
IgE	0–380 IU/mL	0–380 kIU/L
IgG	650–1500 mg/dL	6.5–15 g/L
IgM	40–345 mg/dL	0.4–3.45 g/L
Iron	50–170 µg/dL	9–30 µmol/L
Lactate dehydrogenase, serum	45–90 U/L	45–90 U/L
Luteinizing hormone, serum/ plasma (LH)	Male: 6–23 mIU/mL	6–23 U/L
	Female:	
	Follicular phase, 5–30 mIU/mL	5–30 U/L
	Midcycle, 75–150 mIU/mL	75–150 U/L
	Postmenopause, 30–200 mIU/mL	30–200 U/L
Osmolality, serum	275–295 mOsm/kg	275–295 mOsm/kg
Parathyroid hormone, serum, N-terminal	230–630 pg/mL	230–630 ng/L
Phosphatase (alkaline), serum (p-NPP at 30°C)	20–70 U/L	20–70 U/L
Phosphorus (inorganic), serum	3.0–4.5 mg/dL	1.0–1.5 mmol/L
Prolactin, serum (hPRL)	<20 ng/mL	<20 µg/L
Proteins, serum		
Total (recumbent)	6.0–8.0 g/dL	60–80 g/L
Albumin	3.5–5.5 g/dL	35–55 g/L
Globulin	2.3–3.5 g/dL	23–35 g/L
Thyroid-stimulating hormone, serum or plasma (TSH)	0.5–5.0 µU/mL	0.5–5.0 mU/L
Thyroidal iodine (^{123}I) uptake	8–30% of administered dose/24 hr	0.08–0.30/24 hr
Thyroxine (T_4), serum	4.5–12 µg/dL	58–154 nmol/L
Triglycerides, serum	35–160 mg/dL	0.4–1.81 mmol/L
Triiodothyronine (T_3), serum (RIA)	115–190 ng/dL	1.8–2.9 nmol/L
Triiodothyronine (T_3) resin uptake	25–38%	0.25–0.38
Urea nitrogen, serum (BUN)	7–18 mg/dL	1.2–3.0 mmol urea/L
Uric acid, serum	3.0–8.2 mg/dL	0.18–0.48 mmol/L
Cerebrospinal Fluid		
Cell count	0–5 cells/mm^3	0–5 × 10^6/L
Chloride	118–132 mEq/L	118–132 mmol/L
Gamma globulin	3–12% total proteins	0.03–0.12
Glucose	50–75 mg/dL	2.8–4.2 mmol/L
Pressure	70–180 mm H$_2$O	70–180 mm H$_2$O
Proteins, total	<40 mg/dL	<0.40 g/L
Hematology		
Bleeding time (template)	2–7 min	2–7 min
Erythrocyte count	Male: 4.3–5.9 million/mm^3	4.3–5.9 × 10^{12}/L
	Female: 3.5–5.5 million/mm^3	3.5–5.5 × 10^{12}/L
Erythrocyte sedimentation rate (Westergren)	Male: 0–15 mm/hr	0–15 mm/hr
	Female: 0–20 mm/hr	0–20 mm/hr
Hematocrit (Hct)	Male: 40–54%	0.40–0.54
	Female: 37–47%	0.37–0.47

Test	Conventional Units	SI Units
Hematology—cont'd		
Hemoglobin A$_{1C}$	≤6%	≤ 0.06%
Hemoglobin, blood (Hb)	Male: 13.5–17.5 g/dL	2.09–2.71 mmol/L
	Female: 12.0–16.0 g/dL	1.86–2.48 mmol/L
Hemoglobin, plasma	1–4 mg/dL	0.16–0.62 mmol/L
Leukocyte count and differential		
Leukocyte count	4500–11,000/mm^3	4.5–11.0 × 10^9/L
Segmented neutrophils	54–62%	0.54–0.62
Bands	3–5%	0.03–0.05
Eosinophils	1–3%	0.01–0.03
Basophils	0–0.75%	0–0.0075
Lymphocytes	25–33%	0.25–0.33
Monocytes	3–7%	0.03–0.07
Mean corpuscular hemoglobin (MCH)	25.4–34.6 pg/cell	0.39–0.54 fmol/cell
Mean corpuscular hemoglobin concentration (MCHC)	31–37% Hb/cell	4.81–5.74 mmol Hb/L
Mean corpuscular volume (MCV)	80–100 μm^3	80–100 fl
Partial thromboplastin time (activated) (aPTT)	25–40 sec	25–40 sec
Platelet count	150,000–400,000/mm^3	150–400 × 10^9/L
Prothrombin time (PT)	12–14 sec	12–14 sec
Reticulocyte count	0.5–1.5% of red cells	0.005–0.015
Thrombin time	<2 sec deviation from control	<2 sec deviation from control
Volume		
Plasma	Male: 25–43 mL/kg	0.025–0.043 L/kg
	Female: 28–45 mL/kg	0.028–0.045 L/kg
Red cell	Male: 20–36 mL/kg	0.020–0.036 L/kg
	Female: 19–31 mL/kg	0.019–0.031 L/kg
Sweat		
Chloride	0–35 mmol/L	0–35 mmol/L
Urine		
Calcium	100–300 mg/24 hr	2.5–7.5 mmol/24 hr
Creatinine clearance	Male: 97–137 mL/min	
	Female: 88–128 mL/min	
Estriol, total (in pregnancy)		
30 wk	6–18 mg/24 hr	21–62 μmol/24 hr
35 wk	9–28 mg/24 hr	31–97 μmol/24 hr
40 wk	13–42 mg/24 hr	45–146 μmol/24 hr
17-Hydroxycorticosteroids	Male: 3.0–9.0 mg/24 hr	8.2–25.0 μmol/24 hr
	Female: 2.0–8.0 mg/24 hr	5.5–22.0 μmol/24 hr
17-Ketosteroids, total	Male: 8–22 mg/24 hr	28–76 μmol/24 hr
	Female: 6–15 mg/24 hr	21–52 μmol/24 hr
Osmolality	50–1400 mOsm/kg	
Oxalate	8–40 μg/mL	90–445 μmol/L
Proteins, total	<150 mg/24 hr	<0.15 g/24 hr

questions

DIRECTIONS: Each numbered item or incomplete statement is followed by options arranged in alphabetical or logical order. Select the best answer to each question. Some options may be partially correct, but there is only **ONE BEST** answer.

1. A patient with biliary obstruction and steatorrhea would most likely be deficient in which of the following compounds?
   A. Vitamin C
   B. Vitamin K
   C. Iron
   D. Vitamin B_{12}
   E. Intrinsic factor

2. Hypertensive patients who receive transplanted kidneys from normotensive donors often remain normotensive after the surgery. Which of the following is the most likely explanation of the normalization of blood pressure in these transplant recipients?
   A. Hypoaldosteronism due to immunosuppression
   B. Loss of sympathetic nerve supply to kidneys
   C. Central role of kidneys in long-term blood pressure control
   D. Immune reaction to kidney transplant
   E. Normal stress response after surgery

3. A 69-year-old woman with a history of smoking two packs of cigarettes per day for the past 30 years notes a several-year history of worsening dyspnea with exertion. Pulmonary function testing reveals a reduced ratio of 1-second forced expiratory volume to forced vital capacity (FEV_1/FVC), increased lung volumes (residual volume, functional reserve capacity [FRC], and total lung capacity), and reduced carbon monoxide diffusing capacity. Specialized laboratory testing reveals a deficiency in plasma α_1-antitrypsin. Which of the following best describes normal tidal inspiration in this patient?
   A. Begins at an increased FRC relative to a normal subject
   B. Requires a more negative intrapleural pressure
   C. Involves increased use of internal intercostals
   D. Increased size of FRC means tidal volume can decrease.

4. A 25-year-old man complains of fatigue, occasional bloody stools, and frequent nosebleeds. His mother also suffered from frequent nosebleeds. Physical examination reveals multiple telangiectasias in the oral cavity but is otherwise unremarkable. Laboratory analysis reveals normal prothrombin and partial thromboplastin times and a hemoglobin level of 12 g/dL. Biopsy of the mucous membranes reveals dilated and tortuous blood vessels with very thin walls. Which of the following disorders does this patient most likely have?
   A. Idiopathic thrombocytopenic purpura
   B. Iron deficiency anemia
   C. Cushing's syndrome
   D. Osler-Weber-Rendu disease
   E. Hemolytic uremic syndrome
   F. Celiac disease

5. During an ascent to high altitude, a mountain climber notes that he has a headache. He descends about 2000 m, but the headache remains, although his respiratory rate declines from 25 to 15 breaths per minute. He is taking acetazolamide. Which of the following sentences most accurately describes the physiologic events that may occur at high altitude?
   A. Low blood viscosity is a stronger stimulus for erythropoietin release than hypoxia.
   B. High-altitude pulmonary edema (HAPE) is caused by increased venous pressure.
   C. Cardiac output is diminished at high altitude.
   D. Low atmospheric pressure is the predominant reason for hypocapnia.
   E. Both cerebral and pulmonary edema may occur.

6. The filtration fraction at the glomerulus in a healthy person is approximately 20% of renal plasma flow. Which of the following is normally the most important factor inhibiting filtration at the glomerus.
   A. Glomerular capillary hydrostatic pressure
   B. Bowman's oncotic pressure
   C. Tubuloglomerular feedback
   D. Glomerular capillary oncotic pressure
   E. Bowman's hydrostatic pressure

7. Digitalis, a drug used in the treatment of heart failure, produces its therapeutic effect by inhibition of the sodium-potassium-adenosine triphosphatase (Na^+,K^+-ATPase) pump. Which of the following effects does this inhibition have on the cell?
   A. Increased intracellular potassium concentration
   B. Increased excitability of nerve cells
   C. Decreased intracellular volume
   D. Decreased intracellular sodium concentration
   E. Depolarization of the membrane potential

8. A 65-year-old man is referred to an endocrinologist after his wife notes his increasingly coarse facial features and enlarging hands and feet over the years. The man, who has recently been diagnosed with diabetes, is found to have acromegaly. Which of the following substances will reduce the secretion of growth hormone in this patient?
   A. Insulin
   B. Arginine
   C. Sulfonylurea drugs
   D. Somatostatin
   E. Glucose

9. An 18-year-old male track athlete is warming up for his next race after having eaten a cheeseburger 1 hour earlier. Once the race starts, stimulation of his sympathetic nervous system will result in what response by his digestive system?
   A. Segmental contractions of the proximal colon
   B. Increased rate of gastric emptying
   C. Relaxation of the pyloric sphincter
   D. Inhibition of gut motility and secretory activities
   E. Stimulation of gut motility and secretory activities

10. A 68-year-old patient with severe aortic stenosis is experiencing increasingly severe anginal pain with exertion. He is normotensive, and a recent cardiac catheterization revealed normal coronary arteries. Which of the following physiologic alterations would mostly likely reduce the severity of angina in this patient?
   A. Increasing contractility with epinephrine to increase cardiac output
   B. Increasing diastolic pressures without changing systolic pressures
   C. Increasing preload by means of volume transfusions
   D. Diuresis
   E. Coronary angioplasty

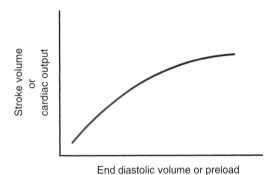

End diastolic volume or preload

11. A 63-year-old woman with a history of vasovagal syncope and atrial fibrillation is admitted to the cardiac floor for observation and cardiac testing after complaints of chest pain and malaise. Cardiac performance testing yields the ventricular function curve shown in the accompanying figure. Assuming no change in afterload, a shift of the curve to the left is most likely to indicate which of the following conditions in this patient?
A. Congestive heart failure
B. Greater stroke work capability for a given preload
C. Increased duration of isometric contraction
D. Increased release of acetylcholine at the sinoatrial node
E. Decreased ventricular ejection fraction

12. The drug verapamil is a calcium channel blocker that reduces the heart rate by antagonizing calcium channels in nodal tissue; it also blocks calcium channels on ventricular myocytes, reducing calcium entry during the plateau of the action potential. Which of the following combination of effects is most likely to occur with administration of verapamil?
A. Decreased preload and contractility
B. Decreased preload and increased contractility
C. Increased preload and decreased contractility
D. Increased preload and contractility

13. The height of the column of blood in the easily identifiable external jugular vein can be used clinically as a rough estimate of right atrial pressure. Deep inspiration results in which of the following consequences?
A. Decreased velocity of blood in the superior vena cava
B. Increased right ventricular stroke volume
C. A rise in the jugular venous column
D. Decreased runoff in the pulmonary artery
E. Increased intrathoracic pressure

14. A 17-year-old female cross-country runner comes to the emergency department with acute-onset shortness of breath and chest discomfort. A chest radiograph confirms the clinical suspicion of a tension pneumothorax. Her blood pressure on arrival is documented at 88/56 mm Hg. Which of the following factors is most likely responsible for the hypotension in this setting?
A. Reduced heart rate
B. Decreased venous return
C. Cardiac tamponade
D. Hypoxemia
E. Hemorrhage

15. A 77-year-old man is evaluated following a fall in which he sustained a forehead laceration. He states that for the last 3 days he has been bumping into furniture with the right side of his body, but he has had no problems with his left side or when staring straight ahead (i.e., macular sparing). An MRI of the brain would most likely show a lesion involving which of the following structures?
A. Left optic nerve
B. Optic chiasm
C. Left optic tract
D. Right optic tract
E. Left geniculocalcarine tract

16. A 70-year-old retired Navy plumber is evaluated for worsening dyspnea. Pulmonary function testing reveals an increased ratio of 1-second forced expiratory volume to forced vital capacity (FEV_1/FVC) of 85% and reduced lung volumes. Arterial blood gas analysis reveals an oxygen tension (PaO_2) of 90 mm Hg and a carbon dioxide tension ($PaCO_2$) of 40 mm Hg. Exercise causes hypoxemia in this patient, most likely through which of the following mechanisms?

A. Increased ratio of residual volume (RV) to total lung capacity (TLC)
B. Increased ventilation/perfusion (V/Q) ratio in the apical lung
C. Diffusion impairment
D. Oxygen desaturation of hemoglobin
E. Hypoventilation

17. A 55-year-old woman with rheumatoid arthritis who is taking penicillamine and ibuprofen is diagnosed with the nephrotic syndrome after a workup for lower extremity edema reveals large amounts of protein in her urine. Although the forces promoting filtration across the glomerulus are altered in this patient, which of the following Starling forces is normally the controlling factor favoring filtration?
A. Glomerular capillary oncotic pressure
B. Hydrostatic pressure in Bowman's space
C. Oncotic pressure in Bowman's space
D. Glomerular capillary hydrostatic pressure

18. An elderly patient comes in for evaluation after several weeks of progressively worsening fatigue, weakness, and shortness of breath with exertion. She also notes a sore tongue. She eats well (her daughter cooks for her). She appears pale and has a shiny, swollen, and "beefy"-appearing tongue. Neurologic examination shows decreased proprioception and vibratory sensation of both lower extremities. Laboratory analysis shows a macrocytic anemia. This woman most likely has which of the following disorders?
A. Anemia of folate deficiency
B. Pernicious anemia
C. Hemolytic anemia
D. Iron deficiency anemia
E. Anemia of chronic disease

19. Cardiac output is evaluated during cardiac catheterization in a 56-year-old man with congestive heart failure. Analysis of mixed venous blood from the right atrium shows an oxygen concentration of 15 mL/dL, whereas a sample of arterial blood from the brachial artery has an oxygen concentration of 20 mL/dL. Oxygen

consumption is measured by analysis of expired gas at a rate of 200 mL oxygen per minute. What is the cardiac output in this patient?
A. 1 L/minute
B. 3 L/minute
C. 4 L/minute
D. 5 L/minute
E. 10 L/minute

20. A 28-year-old woman has an episode of supraventricular tachycardia, which is terminated by applying pressure to the carotid sinus (a vagal maneuver). Vagal stimulation reduces firing frequency in nodal tissues by which of the following mechanisms?
A. Making the maximum diastolic potential more negative
B. Reducing the rate of depolarization of the nodal cells
C. Increasing the threshold for action potential generation
D. All of the above

21. A 52-year-old morbidly obese man is diagnosed with type 2 diabetes after an evaluation for worsening fatigue reveals retinopathy, proteinuria, and a random plasma glucose concentration of 220 mg/dL. A sulfonylurea drug is prescribed. Which of the following statements best describes the mechanism by which this group of drugs helps to treat diabetes?
A. Decreased glucose uptake in muscle
B. Increased insulin sensitivity in the peripheral tissues such as muscle, adipose tissue, and liver
C. Decreased glucose absorption at the brush border
D. Inhibition of hepatic glucose secretion
E. Increased insulin secretion

22. A 71-year-old man, who is recovering from a myocardial infarction sustained 2 days earlier, complains of severe dyspnea. Urine output is noted to be low at 125 mL/day, and plasma levels of atrial natriuretic factor (ANF) are elevated.

Which of the following drugs may be the most appropriate for treating his acute symptoms?
A. Thiazide diuretic
B. Angiotensin-converting enzyme (ACE) inhibitor
C. Potassium-sparing diuretic
D. β-Blocker
E. Loop diuretic

23. A 15-year-old girl with epilepsy undergoes surgery to remove a brain lesion thought to be precipitating her seizures. During recovery the seizures stop, but the girl complains of stomach pain, cramping, and a sense of nausea. Her stool is positive for blood, and radiologic imaging reveals severe duodenal ulceration. If this girl undergoes surgical resection of the duodenum, which of the following functions will be lost?
A. Only those pancreatic secretions controlled by secretin and cholecystokinin (CCK)
B. Contraction of the gallbladder
C. Migrating myoelectric complex
D. Ability to secrete gastrin
E. Ability to secrete secretin and CCK

24. A 58-year-old man with coronary artery disease is found to have a left bundle branch block on electrocardiography, so conduction through the left bundle branch is delayed. Which of the following abnormal auscultatory findings would most likely be caused by this condition?
A. Physiologic inspiratory split of S_2
B. Systolic murmur
C. Paradoxical split of S_2
D. Diastolic murmur

25. A 52-year-old woman complains of dark-appearing urine. She also states that she has been urinating more frequently over the past few months. Urinalysis reveals significant proteinuria and hematuria. Serum creatinine is 1.6 (normal 0.5–1.2). Ultrasound reveals bilaterally enlarged kidneys with multiple cysts. In addition to management of her present symptoms, what other possible diagnosis should be ruled out?
A. Hypertension in upper limbs and hypotension in lower limbs

B. Ventricular septal defect
C. End-systolic click
D. Intracranial berry aneurysm
E. Recent *Streptococcus viridans* infection

26. A 50-year-old woman with a history of severe osteoarthritis of her knees and hands presents with complaints of abdominal pain. The history reveals chronic use of aspirin and nonsteroidal anti-inflammatory drugs (NSAIDs). Upper endoscopy reveals diffuse gastritis but no obvious ulcerations. Chronic use of aspirin and NSAIDs increase the risk of gastritis by causing which of the following effects?
A. Inhibited secretion of gastric mucus and bicarbonate
B. Inhibited secretion of gastric mucus only
C. Inhibited secretion of bicarbonate only
D. Increased secretion of HCl by parietal cells
E. Increased secretion of bicarbonate

27. A 45-year-old alcoholic man is evaluated for multiple recent episodes of hematemesis. On examination, his speech is slurred and there is a sweet odor to his breath, although he appears sober. Laboratory studies reveal an elevated level of ammonia, no ketones, and a normal gastrin level. Which of the following conditions is likely to be associated with these findings?
A. Portal hypertension
B. Diabetic ketoacidosis
C. Thiamine deficiency
D. Pernicious anemia
E. Reduced glomerular filtration rate (GFR)
F. Zollinger-Ellison syndrome

28. A patient with a fasting glucose concentration of 250 mg/dL is seen in the clinic and has a blood pressure of 160/100 mm Hg. He is being treated with an angiotensin-converting enzyme (ACE) inhibitor, insulin, and a β-blocker. What is a possible consequence of this regimen when it is used to treat insulin-dependent diabetes mellitus?
A. Hyperglycemia
B. Hypertonic plasma
C. Hypovolemia
D. Hypotensive crisis
E. Hyperkalemia

29. A patient with moderate hypertension is given hydrochlorothiazide. Two weeks later, an evaluation reveals hypokalemia. An arterial blood gas measurement shows the following: pH, 7.5; partial pressure of carbon dioxide ($PaCO_2$), 50 mm Hg, and bicarbonate (HCO_3^-) concentration, 34 mEq/L. To correct these findings, which of the following drugs might also be given to this patient?
   A. Furosemide
   B. Acetazolamide
   C. Spironolactone
   D. Bumetanide
   E. Mannitol
   F. Intravenous normal saline

30. During the head and neck examination of a 14-year-old boy, the physician asks him to remove his baseball cap so that his scalp can be examined. The boy states that he sometimes forgets he is wearing his cap, and he notices the sensation of wearing it only when he puts it on or takes it off. Which type of sensory receptor is responsible for sensing the putting on and taking off of this boy's baseball cap?
   A. Pacinian corpuscle
   B. Ruffini's corpuscle
   C. Phasic receptor
   D. Photic receptor
   E. Tonic receptor

31. During ovulation, an oocyte is released from the ovary and travels down the fallopian tube toward the uterus. Which of the following events also occurs during this time?
   A. Meiosis I ends to yield haploid 1n oocytes.
   B. Meiosis I resumes and ends to yield a haploid 2n oocyte.
   C. Meiosis II is arrested in metaphase as a haploid 2n oocyte.
   D. Meiosis I is arrested as a diploid 4n oocyte.
   E. Oogonia divide by mitosis.

32. A patient receiving long-term lithium therapy for bipolar disorder is evaluated for symptoms of increased urinary frequency (polyuria) and increased thirst (polydipsia). After a period of fluid restriction, exogenous vasopressin is administered to the patient; this has no clear effect on the symptoms. What is most likely causing the symptoms in this patient?
   A. Syndrome of inappropriate antidiuretic hormone secretion (SIADH)
   B. Hypoparathyroidism
   C. Hypocalcemia
   D. Diabetes insipidus
   E. Orthostatic hypotension
   F. Addison's disease

33. A 32-year-old woman with a history of low blood pressure and fainting spells collapses after waiting for a long time in a line at the grocery store. Which of the following would most likely be an appropriate initial treatment for this woman?
   A. Elevation of the legs above the chest
   B. Administration of epinephrine
   C. Ventricular defibrillation
   D. Cardiopulmonary resuscitation
   E. Administration of intravenous fluids
   F. Elevation of the head above the chest

34. A 7-year-old boy playing in a daycare center abducts both arms to 90 degrees and begins to spin to the right. He starts off slowly and continues to build up rotational speed until he cannot spin faster. Which of the following will occur when the boy suddenly stops spinning and sits down?
   A. His eyes will move slowly to the left.
   B. When asked to point to a target, he will point to the left of the target.
   C. The objects in his visual field will appear to be spinning to the left.
   D. The hair cells in the left semicircular canal will depolarize.
   E. The boy will feel as if the room is spinning to the left.

35. End-stage congestive heart failure is a complex end point of a wide range of cardiovascular disease processes. Which of the following conditions is directly activated by systolic hypotension and is typically associated with most forms of end-stage congestive heart failure?

A. Increased renin secretion
B. Inhibition of the sympathoadrenal axis
C. Decreased levels of atrial natriuretic factor
D. Decreased levels of arginine

36. A 45-year-old man has recent onset of widespread pain in his back, legs, and hips, accompanied by a loss in height of 2 inches. He takes a multivitamin every day, and before the onset of pain, he got adequate exercise by walking a mile each day at lunch. After a trial of high-dose vitamin D, his symptoms remain unchanged. Extensive workup reveals a normal glomerular filtration rate, increased urinary phosphate, and elevated serum calcium and parathyroid hormone (PTH). A whole body bone scan reveals multiple "lytic" lesions in his bones. Which of the following conditions is the most likely cause of the bony changes seen in this patient?

A. Renal failure
B. Mutant vitamin D receptor
C. Vitamin D deficiency
D. Addison's disease
E. X-linked hypophosphatemic rickets
F. Granulomatous disease
G. Malignancy or lesion
H. Cirrhosis

37. A patient with bipolar disorder being treated with lithium begins to notice a profuse increase in the amount of urine he produces every day. Which of the following drugs can be useful in reducing urinary flow in this patient?

A. Vasopressin
B. Angiotensin-converting enzyme (ACE) inhibitors
C. Dopamine
D. Thiazide diuretics
E. Adenosine

38. A 28-year-old woman who has recently delivered her first child is evaluated for fatigue, cold intolerance, and constipation; she is found to have a low plasma level of thyroid-stimulating hormone (TSH). Sheehan's syndrome is suspected, because the delivery was associated with significant blood loss. An MRI of the head reveals ischemic necrosis of the anterior pituitary. To treat secondary hypothyroidism such as this, in which TSH levels are low, TSH would not be used. Which of the following statements best describes the mechanism of action of TSH?

A. It is a glycoprotein hormone that stimulates the intracellular cyclic adenosine monophosphate (cAMP) cascade via binding to the G protein–associated membrane receptor.
B. It is a steroid-like molecule that diffuses into target cells and binds to a cytoplasmic receptor prior to nuclear localization.
C. It is a steroid hormone that binds to a nuclear DNA protein complex and initiates transcription of genes containing a steroid response element.
D. It is a peptide hormone that binds to the β-adrenergic membrane receptor.
E. It is a peptide hormone that acts largely in a paracrine fashion.

39. Patients who suffer a high-level transection of the spinal cord typically recover normal blood pressure within a few weeks, even though direct sympathetic innervation of vascular smooth muscle cells is lost. Which of the following is a reason for this recovery of normal blood pressure?

A. Spinal shock
B. Decreased renin release
C. Renal compensation
D. Baroreceptor reflex
E. Sympathetic nerve "hitchhiking"

40. A 52-year-old woman complains of recent weight loss, difficulty sleeping, muscle tremors, tachycardia, and heat intolerance. Exophthalmos is noted on examination, and laboratory studies show increased plasma levels of thyroid hormone and antibodies to the thyroid-stimulating hormone (TSH) receptor. Which of the following causes best explains the muscle tremors seen in this patient?

A. Upregulation of β-adrenergic receptors on muscle cells

B. Decreased sympathetic outflow

C. Increased parasympathetic outflow

D. Increased plasma levels of catecholamines

41. A patient with aortic stenosis would be expected to have which of the following conditions?

A. Decreased aortic valve opening pressure

B. Raised diastolic pressure

C. Deficits in left coronary artery perfusion

D. Longer isovolumic contraction time

E. Prominent second heart sound

42. A tall, thin 25-year-old man experiences the sudden onset of left-sided chest pain and shortness of breath. Examination reveals that his trachea is noticeably shifted to the right of midline. An ECG is unrevealing but a CT scan of the chest reveals an aneurysmal dilatation at the base of the aortic arch. This patient most likely has which of the following disorders?

A. Myocardial infarction

B. Atrial fibrillation

C. Pneumothorax

D. Congestive heart failure

E. Asthma

43. Which of the following is a theoretical effect of a low-sodium diet?

A. Reduced efferent arteriolar tone in the kidney

B. Reduced renin release

C. Increased blood pressure

D. Reduction in hypertension

E. Reduced efficacy of diuretics

44. A 6-year-old boy is evaluated for pain in the right lower pelvic and inner thigh region. Examination reveals an intact cremasteric reflex on the left, but no testis is seen on the right. An inguinal mass is present on the right side. After a dose of human chorionic gonadotropin (hCG), the testis descends temporarily, accompanied by pain relief. The normal physiologic descent of the testes is triggered by which of the following factors?

A. Gonadotropin-releasing hormone (GnRH) surge at puberty

B. Müllerian inhibiting factor

C. Luteinizing hormone (LH) surge at puberty

D. Testis determining factor

E. Inhibin

45. A drug is developed that stimulates the opening of potassium channels in resting skeletal muscle but does not affect the permeability of other ions. Which of the following effects would this drug have on the cell?

A. The cell hyperpolarizes.

B. The cell depolarizes due to the influx of potassium ions.

C. The cell depolarizes due to the efflux of potassium ions.

D. The membrane potential decreases.

E. The membrane potential remains unchanged.

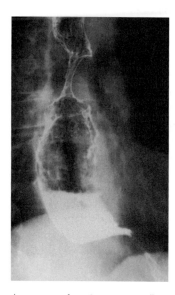

Reproduced with permission from Grainger RG, Allison D, Adam A, Dixon AK: Grainger & Allison's Diagnostic Radiology: A Textbook of Medical Imaging, 4th ed. London, Churchill Livingstone, 2001, Fig. 46-36.

46. A 58-year-old woman complains of a lifelong history of swallowing difficulty (dysphagia) which has recently worsened. She states that the pain until now could be diminished by nitrates.

A contrast study reveals a mass compressing her upper esophagus and an obstruction in the lower esophagus (see the accompanying figure). Biopsy reveals squamous cell carcinoma of the esophagus. Which of the following was most likely the initial cause of this patient's difficulty in swallowing?

A. Boerhaave's syndrome
B. Achalasia
C. Gastroesophageal reflux
D. Angina
E. Zenker's diverticulum
F. Epiphrenic diverticulum
G. Chagas' disease
H. Hiatal hernia

47. It has often been asserted that caffeine and alcohol are diuretics because they antagonize antidiuretic hormone (ADH). Which of the following factors normally promotes the release of ADH from the posterior pituitary?

A. Atrial stretch
B. Angiotensin II
C. Decrease in plasma osmolarity
D. Increased blood urea nitrogen
E. Increased rate of firing of carotid sinus baroreceptor

48. While giving birth to a child after a normal pregnancy, a woman hemorrhages heavily. In the months that follow the birth, she complains of inability to produce breast milk, lack of energy, cold intolerance, and amenorrhea. Which of the following events occurring during parturition is most likely to have caused these symptoms?

A. Lesion of the arcuate nucleus
B. Vasospasm of the superior hypophyseal artery
C. Lesion of pituitary stalk
D. Pituitary adenoma
E. Ischemic necrosis of the posterior pituitary

49. The intensive care unit in a hospital is training a group of residents on the normal operation of a mechanical ventilator. As part of this training, the group discusses optimal settings for tidal volume and functional residual capacity (FRC). In chronic obstructive pulmonary disease, patients breathe at tidal volumes that may start and end at much higher FRCs than in a normal patient. Which of the following conditions is present with a higher FRC?

A. The lung is more compliant.
B. Alveoli at the base of the lung are more compressed.
C. There is less airway resistance.
D. Alveolar vessels are less compressed.
E. Extra-alveolar vessels are compressed.

50. A young girl in Brazil is bitten by the pit viper, *Jararacussu* sp. Initial evaluation reveals a blood pressure of 80/10 mm Hg, but this is stabilized with intravenous fluids and dopamine. Morphine is given for pain. It is later found that the venom of this particular snake contains compounds that inhibit bradykinin degradation as well as an inhibitor of angiotensin-converting enzyme (ACE). Which of the following is the most likely cause of the girl's pain and hypotension?

A. Bradykinin
B. Angiotensin-converting enzyme
C. Angiotensin II
D. Kininase II
E. Kallikrein

answers

1. **B** (vitamin K) is correct. Biliary tract obstruction results in decreased availability of bile salts in the gastrointestinal tract, which leads to the malabsorption of fats and fat-soluble vitamins, weight loss, and steatorrhea. Of the choices available, vitamin K is the only fat-soluble vitamin. Recall that the fat-soluble vitamins include vitamins A, D, E, and K.

    A (vitamin C) is incorrect. Vitamin C is water soluble and is not affected by an obstructed bile duct because it does not depend on bile salts for its absorption.

    C (iron) is incorrect. Iron uptake in the gut is not dependent on bile salts. Iron is absorbed either as a heme complex or as the free ion. In the former case, the activity of heme oxygenase is rate-limiting for removal of iron from heme complexes. In the latter, basolateral combination with transferrin is the rate-limiting step for release into the circulation.

    D (vitamin B_{12}) is incorrect. Absorption of vitamin B_{12} requires intrinsic factor, not bile salts.

    E (intrinsic factor) is incorrect. Intrinsic factor is a glycoprotein secreted from the gastric parietal cells. Intrinsic factor binds to vitamin B_{12} and prevents its degradation in the small intestines. The intrinsic factor–vitamin B_{12} complex is then absorbed in the ileum.

2. **C** (central role of kidneys in long-term blood pressure control) is correct. The kidneys ultimately regulate the "set point" of arterial pressure, through control of sodium and water reabsorption or excretion. This long-term set point is determined by the renal function curve. As long as the kidney functions normally, it can compensate for variations in the volume, pressure, or salt load of the body.

    A (hypoaldosteronism due to immunosuppression) is incorrect. Immunosuppression is used to prevent transplant rejection. This is achieved through the use of steroids, which do not interfere with the function of aldosterone. Aldosterone synthesis is not subject to negative feedback regulation by other steroids at the level of the adrenal cortex.

    B (loss of sympathetic innervation in kidneys) is incorrect. The loss of sympathetic nerve supply to the kidneys might result in an increased glomerular filtration rate (GFR). However, it does not affect the ability of the kidneys to excrete or retain salt.

    D (immune reaction to kidney transplant) is incorrect. The immune reaction to a kidney transplant can be severe. If a hyperacute immune response occurs immediately after surgery, it is usually recognized, and the kidney is removed. The acute rejection is usually managed by immunosuppression. However, the long-term effects of a transplant may include vascular disease that might be expected to result in hypertension.

E (normal stress response after surgery) is incorrect. Although the stress response does act to restore blood pressure through activation of the sympathoadrenal axis, the long-term blood pressure is not primarily determined by this response.

3. **A** (begins at an increased FRC relative to a normal subject) is correct. The FRC is the volume remaining in the lung after a normal tidal volume expiration. This volume is increased in emphysema because the increased compliance of the lung favors inspiration and hinders expiration, and air trapping results. Because the FRC increases, alveolar ventilation must increase to maintain adequate oxygenation of this larger space. This can be achieved by increasing either the volume of each breath or the rate of breathing. Because emphysema is an expiration-limited condition, patients are well oxygenated at rest, because they maintain a pattern of breathing characterized by quick inspirations followed by slow pursed-lip expirations (pink puffers). The increase in compliance in emphysema means that inspiration can occur faster than expiration (bigger volume change for a given pressure change). The slow rate of expiration prevents airway collapse. Overall, patients with emphysema are fairly well ventilated. Although emphysema produces less hypoxemia than chronic bronchitis, adequate ventilation requires increased work of breathing, and the structural lung disease predisposes to structural damage such as pneumothorax. The term "chronic obstructive pulmonary disease" (COPD) encompasses both emphysema and chronic bronchitis. Recall that the definition of chronic bronchitis puts emphasis on the chronic aspect: 3 months of cough productive of sputum over two consecutive years. This patient displays signs more indicative of emphysema. In emphysema, the dyspnea precedes the cough; in chronic bronchitis, the cough precedes the dyspnea.

B (requires a more negative intrapleural pressure) is incorrect. Compliance work is expected to be less in emphysema, and therefore a less negative (more positive) intrapleural pressure would be adequate for inspiration.

C (involves increased use of internal intercostals) is incorrect. The internal intercostals are important in active expiration rather than inspiration.

D (increased size of FRC means tidal volume can decrease) is incorrect. The increased size of the FRC means that more gas is left in the lung at the end of each expiratory cycle. Therefore, the volume of gas that needs to be changed each minute increases.

4. **D** (Osler-Weber-Rendu disease) is correct. This patient's clinical picture most likely represents Osler-Weber-Rendu disease, also known as hereditary hemorrhagic telangiectasia (HHT). It is an autosomal dominant disorder of blood vessels that is characterized by dilation of capillaries and veins throughout the mucous membranes of the oral cavity, nasal mucosa, lips, skin, respiratory tract, gastrointestinal tract, and urinary tract. These weak vessels can rupture, leading to symptoms such as epistaxis, hematuria or bloody stools, and iron deficiency anemia. The family history is also suggestive of this disorder.

A (idiopathic thrombocytopenic purpura) is incorrect. Idiopathic thrombocytopenic purpura (ITP) is an autoimmune disorder in which antiplatelet antibodies are formed that attack platelets. It is most common in women. The clinical picture can resemble Osler-Weber-Rendu disease with epistaxis, hematuria, and melena. However, ITP is characterized by thrombocytopenia, and biopsy of blood vessels in ITP would be unrevealing.

B (iron deficiency anemia) is incorrect. Although the bleeding that occurs in Osler-

Weber-Rendu disease can result in iron deficiency anemia, the anemia does not account for all of the observed signs.

C (Cushing's syndrome) is incorrect. Although excessive steroid levels in Cushing's syndrome can result in structural damage to blood vessels, this patient shows no other signs of Cushing's syndrome (e.g., central obesity, dorsocervical fat pad, hyperglycemia).

E (hemolytic uremic syndrome) is incorrect. Hemolytic uremic syndrome is associated with hemolytic anemia, thrombocytopenia, and acute renal failure in children. It is often triggered by infection with *Escherichia coli.*

F (celiac disease) is incorrect. Celiac disease (celiac sprue) is a malabsorption syndrome caused by the production of antibodies to the protein gluten, which is present in many wheat-containing foods.

5. **E** (both cerebral and pulmonary edema may occur) is correct. The pulmonary edema may be related to hypoxic vasoconstriction. Cerebral blood flow increases in hypoxia due to hypoxic vasodilation. The brain is itself insensitive to hypoxia as a direct stimulus to ventilate. Changes in brain pH are the primary ventilatory stimulus, and these may occur indirectly as a consequence of the effect of hypoxia on cerebral blood flow (increased delivery of carbon dioxide to the brain decreases brain pH).

A (low blood viscosity is a stronger stimulus for erythropoietin release than hypoxia) is incorrect. The major stimulus for erythropoietin release at high altitude is hypoxia. It is unaffected by agents that may thin the blood and reduce its viscosity. This partly explains why aspirin may be helpful at high altitude: it counteracts the increase in blood viscosity and the consequent increased demand on the heart.

B (high-altitude pulmonary edema is caused by increased venous pressure) is incorrect. HAPE

is noncardiogenic in its mechanism; pulmonary venous pressure (left atrial pressure) is not elevated. This partly explains why this edema is not well mobilized by loop diuretics such as furosemide. The exact mechanisms of the edema are uncertain and appear to be multifactorial. It is related in part to the hypoxic vasoconstriction that occurs at high altitude, as well as the increased right heart workload that results from this pulmonary hypertension. Removal of hypoxia generally improves the edema.

C (cardiac output is diminished at high altitude) is incorrect. Cardiac output is defined as the product of heart rate and stroke volume. At sea level, cardiac output is the limiting factor to exercise performance because it determines the amount of oxygen delivered to tissues. This is also true at high altitude. Therefore, the expected response is increased cardiac output. Pulmonary hypertension caused by hypoxic vasoconstriction due to atmospheric and alveolar hypoxia results in an increased demand on the right ventricle. This results in electrocardiographic evidence of right heart strain, such as right axis deviation. HAPE results in tachycardia, most likely as a mechanism to maintain cardiac output in the face of reduced stroke volume caused by impaired flow of blood from the lungs due to the noncardiogenic edema. Colder temperatures increase sympathetic stimulation, and this may increase right heart output, leading to increased pulmonary arterial pressures that may favor edema.

D (low atmospheric pressure is the predominant reason for hypocapnia) is incorrect. Although the atmospheric pressure decreases at high altitude, the production of carbon dioxide in the tissues remains constant. The decline in the partial pressure of carbon dioxide from 40 mm Hg is primarily caused by increased removal of carbon dioxide by ventilation rather than the decreased atmospheric pressure.

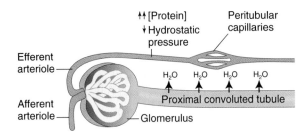

Efferent arteriole

Afferent arteriole

↟↟ [Protein]
↓ Hydrostatic pressure

Peritubular capillaries

H_2O H_2O H_2O H_2O

Proximal convoluted tubule

Glomerulus

6. **D** (glomerular capillary oncotic pressure) is correct. The glomerular capillary oncotic pressure opposes filtration. As filtration proceeds, the osmotic pressure of the fluid in the peritubular capillary becomes ever greater due to the removal of protein-free fluid in the filtrate (see the accompanying figure). This is the force that eventually terminates filtration and causes a fixed fraction of the renal plasma flow to be filtered for a given set of Starling forces. A lower plasma protein concentration results in a reduction in this opposing force and an increase in the filtration fraction. The termination of filtration occurs when the balance of Starling forces reaches zero ("filtration equilibrium").

In diabetics, several factors (e.g., excessive production of nitric oxide, vasodilation of the afferent arteriole) may result in hyperfiltration in some nephrons, contributing to diabetic nephropathy and glomerular sclerosis. Increasing the plasma oncotic pressure might be one way to therapeutically take advantage of this effect. In diabetic patients, filtration is increased because the filtration hydraulic pressure is increased. Although increasing the plasma protein concentration might increase the amount of toxic protein filtered in the kidney, it may be a rational therapy based on physiologic principles in healthy diabetics: it theoretically reduces the balance of forces favoring filtration and thus may ameliorate the thickening of the basement membrane that occurs in diabetes if therapy is instituted

early enough. (The opposite pattern is seen in the nephrotic syndrome, with the reduction in plasma protein oncotic pressure exacerbating the forces favoring filtration.) One objection to the use of albumin therapy in diabetics is that autoregulation would oppose the increased plasma oncotic pressure. However, this could be overcome with angiotensin II antagonists, which are already indicated for diabetics. Further, the hyperosmolarity caused by an increase in plasma albumin has no effect on water balance, because plasma proteins are not exposed to the hypothalamic osmoreceptors.

Note that increasing dietary protein is not the same as increasing plasma protein. In fact, dietary protein restriction is recommended for diabetics. This is related to the reabsorption of dietary amino acids in the proximal tubule with sodium and the effects of tubular sodium on tubuloglomerular feedback and filtration pressure.

A (glomerular capillary hydrostatic pressure) is incorrect. This pressure strongly favors, rather than opposes, glomerular pressure.

B (Bowman's oncotic pressure) is incorrect. This pressure, which is normally of minimal significance, favors rather than opposes glomerular filtration. In conditions such as minimal change disease, however, Bowman's oncotic pressure can become elevated due to filtration of plasma proteins across the glomerular membrane as a result of pathologic changes in the glomerular basement membrane. This results in proteinuria.

C (tubuloglomerular feedback) is incorrect. Tubular glomerular feedback does not have any influence on the filtration fraction; it modifies the amount of renal blood flow, but not the fraction that is filtered.

E (Bowman's hydrostatic pressure) is incorrect. Although this force opposes glomerular filtration, it normally does not play nearly as large a role as does glomerular capillary oncotic pressure.

7. E (depolarization of the membrane potential) is correct. The Na^+,K^+-ATPase pump maintains the resting membrane potential via transport of three sodium ions out of the cell and two potassium ions into the cell. Digitalis, a drug derived from the foxglove plant, inhibits of this pump, causing the ions to move down their respective concentration gradients and eventually reach equilibrium. The cell thus depolarizes due to its inability to maintain the standard resting potential of -60 to $-90\,mV$.

A (increased intracellular potassium concentration) is incorrect. Inhibition of the Na^+,K^+-ATPase pump causes a decrease in the intracellular potassium concentration.

B (increased excitability of cells) is incorrect. The excitability of cells is directly attributable to the resting membrane potential, which is maintained by the Na^+,K^+-ATPase pump. Inactivation of the pump causes the ions to move toward their equilibrium potentials. This decreases the voltage difference across the cell membrane and, hence, the excitability of these cells.

C (decreased intracellular volume) is incorrect. The failure of the Na^+,K^+-ATPase pump causes an increase in the intracellular sodium concentration. The osmotic effect pulls in water, causing the cell to swell.

D (decreased intracellular sodium concentration) is incorrect. The intracellular sodium level increases.

8. D (somatostatin) is correct. Somatostatin is secreted from the hypothalamus and inhibits pituitary secretion of growth hormone. Octreotide, a synthetic somatostatin analogue, is used to treat growth hormone–secreting tumors of the anterior pituitary, as in this patient.

A (insulin) is incorrect. Insulin increases growth hormone release indirectly through its hypoglycemic effect. Because growth hormone has hyperglycemic effects, it can be difficult to treat the diabetes and the growth hormone excess at the same time.

B (arginine) is incorrect. Amino acids in general, and arginine in particular, provide a strong stimulus for the release of growth hormone.

C (sulfonylurea drugs) is incorrect. Sulfonylurea drugs would probably cause increased insulin release and therefore hypoglycemia, leading to growth hormone release.

E (glucose) is incorrect. Glucose in a normal individual reduces the secretion of growth hormone; however, in a person with acromegaly glucose does not have this effect.

9. D (inhibition of gut motility and secretory activities) is correct. Stimulation of the sympathetic system causes inhibition of gut motility and secretory activities. It also causes contraction of intestinal sphincters. All of the other responses listed result from stimulation of the parasympathetic system during rest. Remember that the sympathetic system is responsible for "fight or flight" responses, and the parasympathetic system is responsible for "rest and digest" responses. In this case, the young man should be able to run the race without much difficulty, because his sympathetic system will predominate over his parasympathetic system, although the decreased blood flow to the gastrointestinal tract may cause him to experience a "stitch in his side."

A (segmental contractions of the proximal colon) is incorrect. Contractions of the proximal part of the colon occur in response to stimulation of the parasympathetic system.

B (increased rate of gastric emptying) is incorrect. Gastric emptying increases in response to parasympathetic stimulation of the stomach, rather than sympathetic stimulation.

C (relaxation of the pyloric sphincter) is incorrect. Stimulation of the sympathetic system results in contraction of the pyloric sphincter, which prevents gastric contents from being released into the small intestine.

E (stimulation of gut motility and secretory activities) is incorrect. Stimulation of the sympathetic nervous system results in inhibition of gut motility and secretory activities.

10. **B** (increasing diastolic pressures without changing systolic pressures) is correct. Recall that one of the main determinants of myocardial oxygen supply is diastolic perfusion pressure and that most of the myocardial blood flow occurs during diastole. Increasing the diastolic pressures greatly increases the pressure gradient for blood flow through the coronary arteries during diastole, resulting in increased blood flow to the myocardium.

A (increasing contractility with epinephrine to increase cardiac output) is incorrect. Inotropy is one of the main determinants of myocardial oxygen demand (along with heart rate and wall tension): Increasing contractility increases the demand. Because angina is caused by a myocardial oxygen supply that is insufficient to meet demand, increasing contractility would increase the severity of angina.

C (increasing preload by means of volume transfusions) is incorrect. Increased preload increases the force of ventricular contraction,

which requires greater oxygen consumption. This increased demand would increase the severity of angina.

D (diuresis) is incorrect. Diuresis depletes the plasma volume and may even decrease the diastolic perfusion pressure, which would reduce coronary perfusion. Although diuresis may reduce systolic blood pressure, which is a component of afterload, this patient is normotensive, and most of his increased afterload comes from the stenotic aortic valve.

E (coronary angioplasty) is incorrect. Although the resistance of the coronary vessels is a major determinant of myocardial perfusion and oxygen supply, this patient has normal (not constricted) coronary arteries.

11. **B** (greater stroke work capability for a given preload) is correct. A ventricular function curve provides information on cardiac performance by relating ventricular preload (end-diastolic volume) and stroke work (total energy spent by the ventricle during isometric and isotonic contraction of systole). Because end-diastolic volume and stroke work can be difficult to measure, end-diastolic pressure or atrial pressures can be used in place of preload and stroke volume or cardiac output in place of stroke work.

A shift to the left indicates increased contractility of the ventricle, such that, for a given preload, the ventricle performs more work. If afterload remains constant, increased contractility (e.g., sympathetic innervation) will result in a greater ejection fraction because more time is spent in the isotonic phase of contraction. If afterload increases, increased contraction will cause the ventricle to spend more energy in the isometric phase of contraction because sufficient energy must be produced to overcome the increased afterload. Therefore, even with a shift of the ventricular function curve to the left, a markedly increased afterload can still cause the ejection fraction to decline (e.g., in congestive heart failure).

A (congestive heart failure) is incorrect. Congestive heart failure is characterized by a shift to the right in the ventricular function curve because, for a given preload, the heart has a decreased stroke work capacity (relative to normal).

C (increased duration of isometric contraction) is incorrect. Increased time spent in isometric contraction would occur only with an elevated afterload.

D (increased release of acetylcholine at the sinoatrial node) is incorrect. A left shift of the ventricular function curve indicates increased cardiac performance. Vagal input to the sinoatrial node would have a negative inotropic effect on the heart, leading to decreased cardiac performance.

E (decreased ventricular ejection fraction) is incorrect. Assuming a constant afterload, a left shift of the ventricular function curve would result in an increased ejection fraction.

12. **C** (increased preload and decreased contractility) is correct. Reduction of heart rate by verapamil increases ventricular filling during a prolonged diastole, which increases preload. Additionally, because verapamil blocks calcium entry during the plateau phase of the ventricular action potential, calcium-induced calcium release, and therefore contractility, is reduced. Verapamil is used clinically in patients with hypertension, atrial fibrillation, hypertrophic cardiomyopathy, or Prinzmetal's angina (coronary artery spasm).

A (decreased preload and contractility) is incorrect. Calcium channel blockers such as verapamil slow the heart rate and result in increased ventricular filling, thereby increasing preload.

B (increased contractility and decreased preload) is incorrect. Calcium channel blockers such as verapamil have negative inotropic and chronotropic effects. The negative inotropic effect reduces contractility, and the negative

chronotropic effect increases ventricular filling and thereby increases preload.

D (increased preload and contractility) is incorrect. Although calcium channel blockers such as verapamil do increase preload, they decrease cardiac contractility.

13. **B** (increased right ventricular stroke volume) is correct. Both the inferior displacement of the diaphragm and the outward expansion of the chest wall during inspiration cause a decrease in intrathoracic pressure. This dilates the pulmonary vasculature and decreases pulmonary vascular resistance (i.e., reduces the work of the right ventricle); the result is increased right ventricular filling and, therefore, increased right ventricular stroke volume. Because right ventricular filling increases, the height of the column of blood in the jugular vein should fall during deep inspiration. Elevated neck veins can often be appreciated in patients with right-sided heart failure, because the failing right ventricle is unable to eject a normal stroke volume (or can do so only at elevated filling pressures), resulting in back-pressure and elevated neck veins.

A (decreased velocity of blood in the superior vena cava) is incorrect. The combination of increased ejection of blood from the right ventricle and dilation of the superior vena cava (SVC) due to reduced intrathoracic pressure results in higher than normal velocity of blood flow through the SVC.

C (a rise in the jugular venous column) is incorrect. Deep inspiration increases the movement of blood through the right side of the heart. Therefore, the pool of blood in the jugular vein should fall with deep inspiration.

D (decreased runoff in the pulmonary artery) is incorrect. The decrease in intrathoracic pressure dilates the pulmonary vasculature and decreases pulmonary resistance, leading to an increased arterial runoff.

E (increased intrathoracic pressure) is incorrect. Inspiration causes a decrease in intrathoracic pressure. This results in movement of blood into the thorax and a consequent fall in the height of the venous column. An easy way to remember how intrathoracic pressure changes with inspiration is to think of the venous column as a cardiothoracic manometer.

14. **B** (decreased venous return) is correct. In a tension pneumothorax, accumulation of air within the pleural cavity substantially increases intrathoracic pressure. This reduces the pressure gradient for venous return from the systemic veins to the right atrium. The intrathoracic pressure can be so great that the superior and inferior vena cavae collapse. Decrease in venous blood return to the heart causes a dramatic reduction in preload, and consequently reductions in stroke volume and cardiac output, leading to hypotension.

A (reduced heart rate) is incorrect. Because of the hypotension caused by decreased venous return in a tension pneumothorax, the baroreceptor reflex is activated, causing tachycardia.

C (cardiac tamponade) is incorrect. Cardiac tamponade occurs when fluid accumulates in the pericardial space, restricting ventricular filling during diastole. Tension pneumothorax and cardiac tamponade may both occur after penetrating injuries to the chest, but they do not cause one another.

D (hypoxemia) is incorrect. Hypoxemia activates the sympathetic nervous system, which increases heart rate and contractility, and these mechanisms initially counteract decreasing oxygen supply to the tissues while possibly elevating blood pressure. If hypoxemia were prolonged, it could reduce myocardial oxygen delivery and compromise cardiac function, resulting in hypotension.

E (hemorrhage) is incorrect. A tension pneumothorax is not necessarily accompanied by hemorrhage. Vessel rupture and hemorrhage are not typically responsible for the hemodynamic complications of tension pneumothorax.

15. **E** (left geniculocalcarine tract) is correct. A lesion involving the left geniculocalcarine tract causes a right homonymous hemianopia with macular sparing. The fibers of the left geniculocalcarine tract carry visual information from the right side of the visual field. Because the geniculocalcarine tract is found downstream from the lateral geniculate body (which receives fibers from the macula, or center of the visual field), visual acuity in the center of the visual field is retained.

A (left optic nerve) is incorrect. A lesion involving the left optic nerve causes blindness in the ipsilateral (left) eye. This results in inability to see out of the left eye, as well as a loss of depth perception.

B (optic chiasm) is incorrect. A lesion involving the optic chiasm causes a bitemporal hemianopia. Central visual acuity is spared, because fibers from the lateral area of the eye do not cross the optic chiasm. Lesion of the optic chiasm causes tunnel vision, because the lateral visual fields of both eyes are lost.

C (left optic tract) is incorrect. A lesion involving the left optic tract causes a pure right homonymous hemianopia that includes the fibers from the macula (i.e., the center of the visual field). Because this patient retained vision in the center of his visual field, the optic tracts must be intact.

D (right optic tract) is incorrect. A lesion involving the right optic tract causes a pure left homonymous hemianopia. The right optic tract includes fibers that originate in the left nasal and right temporal areas of the eye, corresponding to vision from the right side of the body.

16. **C** (diffusion impairment) is correct. Based on the history and the results of pulmonary function testing, this man most likely has a restrictive lung disease. The hypoxia in restrictive disorders may be the result of decreased oxygen diffusion across the pulmonary membrane. This causes decreased arterial oxygen partial pressure on exercise, because the increased blood flow to the lung results in a switch from perfusion-limited transfer of oxygen (at low blood flow rates when at rest) to diffusion-limited transfer. The limiting factor for oxygen transfer is the blood flow, but once pulmonary blood flow increases during exertion, the transfer becomes diffusion-limited, because oxygen diffusion cannot match the increase in perfusion.

In this situation, exercise increases the arterial-alveolar oxygen partial pressure gradient. However, this increase can be blocked by concurrent oxygen administration, which would not be true if a shunt were present. A high alveolar-arterial oxygen partial pressure gradient does not mean that diffusion is normal (even though the gradient for diffusion is increased). Although the lung segments are well ventilated and well perfused, the oxygen cannot reach the blood because of the impairment in diffusion. This has the same functional consequences as if the segments were perfused but poorly ventilated in the presence of normal diffusion: the result is arterial hypoxia.

A (increased ratio of residual volume to total lung capacity) is incorrect. In restrictive disorders, most lung volumes remain proportional to each other. Although the vital capacity is a normal fraction of the TLC, it is still reduced (compared with a healthy individual), and more effort is required to achieve it due to the loss of compliance in the lung. The ratio of RV to TLC increases in obstructive disease, in which hyperinflation is observed, and exercise capacity is limited by the reduced vital capacity.

B (increased ventilation/perfusion ratio in the apical lung) is incorrect. Because the blood flow to the apex of the lung increases with exercise, the V/Q ratio in the apex falls slightly. Exercise equalizes the V/Q ratios throughout the lung.

D (oxygen desaturation of hemoglobin) is incorrect. Recall that oxygen desaturation of hemoglobin occurs when the hemoglobin-O_2 dissociation curve shifts to the right. This occurs in the venous system (Bohr effect) in response to products of metabolism, such as low pH, high CO_2, and 2,3-diphosphoglycerate (DPG). Desaturation increases during exercise to allow increased venous extraction. However, if the hemoglobin is not initially saturated in the lungs due to a diffusion impairment, venous desaturation would start from an abnormally low level of oxygen in hemoglobin. The diffusion impairment would have to be severe to cause this, because the flattening of the hemoglobin curve at the upper levels of oxygen pressure is a protection against just this effect.

E (hypoventilation) is incorrect. Alveolar ventilation increases with exercise, increasing the alveolar oxygen tension.

17. **D** (glomerular capillary hydrostatic pressure) is correct. The plasma hydrostatic pressure in the glomerular capillaries is normally twice that of capillaries elsewhere in the body. This favors filtration. In the nephrotic syndrome, the permeability characteristics of the ultrafiltration barrier are altered, and molecules of abnormally large size or negative charge can cross the barrier. This patient probably has membranous glomerulonephritis, which is associated with the use of nonsteroidal anti-inflammatory drugs (NSAIDs) and penicillamine. An inflammatory process, mediated probably by complement and immunoglobulin deposition, leads to altered integrity of the filtration apparatus.

A (glomerular capillary oncotic pressure) is incorrect. The loss of plasma proteins through the glomerulus means that there is a reduction in the plasma oncotic pressure, which normally opposes filtration. This opposition is reduced in the case of nephrotic syndrome, but the main force driving filtration is the plasma hydrostatic pressure.

B (hydrostatic pressure in Bowman's space) is incorrect. The hydrostatic pressure in Bowman's space opposes filtration whether the patient has nephrotic syndrome or not.

C (oncotic pressure in Bowman's space) is incorrect. The increased flux of protein through the glomerulus means that the oncotic pressure in Bowman's space, which normally is almost zero and does not contribute to filtration, rises slightly. Despite this rise, the major force favoring filtration is the plasma hydrostatic pressure.

18. **B** (pernicious anemia) is the correct choice. This patient displays the typical symptoms of vitamin B_{12} deficiency: paresthesias, weakness, macrocytic anemia, and sore tongue. An important cause of B_{12} deficiency in the elderly is pernicious anemia. Pernicious anemia results from autoimmune destruction of the gastric mucosa, which leads to a failure of the production of intrinsic factor by the parietal cells. Without intrinsic factor, vitamin B_{12} cannot be absorbed in the ileum, resulting in a macrocytic anemia, macroglossia, and neurologic signs. This type of anemia has an insidious onset.

A (anemia of folate deficiency) is incorrect. Although anemia of folate deficiency does result in a macrocytic anemia, the neurologic changes seen in anemia of vitamin B_{12} deficiency do not occur.

C (hemolytic anemia) is incorrect. This patient has no other symptoms of hemolytic anemia, and she has a macrocytic anemia, not a hemolytic anemia.

D (iron deficiency anemia) is incorrect. Although iron deficiency anemia can occur in the elderly, it produces a microcytic hypochromic anemia.

E (anemia of chronic disease) is incorrect. Although anemia of chronic disease can cause anemia in an elderly patient, it is typically a normocytic or microcytic anemia.

19. **C** (4 L/minute) is correct. Calculation of cardiac output (CO) exploits the principle that the rate of oxygen consumption (in this case, 200 mL/minute) is equal to the rate of oxygen supplied to the tissue in arterial blood minus the rate of oxygen returned to the heart in venous blood. The rate of oxygen supply is equal to the arterial oxygen concentration times the blood flow in the arteries (i.e., the CO). Assuming that arterial and venous blood flow rates are the same:

$$O_2 \text{ consumption} = (\text{Arterial } [O_2] \times CO) - (\text{Venous } [O_2] \times CO)$$

$$200\,\text{mL/min} = CO \times \left[\left(\frac{20\,\text{mL O}_2}{100\,\text{mL blood}} \right) - \left(\frac{15\,\text{mL O}_2}{100\,\text{mL blood}} \right) \right]$$

Therefore, CO = 200 ÷ 0.05 = 4000 mL/minute. Four liters of blood per minute is being pumped through the vasculature.

The CO calculated in this manner utilizes the Fick equation, which is based on the concept of conservation of mass. The Fick equation states the same concept mathematically as follows:

$$CO(\text{mL blood/min}) = \frac{\text{Rate of oxygen consumption} \ (\text{mL O}_2/\text{min})}{\text{Arteriovenous oxygen difference} \ (\text{mL O}_2/\text{mL blood})}$$

A (1 L/minute) is incorrect. Clearly, if 5 mL of O_2 is used from every 100 mL of blood, 1000 mL of blood provides only 10×5 or 50 mL of O_2. It takes 40×100 mL, or a CO of 4 L/min, to provide 200 mL of O_2 in 1 minute.

B (3 L/minute) is incorrect. If 5 mL of O_2 is used for every 100 mL of blood pumped through the vessels, 30 sets of 100 mL provides only 150 mL O_2, far less than the required amount.

D (5 L/minute) is incorrect. If 5 L of blood were pumped per minute, the rate of O_2 consumption in this case would be 5000 mL $\times$ 5 mL O_2 per 100 mL blood, or 250 mL of O_2 per minute, not 200 mL.

E (10 L/minute) is incorrect. Clearly, if 5 mL of O_2 is used for every 100 mL of blood (obtained from the arteriovenous gradient), pumping of 10 L/minute would result in the use of 500 mL of O_2 per minute, a prodigious amount.

20. **D** (all of the above) is correct. Vagal stimulation exploits several mechanisms to slow the firing frequency in nodal tissues. Making the maximum diastolic potential more negative increases the time between action potentials because a greater depolarization must be achieved to reach threshold. The rate of depolarization during phase 4 is reduced because of the effects on ion permeability and fluxes across the nodal cell membrane, and this also increases the time required to reach threshold. Finally, the threshold for generating an action potential is raised, further slowing the firing frequency.

A (making the maximum diastolic potential more negative) is incorrect. This option is a correct response but is not the correct full answer to the question.

B (reducing the rate of depolarization of the nodal cells) is incorrect. This option is a correct response but is not the correct full answer to the question.

C (increasing the threshold for action potential generation) is incorrect. This option is a correct response but is not the correct full answer to the question.

21. **E** (increased insulin secretion) is correct. One way to reduce plasma glucose is to stimulate the β cells to secrete more insulin. The sulfonylurea drugs (e.g., tolbutamide, glyburide) stimulate insulin secretion by closing membrane-spanning K^+ channels on pancreatic β cells, resulting in depolarization; the resulting calcium influx triggers insulin secretion. These drugs are primarily useful in type 2 diabetes, because their mechanism of action is dependent on the presence of functional β cells. These drugs carry a significant risk of hypoglycemia.

A (decreased glucose uptake in muscle) is incorrect. The goal in treating diabetes is to decrease the level of blood glucose. An agent that decreased glucose uptake into muscles would worsen or increase blood glucose levels.

B (increased insulin sensitivity in the peripheral tissues including muscle, adipose tissue, and liver) is incorrect. The group of medicines that function in this manner to treat diabetes is the thiazolidinediones.

C (decreased glucose absorption at the brush border) is incorrect. The sulfonylureas, in contrast to other classes of oral agents, have no effects on the absorption of glucose. Inhibitors of α-glucosidase (e.g., acarbose, miglitol) do inhibit absorption of glucose.

D (inhibition of hepatic glucose secretion) is incorrect. The agent metformin inhibits hepatic glucose secretion and thereby decreases blood glucose levels. It also stimulates glucose uptake in peripheral tissues.

22. **E** (loop diuretic) is correct. Principally because of their site of action, loop diuretics such as furosemide are the most powerful type of diuretics available. Loop diuretics inhibit the sodium-potassium-chloride cotransporter of the thick limb of Henle's loop, thereby increasing the percentage of filtrate lost in the urine by as much as 20- to 30-fold. A patient with congestive heart failure and pulmonary edema typically has a very small rate of urine production because of renal hypoperfusion due to inadequate cardiac output. Administration of furosemide results in an explosive production of urine, thereby reducing extracellular fluid volume and alleviating the pulmonary edema. However, the use of loop diuretics is typically reserved for the acute setting.

A (thiazide diuretic) is incorrect. Thiazide diuretics act on the Na-Cl cotransporter of the distal tubule. They are not typically used for acute symptoms such as dyspnea and pulmonary edema.

B (angiotensin-converting enzyme inhibitor) is incorrect. ACE inhibitors such as captopril are commonly used for hypertension and congestive heart failure, but not typically for acute symptoms such as dyspnea and pulmonary edema, although they can be used acutely as afterload reducers in diastolic heart failure.

C (potassium-sparing diuretic) is incorrect. Potassium-sparing diuretics such as amiloride are typically given to patients along with thiazide diuretics, to counteract the potassium-losing effects of these drugs.

D (β-blocker) is incorrect. Although β-blockers are indicated for the long-term treatment of heart failure after myocardial infarction, they are not indicated for an acute exacerbation of heart failure.

23. **E** (ability to secrete secretin and cholecystokinin) is correct. Ulcers are associated with intracranial trauma as well as intracranial surgery. This may be related to stimulatory effects of the vagus nerve on acid secretion. The ulcers, known as Cushing's ulcers, may affect the duodenum, the stomach, or the esophagus. The secretion of secretin and CCK occurs in the duodenum. Secretin primarily stimulates the secretion of pancreatic enzymes, whereas CCK primarily stimulates gallbladder contraction. Both secretory capabilities are lost with surgical resection of the duodenum. Curling's ulcers, by contrast, are associated with severe burns or trauma and typically occur in the proximal duodenum.

A (only those pancreatic secretions controlled by secretin and cholecystokinin) is incorrect. Secretin and CCK have multiple actions. For example, secretin stimulates the secretion of bile from the liver, and CCK is the major stimulus for contraction of the gallbladder. Both stimulate insulin secretion. All actions of secretin and CCK are lost with surgical resection of the duodenum.

B (contraction of the gallbladder) is incorrect. The gallbladder can also contract in response to a vagal reflex.

C (migrating myoelectric complex) is incorrect. The migrating myoelectric complex is stimulated by motilin and begins in the stomach, moving to the ileum approximately every 90 minutes.

D (ability to secrete gastrin) is incorrect. The duodenum does not secrete gastrin, although, in some circumstances, a gastrinoma can occur there. Gastrin is normally secreted by the G cells in the pyloric glands of the distal stomach.

24. **C** (paradoxical split of S_2) is correct. Because conduction to the left ventricle is delayed, contraction of the left ventricle is delayed in relation to contraction of the right ventricle. Consequently, the left ventricle finishes ejecting blood into the aorta after the right ventricle has already finished pumping blood out. Therefore, the aortic valve closes after the pulmonic valve. Because the pulmonic valve normally closes slightly after the aortic, especially during inspiration, the splitting observed in left bundle branch block is considered paradoxical.

A (physiologic inspiratory split of S_2) is incorrect. A physiologic inspiratory split of S_2 is a normal finding. During inspiration, the decreased intrathoracic pressure increases the pressure gradient for venous return to the right atrium and ventricle. The resulting increased end-diastolic volume in the right ventricle during inspiration requires longer to eject, so the pulmonic valve closes after the aortic valve.

B (systolic murmur) is incorrect. Murmurs occur because of turbulent blood flow. Delay in conduction to and contraction of the left ventricle does not create any turbulent flow.

D (diastolic murmur) is incorrect. Murmurs occur because of turbulent blood flow. Delay in conduction to and contraction of the left ventricle does not create any turbulent flow.

25. **D** (intracranial berry aneurysm) is correct. The patient has classic symptoms and findings suggestive of adult polycystic kidney disease, an autosomal dominant disorder that has multiple pathophysiologic manifestations, including a slow decline in renal function and increasing risk of renal failure with age. The disorder is associated with an increased risk of berry aneurysms. Approximately 15% of patients with this disorder die of a ruptured berry aneurysm, resulting in a subarachnoid hemorrhage.

In addition to the kidney, the heart and liver are also affected. There is increased incidence of mitral valve prolapse, which results in a midsystolic click correlating with the snapping shut of the mitral valve chordae tendineae during systole. Like the kidneys, the liver can have multiple cysts.

A (hypertension in upper limbs and hypotension in lower limbs) is incorrect. Hypertension in the upper limbs with hypotension in the lower limbs indicates coarctation, or narrowing, of the aorta. Coarctation of the aorta is also associated with a systolic murmur and with increased risk of berry aneurysms. However, renal and hepatic manifestations are absent.

B (ventricular septal defect) is incorrect. Ventricular septal defect is the most common congenital cardiac abnormality. It is associated with pulmonary hypertension and a systolic murmur. However, the renal manifestations are expected.

C (end-systolic click) is incorrect. A click correlates with snapping shut of the atrioventricular valves, which are anchored to the ventricular wall by ligaments. These are not present in the aortic and pulmonary valves, which close at the onset of diastole. Therefore, a sound at the end of systole is more likely to be a snap than a click.

E (recent *Streptococcus viridans* infection) is incorrect. A differential diagnosis of this patient's symptoms should probably include rheumatic fever and other poststreptococcal sequelae, which also commonly involve the mitral valve and can have renal manifestations as well. However, these conditions are caused by β-hemolytic group A streptococci rather than *Streptococcus viridans*. The former organisms, among others, also are associated with endocarditis after dental procedures.

26. **A** (inhibited secretion of gastric mucus and bicarbonate) is correct. Aspirin and NSAIDs are both cyclo-oxygenase 1 (COX-1) and COX-2 inhibitors. Unlike NSAIDs that reversibly inhibit COX-1 and COX-2, aspirin irreversibly inhibits these enzymes. COX-1 normally acts to increase mucus and bicarbonate secretions as well as decreasing stomach acid secretions. COX-2 is associated with pain and inflammation. Therefore, because they inhibit COX-1, aspirin and NSAIDs can lead to an increase risk of gastritis or even gastric ulceration via decreased mucus and bicarbonate secretions as well as increased HCl production.

B (inhibited secretion of gastric mucus only) is incorrect. Aspirin and NSAIDs inhibit the secretion of *both* gastric mucus and bicarbonate.

C (inhibited secretion of bicarbonate only) is incorrect. Aspirin and NSAIDs inhibit the secretion of *both* gastric mucus and bicarbonate.

D (increased secretion of HCl by parietal cells) is incorrect. Aspirin and NSAIDs act to inhibit COX-1 enzyme, which leads to decreased secretion of HCl by the parietal cells.

E (increased secretion of bicarbonate) is incorrect. Aspirin and NSAIDs lead to decreased production of bicarbonate through inhibition of COX-1 enzyme.

27. **A** (portal hypertension) is correct. The findings described are most likely consequences of alcoholic cirrhosis resulting in portal hypertension. Cirrhosis of the liver is the most common cause of portal hypertension, which can result in ascites, splenomegaly, hepatic encephalopathy, and portosystemic venous shunts. Hepatic encephalopathy results in confusion, asterixis, rigidity, and hyperreflexia; the reasons for these symptoms are unclear but increased levels of blood ammonia do play a role. Portosystemic venous shunts can result in hemorrhoids and esophageal varices. The sweet-smelling breath of this patient is known as *fetor hepaticus,* a characteristic feature of hepatic failure and cirrhosis.

B (diabetic ketoacidosis) is incorrect. The sweet-smelling breath could incorrectly be thought to indicate diabetic ketoacidosis. However, in diabetic ketoacidosis an increased ammonia level, ketosis, and glycosuria are expected.

C (thiamine deficiency) is incorrect. Although this patient is at increased risk of thiamine deficiency due to alcoholism (which is associated with decreased intake, impaired absorption, and an increased requirement of thiamine), the clinical scenario does not describe typical features of thiamine deficiency.

D (pernicious anemia) is incorrect. Pernicious anemia usually results from an inflammation of the stomach that leads to impaired absorption of vitamin B_{12} due to decreased production of intrinsic factor and lack of acid secretion. Although neurologic signs (tremor) may accompany vitamin B_{12} deficiency, this does not adequately explain the entire clinical presentation.

E (Reduced glomerular filtration rate) is incorrect. Renal failure could result in increased concentrations of toxic metabolites such as ammonia and possible neurologic sequelae. However, renal failure alone does not adequately explain the entire clinical presentation.

F (Zollinger-Ellison syndrome) is incorrect. Ulceration and bleeding would be expected if a tumor secreting excess gastrin were present. However, this patient has a normal serum gastrin level. Also, Zollinger-Ellison syndrome does not explain the rest of the patient's symptoms.

28. **E** (hyperkalemia) is correct. Adrenergic β-receptors and insulin are critical for the movement of potassium into cells after a meal. It should be recalled that glucose is cotransported along with potassium into cells, so a lack of insulin could precipitate hyperkalemia. Additionally, ACE inhibitors are expected to lower levels of aldosterone, a critical hormone in the excretion of potassium, thereby contributing to hyperkalemia. Of note, β-blockers are relatively contraindicated in diabetics because they can mask the warning symptoms of severe hypoglycemia (e.g., tremors, palpitations) caused by the administration of excessive insulin.

A (hyperglycemia) is incorrect. Hyperglycemia is not expected as long as tight control of plasma glucose is maintained. One risk of β-blockade is hypoglycemia.

B (hypertonic plasma) is incorrect. The usual cause of hypertonic plasma in patients with diabetes is uncontrolled hyperglycemia.

C (hypovolemia) is incorrect. One risk in uncontrolled diabetes is the loss of fluid caused by hyperglycemia and the resulting osmotic diuresis. However, in a patient whose insulin and glucose are well controlled, this is less of a concern.

D (hypotensive crisis) is incorrect. In a patient with hypertension and diabetes, the risk of long-term vascular complications is increased, so hypertension should be managed aggressively. However, β-blockers carry certain risks in diabetic patients, such as the risk of hypoglycemia, and other possible therapies might be considered.

29. **C** (spironolactone) is correct. Hydrochlorothiazide is a thiazide diuretic that can cause hypokalemia and, rarely, metabolic alkalosis. Spironolactone is a potassium-sparing diuretic that acts as a competitive antagonist of aldosterone. Because aldosterone increases renal excretion of potassium, the administration of spironolactone with a potassium-losing diuretic such as hydrochlorothiazide should help prevent hypokalemia from developing. Aldosterone is also a critical element of acid secretion. Inhibiting the effects of aldosterone also ameliorates some of the alkalotic effects of the thiazide. Unwanted steroidal side effects of spironolactone include gynecomastia.

A (furosemide) is incorrect. Furosemide is a loop diuretic that causes potassium wasting and a metabolic alkalosis. The combination of furosemide with hydrochlorothiazide is reserved for more severe, diuretic-unresponsive cases.

B (acetazolamide) is incorrect. Acetazolamide is a carbonic anhydrase inhibitor that produces the same effect as proximal tubule acidosis: Inhibition of carbonic anhydrase prevents reabsorption of bicarbonate and acidosis ensues. Because there is also a diuresis that increases the bicarbonate load to the distal tubule, acetazolamide also causes increased potassium excretion due to enhancement of the negative lumen in the collecting duct. Although the alkalosis is corrected, the hypokalemia is not.

D (bumetanide) is incorrect. Bumetanide is a loop diuretic that causes potassium wasting and metabolic alkalosis.

E (mannitol) is incorrect. Mannitol is an osmotic diuretic. Because it exerts an osmotic effect, it is often used to reduce intracranial pressure. It causes an osmotic diuresis that does not significantly affect the electrolyte status of the filtrate, so hypokalemia is not affected.

F (intravenous normal saline) is incorrect. Intravenous saline may be used in combination with loop diuretics to treat hypercalcemia, because these diuretics inhibit calcium reabsorption in the loop (but not in the distal tubule). In contrast, thiazide diuretics have the opposite effect: They stimulate calcium reabsorption in the distal tubule and may be useful for dissolving renal calcium stones. Intravenous saline does not correct hypokalemia or hypertension.

30. **C** (phasic receptor) is correct. Rapidly adapting (phasic, dynamic) receptors fire action potentials at a decreasing rate during the application of a stimulus.

A (pacinian corpuscle) is incorrect. Pacinian corpuscles respond to vibratory stimuli on the skin.

B (Ruffini's corpuscle) is incorrect. Ruffini's corpuscles respond to pressure applied to the skin.

D (photic receptor) is incorrect. The term "photic receptor" applies generally to any receptor that is stimulated by light.

E (tonic receptor) is incorrect. Slowly adapting (tonic, static) receptors fire action potentials continuously during stimulus application.

31. **B** (meiosis I resumes and ends to yield a haploid 2n oocyte) is correct. At the time of ovulation, triggered by the surge in luteinizing hormone, the primary oocytes complete the first meiotic stage, moving from the diplotene stage (diploid 4n DNA) to complete meiosis I, expelling the polar body, and becoming haploid 2n oocytes. After ovulation, these oocytes become secondary oocytes. Recall that the purpose of meiosis I is to separate the pairs of homologous chromosomes into two distinct sets, and that crossing over occurs in meiosis I. If meiosis I in the mother does not proceed properly, the zygote can have one normal complement of chromosomes from the father, with either a missing chromosome or two homologous chromosomes from the mother (a nondisjunction). Therefore, important genetic events occur coincidentally with ovulation.

A (meiosis I ends to yield haploid 1n oocytes) is incorrect. At the end of meiosis I, the oocytes

are haploid 2n, having expelled the first Barr body, which was haploid 2n as well. Meiosis I goes from diploid 4n to haploid 2n; meiosis II goes from haploid 2n to haploid 1n.

C (meiosis II is arrested in metaphase as a haploid 2n oocyte) is incorrect. After ovulation, the oocytes finish meiosis I and enter meiosis II; they are arrested in meiosis II and cannot complete it until they are fertilized. At the time of fertilization, the ovum has a metaphase spread of two haploid 1n oocytes, one of which is released as the second Barr body if fertilization is successful.

D (meiosis I is arrested as a diploid 4n oocyte) is incorrect. Shortly after oogonia become primary oocytes by beginning meiosis I in the embryo, they are arrested at that stage and stay arrested until ovulation. Puberty, caused by the surge in gonadotropin-releasing hormone, causes changes only in the structures of the ovary, as several primordial follicles become selected each month to become primary follicles.

E (oogonia divide by mitosis) is incorrect. Oogonia exist only before the mother is born; once the oogonium begins the first meiotic division, it is a primary oocyte. When a female is born, all of her oocytes are primary oocytes arrested in the first meiotic division.

32. **D** (diabetes insipidus) is correct. Lithium nephrotoxicity can cause nephrogenic diabetes insipidus, in which the kidney is no longer capable of responding to circulating ADH (vasopressin), resulting in free water loss by the kidneys. The collecting ducts normally increase water reabsorption in the presence of ADH, which is released from the posterior pituitary. The lack of responsiveness in nephrogenic diabetes insipidus may be caused by a defect in the ADH receptor itself or in the aquaporin water channels that are normally inserted into the luminal membrane in response to ADH.

Lithium can also stimulate excessive secretion of parathyroid hormone (PTH) and thereby cause hypercalcemia, which can then contribute to the polyuria.

A (syndrome of inappropriate antidiuretic hormone secretion) is incorrect. SIADH is not associated with polyuria or polydipsia. The lack of response of the kidney to ADH in nephrogenic insipidus also elevates secretion of ADH, because the negative feedback cutoff of ADH levels is mediated by the osmolality of the plasma, not by the absolute level of ADH. The distinction between central and nephrogenic diabetes insipidus is made by administration of ADH (vasopressin); the distinction between SIADH and nephrogenic insipidus (both of which exhibit high ADH levels) is made on clinical grounds.

B (hypoparathyroidism) is incorrect. Lithium increases secretion of parathyroid hormone (PTH), which can result in hypercalcemia, associated with nephrogenic diabetes insipidus.

C (hypocalcemia) is incorrect. Lithium stimulates secretion of parathyroid hormone (PTH), which can result in hypercalcemia. Hypercalcemia can also cause nephrogenic diabetes insipidus.

E (orthostatic hypotension) is incorrect. Hypotension after assumption of the upright posture indicates malfunction of the baroreceptor reflex that regulates blood pressure in the short term.

F (Addison's disease) is incorrect. Addison's disease is manifested in the kidneys by a lack of aldosterone that results in hypovolemia. Both aldosterone and ADH exert their effects at the collecting duct. Addison's disease in a patient with nephrogenic diabetes insipidus has severe effects, a point to consider in long-term lithium therapy for a patient with compromised adrenal function.

33. **A** (elevation of the legs above the chest) is the correct choice. This woman most likely fainted because of inadequate cardiac output caused by reduced venous return to the heart. Long periods of standing still can reduce venous return to the heart because, when the lower limbs are not moving, the skeletal muscle pump does not assist venous return. Because the veins of the lower limbs act as high-capacity storage vessels (and approximately two thirds of blood in the circulatory system is located in veins), elevation of the legs above the chest immediately increases venous return to the heart and should provide sufficient cerebral blood flow to restore consciousness.

B (administration of epinephrine) is incorrect. Epinephrine would increase cardiac output and cerebral perfusion in this patient. However, administration of epinephrine would be appropriate only at a later stage. If the woman does not recover consciousness after venous return is increased by elevation of her legs above her chest, it might then be appropriate to consider the use of epinephrine.

C (ventricular defibrillation) is incorrect. This patient has most likely fainted due to poor cerebral perfusion. Cardiac arrhythmias are less likely.

D (cardiopulmonary resuscitation) is incorrect. This patient most likely has fainted due to cerebral hypoperfusion, but she should be breathing and her heart should still be pumping. Therefore, cardiopulmonary resuscitation is not needed.

E (administration of intravenous fluids) is incorrect. The woman may be dehydrated, in which case administration of an isotonic electrolyte solution to increase plasma volume would be appropriate. However, proper positioning is a more appropriate initial intervention.

F (elevation of the head above the chest) is incorrect. Elevation of the head above the chest would further reduce cerebral perfusion and therefore would be inappropriate for this patient.

34. **D** (the hair cells in the left semicircular canal will depolarize) is correct. When the head is rotating toward the right, the endolymph within the semicircular canals begins to flow in the direction opposite the rotational force. The flow of endolymph causes the cilia contained within both the right and left cupola to bend toward the left. This is significant because when the stereocilia are bent towards the kinocilium, the hair cell depolarizes, and when the stereocilia are bent away from the kinocilium, the hair cell hyperpolarizes. When rotation stops, the endolymph continues to move, and in effect pushes the cilia in the opposite direction. In this scenario, the hair cells in the right semicircular canal depolarize and those in the left semicircular canal hyperpolarize while the child is spinning. When the child stops spinning, the hair cells in the left semicircular canal depolarize, and those in the right semicircular canal hyperpolarize.

A (his eyes will move slowly to the left) is incorrect. When the child stops spinning, the flow of endolymph reverses, resulting in depolarization of the left semicircular canal and the left vestibular nerve, which causes the eyes to deviate to the right.

B (when asked to point to a target, he will point to the left of the target) is incorrect. Excitation of the left vestibular nerve causes the eyes to deviate to the right. As a result, when the boy stops rotating, he feels as if he is spinning to the left (due reversal of the flow of endolymph), or that the room is spinning to the right. Therefore, when asked to point to a target, the boy will sense that the object is moving toward the right and will mistakenly point to the right of the object.

C (the objects in his visual field will appear to be spinning to the left) is incorrect. The objects in his visual field will appear to be spinning to the right.

E (the boy will feel as if the room is spinning to the left) is incorrect. The boy will feel as if he were spinning to the left or as if the room were spinning to the right.

35. **A** (increased renin secretion) is correct. The factors that stimulate renin secretion from the juxtaglomerular apparatus of the nephron are decreased renal perfusion pressure, activation of sympathetic nerves, and decreased sodium chloride delivery to the macula densa. All of these factors may occur in heart failure.

B (inhibition of the sympathoadrenal axis) is incorrect. The sympathoadrenal axis consists of the sympathetic nervous system as well as the renin-angiotensin-aldosterone system. This axis is stimulated, not inhibited, by hypotension.

C (increased levels of atrial natriuretic factor) is incorrect. Atrial natriuretic factor (ANF) is released from the cardiac atria under situations of increased atrial distention. If there is a fall in systolic blood pressure, the secretion of ANF usually is not stimulated, unless hypervolemia is present. Hypotension itself does not stimulate ANF release. ANF stimulates renal diuresis and also promotes vasodilation.

D (decreased levels of arginine vasopressin) is incorrect. Secretion of arginine vasopressin is increased by hypotension. Vasopressin stimulates volume expansion (through the kidneys) and systemic arteriolar vasoconstriction.

36. **G** (malignancy or lesion) is correct. The patient has adequate exposure to sunlight and takes a multivitamin, which usually rules out any sort of deficiency state, and the presence of normal health before the onset of symptoms rules out a congenital cause. A malignancy is likely in this man, and one such as multiple myeloma should be suspected whenever x-rays or bone scans reveal multiple "lytic" lesions. Other malignancy-related possibilities are paraneoplastic syndromes, such as that caused by excessive secretion of parathyroid hormone-related protein (PTHrP) from a small cell carcinoma of the lung. Another possibility is primary hyperparathyroidism secondary to a hypersecreting tumor of the parathyroid glands. Note that secondary hyperparathyroidism is typically caused by renal failure and is accompanied by low serum calcium and raised serum phosphate.

A (renal failure) is incorrect. This patient has normal renal function, which rules out renal failure. The spectrum of disorders associated with renal failure includes osteomalacia, osteitis fibrosa cystica, osteoporosis, and metastatic calcification. These are generally associated with increased serum PTH, raised serum phosphate, low serum calcium, and lowered 1,25-vitamin D_3. In chronic renal failure, the kidney does not reabsorb phosphate, the level of vitamin D_3 falls, and the serum calcium concentration falls as a consequence of increased binding to phosphate and lack of vitamin D_3 effect.

B (mutant vitamin D receptor) is incorrect. If this were the case, the pattern of adult onset would not be expected.

C (vitamin D deficiency) is incorrect. A vitamin D deficiency should have been reversed by the high-dose vitamin D therapy.

D (Addison's disease) is incorrect. In Addison's disease, the reabsorption of phosphates is impaired, so these patients tend to have elevated serum phosphate concentrations.

E (X-linked hypophosphatemic rickets) is incorrect. Although X-linked hypophosphatemic rickets results in a loss of phosphate in the urine and symptoms similar

to those of osteomalacia, it is a congenital disease and does not manifest in middle adulthood.

F (granulomatous disease) is incorrect. Granulomatous disease results in increased synthesis of vitamin D_3, which causes increased serum calcium, and this clinical picture does not fit with the elevated PTH level observed in this patient.

H (cirrhosis) is incorrect. Although the liver is critical in the metabolism of vitamin D, high-dose vitamin D should reverse any related liver dysfunction.

37. **D** (thiazide diuretics) is correct. Long-term lithium therapy can inhibit the actions of vasopressin (ADH) on the kidneys, resulting in the production of large amounts of dilute urine and polydipsia. The addition of a thiazide diuretic may be helpful in this scenario. The thiazide diuretics cause a reduction of effective circulating volume, which in turn reduces the glomerular filtration rate (GFR) and the amount of fluid presented to the kidney. This reduces the maximum amount of dilute urine that can be produced, thus reducing the polyuria. This approach is not without its side effects, because thiazide diuretics can increase lithium toxicity. An alternative drug is the potassium-sparing diuretic amiloride, which can also partially correct the effect of lithium on vasopressin.

A (vasopressin) is incorrect. Vasopressin is also known as antidiuretic hormone (ADH). It is responsible for stimulating water uptake in the distal collecting duct and is ineffective in reabsorbing water in the collecting duct in the presence of lithium.

B (angiotensin-converting enzyme inhibitors) is incorrect. ACE inhibitors do not reduce urinary flow, because they increase the glomerular filtration rate (GFR).

C (dopamine) is incorrect. Dopamine is released endogenously by the kidney. It increases the glomerular flow rate (GFR) and dilates the afferent arteriole. Therefore, it would not be expected to reduce urinary flow.

E (adenosine) is incorrect. Adenosine has been advanced as a mediator responsible for tubuloglomerular feedback, constricting the afferent arteriole and possibly reducing urinary flow. It is not used clinically except in cardiac applications, because of its extremely short half-life.

38. A (it is a glycoprotein hormone that stimulates the intracellular cyclic adenosine monophosphate cascade via binding to the G protein–associated membrane receptor) is correct. TSH, also known as thyrotropin, is a glycoprotein hormone (MW 28,000) that binds to a G protein–associated membrane receptor on the follicular cells of the thyroid gland, stimulating increased production of intracellular cAMP and activation of protein kinase A. (The inositol triphosphate (IP$_3$)/calcium pathway may also be important.) It does not bind to β-adrenergic receptors, which are typically occupied by monoamine substances such as the adrenal catecholamines. The rise in cAMP increases the level of iodide uptake by the thyroid gland. Indeed, TSH stimulates all aspects of thyroid function, including upregulation of iodide transport, increased iodination of thyroglobulin, increased follicular growth, increased colloid resorption, and increased secretion of triiodothyronine (T$_3$) and thyroxine (T$_4$). Although TSH might appear to be a logical choice for therapy, in practice thyroxine is used, because of the breakdown of TSH, the difficulty of titrating dosage to avoid toxic effects, and the expense of peptides as therapeutic tools. Some cases of postpartum pituitary necrosis differ from this one in that the levels of TSH are paradoxically elevated even though hypothyroidism is present; this may be a result of reduced bioactivity of the TSH.

B (it is a steroid-like molecule that diffuses into target cells and binds to a cytoplasmic receptor prior to nuclear localization) is incorrect. The steroid receptor superfamily includes receptors for thyroid hormone, as well as estrogens, prostaglandins, vitamin A, and glucocorticoids. All of these receptors have a nuclear localization sequence and also bind a complex of repressors and other proteins that control transcription through a DNA binding region.

C (it is a steroid hormone that binds to a nuclear DNA protein complex and initiates transcription of genes containing a steroid response element) is incorrect. As a first approximation, both steroids and thyroid hormone act in a similar manner: They bind to receptors, eventually forming a complex bound to DNA.

D (it is a peptide hormone that binds to the β-adrenergic membrane receptor) is incorrect. TSH does not bind the β-adrenergic receptor, although both receptors increase the production of cAMP. The adrenergic effects of thyroid hormone (not TSH) may be caused by increased numbers of adrenergic receptors.

E (it is a peptide hormone that acts largely acts in a paracrine fashion) is incorrect. Prostaglandins are an example of substances that act in a paracrine fashion. These substances act largely on adjacent cells and tissues. Because of their short half-life, prostaglandins do not typically act on distant sites in the body. Peptides usually have a long enough half-life to be classified as hormones.

39. C (renal compensation) is correct. The sympathetic nervous system is important in the maintenance of blood pressure. Basal sympathetic outflow from the vasomotor center maintains tonic constriction of systemic arterioles. It is thought that resistance vessels are constricted to approximately 50% of their maximal diameter as a result of this sympathetic tone, and this explains the marked hypotension that occurs with spinal shock, when sympathetic outflow ceases. However, the long-term control of blood pressure is primarily determined by the ability of the kidney to excrete or retain salt. Because the sympathetic nervous system vasoconstricts the afferent arteriole, loss of sympathetic innervation increases blood flow through the glomerulus, and the glomerular filtration rate (GFR) is preserved. In addition, the reduced pressure at the mesangial cells leads to activation of the renin-angiotensin-aldosterone system, which acts to restore blood pressure. If the renin-angiotensin-aldosterone system is blocked, blood pressure after hemorrhage returns only halfway to normal levels, illustrating the importance of this system in long-term regulation of blood pressure.

A (spinal shock) is incorrect. Spinal shock refers to the loss of all functions of the spinal cord after transection of the upper (e.g., cervical) cord. The hypotension that accompanies spinal shock, caused by the loss of sympathetic reflexes, is abolished within a few days, much earlier than the expected recovery of spinal function, indicating that compensation must occur in the absence of sympathetic control.

B (decreased renin release) is incorrect. Renin release does not decrease but increases in response to hypotension.

D (baroreceptor reflex) is incorrect. The baroreceptor reflexes to control blood pressure depend on the activity of the sympathetic nervous system for their efferent limb. The baroreceptor reflex, although critical for responding to rapid changes in blood pressure (e.g., recumbent to supine position), has little to do with its long-term maintenance.

E (sympathetic nerve "hitchhiking") is incorrect. The sympathetic nervous system is also known as the thoracolumbar system, because all nerves exit the spinal cord in the thoracic and lumbar segments. This means that sympathetic nerve fibers are often found "hitchhiking" with cranial nerves as well as blood vessels, particularly in the head. However, all of the sympathetic impulses must pass through the thoracic or lumbar spinal cord. Because an upper spinal cord lesion does interrupt these pathways, sympathetic nerve "hitchhiking" cannot create accessory pathways for the sympathetic outflow.

40. **A** (upregulation of β-adrenergic receptors on muscle cells) is correct. This patient has Graves' disease, which is characterized by hyperthyroidism secondary to stimulation of anti-TSH receptor antibodies. Thyroxine hormone stimulates upregulation of adrenergic receptors in target tissues, which causes increased sensitivity to circulating catecholamines, leading to muscle tremors. This is part of the reason that β-blockers may be helpful in controlling the symptoms of hyperthyroidism.

B (decreased sympathetic outflow) is incorrect. Decreased sympathetic outflow does not occur in Graves' disease.

C (increased parasympathetic outflow) is incorrect. Increased parasympathetic outflow does not cause muscle tremors.

D (increased plasma levels of catecholamines) is incorrect. It is primarily the increased responsiveness of muscle cells to circulating catecholamines that causes muscle tremors, rather than a significant increase in levels of catecholamines.

41. **C** (deficits in coronary artery perfusion) is correct. Because the left coronary arteries receive most of their blood flow during diastole, this blood flow is dependent on the diastolic perfusion pressure. In aortic stenosis, most of the energy of ejection goes into pushing blood through the narrowed aortic valve, resulting in low diastolic perfusion pressure, episodes of syncope, and dyspnea with exertion.

In contrast to the left ventricle, the right ventricle receives much of its blood flow during systole, because the extravascular pressures generated during systole are much lower in the right ventricle than in the left.

A (decreased aortic valve opening pressure) is incorrect. The pressure required to open the aortic valve in systole is commonly conceptualized as the afterload. The increase in afterload in aortic stenosis occurs, not because of high peripheral systemic vascular resistance, but rather because of the narrowing of the aortic valve and the resistance to flow through it.

B (raised diastolic pressure) is incorrect. Because much of the energy of left ventricular contraction is expended in overcoming the resistance of the narrowed aortic valve, the diastolic pressure is reduced. In contrast, in conditions in which afterload is elevated due to high peripheral resistance, the aorta retains the ability to elastically release the energy stored in it during systole and thereby maintain an elevated diastolic pressure.

D (longer isovolumic contraction time) is incorrect. The isovolumic contraction time would lengthen only if the aortic pressure in systole were increased. Because diastolic pressure is low, the aortic valve opens faster, and isovolumic contraction is not prolonged. In contrast, there is a delay in the carotid pulse that is easily palpable and results from the prolonged ejection time caused by the narrow aorta.

E (prominent second heart sound) is incorrect. The second heart sound, representing closure of the aortic and pulmonary valves at the end of systole, is softer because the closure of the aortic valve is abnormal owing to the altered hemodynamics of ejection and the substantial transvalvular pressure gradient.

42. **C** (pneumothorax) is the correct choice. Based on the patient's stature and the presence of an aortic aneurysm, it is likely that he has Marfan's syndrome, an inherited disorder of connective tissue. Patients with Marfan's syndrome are at higher risk of spontaneous pneumothorax.

A (myocardial infarction) is incorrect. In myocardial infarction, ECG changes (e.g., ST elevation), as well as increased levels of creatine kinase isoenzyme MB (CK-MB) and cardiac troponin I, would be expected.

B (atrial fibrillation) is incorrect. ECG analysis in a patient with atrial fibrillation would show the absence of P waves.

D (congestive heart failure) is incorrect. Symptoms of congestive heart failure occur gradually, and acute symptoms would not be expected in a previously healthy 25-year-old man. Additionally, ECG changes related to cardiac ischemia would most likely be apparent in congestive heart failure.

E (asthma) is incorrect. Asthma is an obstructive pulmonary disease characterized by airway hypersensitivity. The symptoms experienced by this patient are not consistent with an asthmatic attack.

43. **D** (reduction in hypertension) is correct. Sodium is an important determinant of the circulating volume. Low sodium intake can result in a decline in circulating blood volume and a consequent reduction in both systolic and diastolic blood pressure. This dietary modification has been found to be particularly efficacious for the lowering of blood pressure in African Americans, specifically those who have a low renin level. Restriction of sodium in these patients tends not to lead to compensatory stimulation of the renin-angiotensin system and therefore can have a potent antihypertensive effect.

A (reduced efferent arteriolar tone in the kidney) is incorrect. Low sodium intake results in a decline in the circulating volume, which activates the renin-angiotensin system. This constricts the efferent arteriole, increasing its tone.

B (reduced renin release) is incorrect. Low sodium intake activates the renin-angiotensin system and thus increases renin release.

C (increased blood pressure) is incorrect. Sodium restriction tends to decrease blood pressure.

E (reduced efficacy of diuretics) is incorrect. Diuretic efficacy is enhanced by low sodium intake. In fact, the effect of diuretics can be completely blocked by a high sodium intake, in part because diuretics can result in a compensatory increase in sodium reabsorption in the tubules.

44. **B** (müllerian inhibiting factor) is correct. The descent of the testes from their original retroperitoneal location occurs in two phases. The first phase is triggered by müllerian inhibiting substance. The second phase may occur in response to release of calcitonin gene-related peptide from the genitofemoral nerve by androgens. The only sign may be pain in the lower abdominal and testicular region. The other disorder to include in the differential diagnosis is testicular torsion, which may manifest as unilateral testicular pain. Other unilateral testicular disorders include varicocele, which is more common on the left side because of the downstream connection of the left testicular vein to the high-pressure left renal vein (compared with the right testicular vein, which drains into the inferior vena cava). A left-sided varicocele may be a sentinel feature of a renal malignancy.

A (gonadotropin-releasing hormone surge at puberty) is incorrect. The GnRH surge at puberty plays an important role in promoting testosterone production and development of secondary sexual characteristics. However, it does not play a role in descent of the testes.

C (luteinizing hormone surge at puberty) is incorrect. The normal physiologic descent of the testes may be related to the in utero surge of LH and/or androgens, but it is not related to the LH surge at puberty.

D (testis determining factor) is incorrect. Testis determining factor is encoded on the Y chromosome and is required for development of the testes. It plays no role in descent of the testes.

E (inhibin) is incorrect. Inhibin is secreted by the Sertoli cells and decreases secretion of follicle-stimulating hormone (in contrast to testosterone and dihydrotestosterone, which have little negative feedback effect unless administered in very high, supraphysiologic doses).

45. **A** (the cell hyperpolarizes) is correct. The resting membrane potential, which is maintained by the sodium-potassium-adenosine triphosphatase (Na^+,K^+-ATPase) pump, keeps the intracellular concentration of potassium high while maintaining the high extracellular concentration of sodium. Because the drug preferentially opens potassium channels, the potassium ions move down their concentration gradient, which in the case of a resting skeletal muscle causes an efflux of potassium ions. The loss of positive charges from the inside of the cell hyperpolarizes the cell by increasing the membrane potential.

B (the cell depolarizes due to the influx of potassium ions) is incorrect. The opening of the channel causes a hyperpolarization of the cell due to the efflux of potassium ions.

C (the cell depolarizes due to the efflux of potassium ions) is incorrect. Although there is an efflux of potassium ions, it causes a hyperpolarization, not a depolarization.

D (the membrane potential decreases) is incorrect. The efflux of potassium ions causes an increase in the membrane potential.

E (the membrane potential remains unchanged) is incorrect. The membrane potential increases due to the effect of the drug.

46. **B** (achalasia) is correct. Achalasia is a rare disorder of the esophagus in which the function of the lower esophageal sphincter (LES) is impaired and the sphincter does not relax. The radiologic finding in this case shows the characteristic "bird beak" opening as the increased esophageal pressure occasionally allows a small amount of barium to leak through the sphincter. Achalasia leads to a 5% increased risk of esophageal squamous cell carcinoma; aspiration pneumonia may also occur. The stricture in the upper esophagus of this patient is the result of a carcinoma.

A (Boerhaave's syndrome) is incorrect. Boerhaave's syndrome is a rupture of the esophagus, which may occur after predisposing Mallory-Weiss tears of the esophagogastric junction or prolonged vomiting or retching. It does not lead to an increased risk of esophageal cancer.

C (gastroesophageal reflux) is incorrect. Gastroesophageal reflux (GERD) typically does not cause difficulty in swallowing. GERD can lead to an increased risk of Barrett's esophagus, which can predispose to adenocarcinoma.

D (angina) is incorrect. Angina may be confused with achalasia because both can result in chest pain that is relieved by nitrates. The radiograph in this case that suggests angina is not the most likely cause of the pain.

E (Zenker's diverticulum) is incorrect. A Zenker's diverticulum (pharyngeal pouch) may form above the upper esophageal sphincter due to a weakness in the pharyngeal wall. It causes accumulation of food, which may result in regurgitation without dysphagia and a risk of aspiration pneumonia, as well as foul-smelling breath.

F (epiphrenic diverticulum) is incorrect. An epiphrenic diverticulum is an outpouching of the esophagus above the lower esophageal sphincter. The most telling sign of an epiphrenic diverticulum is regurgitation of fluid at night. The radiographic finding in this case is not supportive of a diverticulum.

G (Chagas' disease) is incorrect. Chagas' disease, an infectious disease common in Central and South America, may result in secondary achalasia. However, the disease also affects other parts of the gastrointestinal tract due to the acquired destruction of the myenteric plexus by the parasite *Trypanosoma cruzi*.

H (hiatal hernia) is incorrect. Hiatal hernia is a condition that occurs when a portion of the stomach herniates through the diaphragm into the mediastinum. It is associated with incompetence of the lower esophageal sphincter and reflux rather than dysphagia. The radiograph does not support a diagnosis of hiatal hernia.

47. **B** (angiotensin II) is correct. Angiotensin II stimulates the release of ADH as part of actions to increase circulating volume. Angiotensin II is increased primarily in response to decreased perfusion pressure of the renal artery, which leads to release of renin and stimulation of the renin-angiotensin-aldosterone system. Therefore, angiotensin is primarily responsive to changes in blood pressure. In contrast, the most important stimulus for release of ADH is an increase in plasma osmolarity, which occurs via active osmoreceptors in the hypothalamus. However, ADH can also be stimulated by a fall in blood volume, both by baroreceptors and by angiotensin II, providing a safety factor for maintenance of blood pressure. Note that each stimulus alters the opposite variable. Although osmolarity is the most important stimulus for ADH, the most significant effect is on body water. In contrast, angiotensin II is primarily stimulated by a decline in circulating volume but exerts its effect on reabsorption of sodium.

A (atrial stretch) is incorrect. Atrial stretch results in the release of atrial natriuretic factor, which acts to diminish circulating blood volume and sodium.

C (decrease in plasma osmolarity) is incorrect. ADH release is inhibited by a decrease in plasma osmolarity.

D (increased blood urea nitrogen) is incorrect. Although an increase in blood urea nitrogen is a sign of impending renal failure, ADH is insensitive to urea. This is because urea is not an effective osmole in the central nervous system and cannot activate osmoreceptors.

E (increased rate of firing of carotid sinus baroreceptor) is incorrect. The carotid sinus baroreceptor stimulates ADH release only when blood pressure falls and the rate of firing is decreased.

48. **B** (vasospasm of the superior hypophyseal artery) is correct. This woman's symptoms (amenorrhea, inability to lactate, fatigue, cold intolerance) are characteristic of hypopituitarism from decreased secretion of anterior pituitary hormones. This can occur in Sheehan's syndrome due to ischemic necrosis of the anterior pituitary after a hemorrhagic delivery. The anterior pituitary is supplied by the superior hypophyseal artery, which normally enlarges substantially during pregnancy (primarily as a result of lactotroph proliferation). However, if hemorrhage occurs, blood supply is reduced; this causes vasospasm of the artery which leads to ischemic necrosis of the anterior pituitary.

A (lesion of the arcuate nucleus) is incorrect. The arcuate nucleus in the hypothalamus is the site of dopamine synthesis, which inhibits prolactin, so the expected consequence of a lesion of the arcuate nucleus is increased prolactin. Unless accompanied by failure to secrete oxytocin, increased levels of prolactin would not account for the failure to lactate. However, a lesion of the arcuate nucleus could cause amenorrhea, because it is the site

of release of gonadotropin-releasing hormone (GnRH). Note that amenorrhea is normal after parturition due to the effect of prolactin, which suppresses secretion of luteinizing hormone. The general endocrine defects in this case point to the anterior pituitary rather than the arcuate nucleus as the source of the problem.

C (lesion of the pituitary stalk) is incorrect. The lack of oxytocin that accompanies a lesion of the pituitary stalk (causing lack of breast milk ejection) makes it difficult to rule out this possibility unless antidiuretic hormone (and, hence, urine volumes) were normal. However, lack of prolactin secretion could also account for a failure to produce breast milk, and this could occur with damage to the anterior pituitary.

D (pituitary adenoma) is incorrect. Bleeding can occur into a pituitary adenoma, which can result in hypopituitarism identical to that seen here. However, there is no evidence that this patient had a previously existing pituitary adenoma.

E (ischemic necrosis of the posterior pituitary) is incorrect. The posterior pituitary is typically spared in Sheehan's syndrome, because it has a different blood supply than the anterior pituitary. Recall that the anterior and posterior pituitary have different embryologic origins, and therefore different blood supplies.

49. **C** (there is less airway resistance) is correct. Less airway resistance occurs at higher lung volumes, probably because the average diameter of airways is increased. Although most of the resistance is in the larger airways and Poiseuille's law does not apply to the nonlaminar flow there, the increased airway diameter probably decreases overall resistance, because Poiseuille's law states that the resistance is inversely related to the fourth power of the radius.

A (the lung is more compliant) is incorrect. The lung is usually less compliant at higher volumes.

B (alveoli at the base of the lung are more compressed) is incorrect. Alveoli at the base of the lung are less compressed at higher volumes.

D (alveolar vessels are less compressed) is incorrect. The alveolar vessels are more compressed at higher lung volumes, because the lung expands and compresses them. This occurs because a higher distending pressure is required at higher lung volumes, and the alveolar pressure is therefore more capable of compressing the thin-walled capillaries.

E (extra-alveolar vessels are compressed) is incorrect. The extra-alveolar vessels are the bronchial arteries and arterioles, which do not participate in gas exchange, and the pulmonary veins. Recall that pulmonary veins do not follow the same branching pattern as the pulmonary arteries, arterioles, and alveoli (which all branch in the same pattern). The extra-alveolar vessels therefore are not exposed to the increased alveolar pressures required to distend the lung, and at higher volumes they actually expand.

50. **A** (bradykinin) is correct. Bradykinin is a vasodilator peptide formed from the cleavage of kininogens by kallikrein. It is an arteriolar vasodilator and a venous vasoconstrictor; it increases vascular permeability and produces pain. Bradykinin is also involved in regulation of sweating and in the production of saliva. It is normally degraded by kininase II, which is an isoform of ACE. Therefore, inhibition of bradykinin degradation results in vasodilation directly mediated by bradykinin. Inhibition of ACE also results in a loss of vasoconstriction normally regulated via angiotensin II.

The hypotensive effects of ACE inhibitors may possibly be a combination of angiotensin II blockade and bradykinin potentiation.

B (angiotensin converting enzyme) is incorrect. The effect of ACE is to activate angiotensin II, which is a potent vasoconstrictor. ACE also inactivates bradykinin, a vasodilator.

C (angiotensin II) is incorrect. Angiotensin II is a vasoconstrictor and does not produce hypotension.

D (kininase II) is incorrect. Kininase II is an isoform of ACE. It degrades bradykinin and does not produce hypotension.

E (kallikrein) is incorrect. Kallikrein is a protease formed from prekallikrein by contact with Hageman factor (factor XII). Kallikrein cleaves bradykinin from high-molecular-weight kininogen. Kallikrein has other functions besides being responsible for the activation of bradykinin; these include activation of complement (conversion of C5 to C5a).

questions

DIRECTIONS: Each numbered item or incomplete statement is followed by options arranged in alphabetical or logical order. Select the best answer to each question. Some options may be partially correct, but there is only **ONE BEST** answer.

1. A 48-year-old woman with a history of rheumatic fever is evaluated for worsening dyspnea with exertion. Examination reveals normal vital signs and a normal pulse pressure, but cardiac auscultation is significant for a loud diastolic murmur over the apex. Which of the following valvular disorders is most likely responsible for this woman's complaints?
A. Aortic stenosis
B. Aortic regurgitation
C. Mitral regurgitation
D. Mitral stenosis

2. An arterial blood gas measurement in a patient with renal failure reveals the following: pH, 7.3; partial pressure of carbon dioxide (Pa_{CO_2}), 30 mm Hg; and bicarbonate (HCO_3^-), 18 mmol/L (normal 24–30). Administration of which of the following agents could potentially worsen the existing metabolic acidosis?
A. Bumetanide
B. Acetazolamide
C. Furosemide
D. Ethacrynic acid
E. Hydrochlorothiazide

3. A 53-year-old woman has symptoms of early stages of volume-overload hypertension, including headaches and microalbuminuria. Which of the following endogenous hormones acts to limit increases in blood pressure by stimulating diuresis?

A. Arginine vasopressin
B. Angiotensin II
C. Atrial natriuretic peptide
D. Aldosterone
E. Antidiuretic hormone

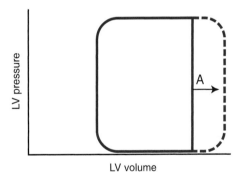

4. In the left ventricular (LV) pressure-volume loop shown in the accompanying figure, a shift of line A to the right is associated with which of the following effects?
A. Less compliant ventricle in hypertension
B. Increased afterload in hypertension
C. Increased preload after brief exercise
D. Increased contractility with increased heart rate
E. The effect of afterload reduction therapy

5. A 28-year-old man has mild hypertension. Because of his age, specialized testing is performed to determine whether a treatable secondary cause for his hypertension can be identified. Workup reveals elevated levels of plasma aldosterone, and a computed tomographic scan of the abdomen confirms the presence of a mass on his left adrenal gland. What physiologic mechanism ensures that this patient is only mildly hypertensive?

A. Target tissue insensitivity to aldosterone
B. Decreased atrial natriuretic peptide
C. Feedback inhibition of angiotensin-converting enzyme by aldosterone
D. Pressure diuresis
E. Increased baroreceptor-mediated sympathetic outflow

6. A 4-year-old girl is evaluated after a 3-month history of diarrhea, fatigue, and weight loss. The diarrhea is nonbloody and seems to improve if she eats less breads and grains. She tolerates milk well. The mother denies any recent history of fever, nausea, or vomiting. Physical examination and vital signs are completely normal. Small bowel biopsy shows flattening of the villi and deepening of the crypts. What is the most likely explanation of this girl's symptoms?

A. Whipple's disease
B. Celiac sprue
C. Lactase deficiency
D. Pseudomembranous colitis
E. Viral gastroenteritis

7. A 34-year-old woman comes in for evaluation of weight gain, depression, and newly diagnosed hypertension. Examination reveals truncal obesity and accumulation of fat in the posterior neck and back. Laboratory testing reveals increased levels glucose and cortisol in the blood. A dexamethasone suppression test shows no change in plasma cortisol or adrenocorticotropic hormone (ACTH) after low-dose dexamethasone but a substantial drop in ACTH and cortisol after administration of high-dose dexamethasone. This woman's symptoms are most likely due to which of the following disorders?

A. Thyroid adenoma
B. Adrenocorticotropic hormone–secreting pituitary adenoma

C. Ectopic secretion of adrenocorticotropic hormone
D. Adrenal tumor
E. Congenital adrenal hyperplasia

8. A patient with an arrhythmia is given a drug that blocks the potassium channels that are involved in membrane repolarization. Which of the following effects on the action potential in myocytes is most likely to occur with administration of this drug?

A. Shortening of phase 0
B. Prolonging of phase 3
C. Shortening of phase 3
D. Prolonging of phase 0

9. Which characteristic is better encoded by the phasic receptor than by the tonic receptor?

A. Strength of stimulus
B. Duration of stimulus
C. Quality of stimulus
D. How rapidly the stimulus is applied
E. Location of stimulus

10. A 58-year-old, moderately obese woman works in a job that requires her to stand for long hours. Her feet have recently developed nonhealing ulcers that she is unable to treat with over-the-counter medications. She also complains of increased thirst, urinary frequency, and fatigue. How does the hormone that has most likely caused these symptoms exert its effect on cells?

A. Activates tyrosine-specific protein kinase autophosphorylation
B. Activates adenyl cyclase
C. Activates phospholipase C
D. Binds to intracellular receptors, which then bind regulatory elements on DNA
E. Activates guanylate cyclase

11. Release of which of the following hormones best illustrates neuroendocrine secretion?

A. Cortisol by the adrenal cortex
B. Oxytocin by the hypothalamus
C. Corticotropin-releasing hormone (CRH) by the neurohypophysis

D. Thyroid-stimulating hormone (TSH) by the anterior pituitary

E. Insulin by pancreatic β-cells

12. A friend has decided to move to the Andes Mountains and asks you what physiologic responses he can expect due to the change in altitude. You tell him that he will most likely experience which of the following?

A. A decrease in erythropoietin

B. A decrease in 2,3-DPG

C. An acute decrease in ventilatory rate

D. A chronic decrease in ventilatory rate

E. An increase in the renal excretion of bicarbonate

13. A 15-year-old boy is evaluated for undescended testis (cryptorchidism) and delayed pubertal development. Ultrasonography of the abdomen and pelvis reveals what appear to be testicular structures in the lower pelvis, as well as agenesis of the right kidney. A detailed neurologic examination is significant for the finding of anosmia. The boy's height falls within normal predicted values for his age, although a bone scan shows decreased bone density. In this patient, the developmental delay can be treated by exogenous administration of which of the following drugs?

A. Human chorionic gonadotropin (hCG)

B. Growth hormone (GH)

C. Gonadotropin-releasing hormone (GnRH)

D. Clomiphene

E. Follicle-stimulating hormone (FSH)

14. A medical student is asked to assess a man who has been brought to the emergency department after being found comatose in his apartment. During the physical examination, the student notices a fruity odor on the patient's breath. His respiratory rate is 30 breaths per minute, and he seems to be taking very deep breaths. When the attending physician asks the student to name the respiratory response, the correct response is

A. Cheyne-Stokes respiration

B. Biot's breathing

C. Apneustic breathing

D. Kussmaul's respiration

E. Normal respiration

15. A 42-year-old man has hypertension that has been refractory to all commonly employed antihypertensives. Angiography of the renal artery is performed, and the results suggest a diagnosis of secondary hypertension. Which of the following conditions would most likely be found in this patient?

A. Renal hyperperfusion

B. Low plasma renin activity

C. Expanded plasma volume

D. Decreased total peripheral resistance

16. A male infant is born without complication. However, shortly thereafter nurses note that he has failed to pass meconium, has bilious vomiting, and a distended abdomen. Barium enema shows a dilated proximal segment of large bowel followed by a narrow distal segment. Biopsy of the large bowel would most likely show

A. Absence of Auerbach's plexus only

B. Absence of Meissner's plexus only

C. Absence of all ganglion cells in the affected segment of bowel

D. Failure of involution of the vitelline duct

E. Absence of pathology, because failure to pass meconium is normal for a newborn

17. In terms of its effects on venous return, which of the following conditions is hemodynamically most similar to venoconstriction?

A. Arterial vasoconstriction

B. Transfusion

C. Hemorrhage

D. Diuresis

18. An 80-year-old man has hypertension and left-sided heart failure that has been managed for years with hydrochlorothiazide. However, due to recent progression of his symptoms, it is decided that an additional drug should be added to his chronic heart failure regimen, and he is started on digitalis. What side effect is possible if digitalis is given in addition to the hydrochlorothiazide?

A. Hyperkalemia
B. Hypouricemia
C. Hypoglycemia
D. Ventricular arrhythmia
E. Hypocalcemia

19. A 52-year-old woman comes in for evaluation after a several-month history of hot flashes that are making it difficult for her to sleep at night. Her last menstrual period was 1 year ago. She also says she has been more irritable in recent months. Which of the following endocrine findings would be predicted in this patient?

A. Lack of pulsatile secretion of gonadotropin-releasing hormone (GnRH)
B. Complete loss of estrogen production
C. Increased levels of luteinizing hormone (LH) and follicle-simulating hormone (FSH)
D. Monthly cycle in which a high ratio of LH to FSH is maintained
E. Decline in estrogen production only

20. In an attempt to find a cure for Parkinson's disease, a neuroscientist inserts an electrical probe into a rat's brain and intends to monitor the subsequent release of dopamine from the cells. After several minutes, the scientist measures the levels of all substances released and finds an abnormally high concentration of norepinephrine. Into which structure of the brain did the scientist actually place the probe?

A. Basal nucleus of Meynert
B. Locus ceruleus
C. Raphe nucleus
D. Substantia nigra
E. Caudate nucleus

21. A 34-year-old woman who is a vegetarian and a native of India complains of malaise and tingling sensations (paresthesias) in her extremities for the past 6 months. A complete blood count reveals a hematocrit of 25% and a hemoglobin level of 9 g/dL. Peripheral blood smear reveals enlarged red blood cells and hypersegmented polymorphonuclear cells. A neurologic

examination is remarkable for decreased proprioception, fine touch, and vibratory sensations. Which of the following substances is most likely to be abnormally low in this patient?

A. Vitamin B_1
B. Intrinsic factor
C. Iron
D. Vitamin B_{12}
E. Pyridoxine

22. In which of the following settings is diuretic therapy appropriate for the treatment of edema?

A. Lymphedema
B. Laryngeal edema
C. Adult respiratory distress syndrome
D. Myxedema
E. Acute cardiogenic pulmonary edema

23. A 65-year-old construction worker with a 40-year history of smoking two packs of cigarettes per day is evaluated for worsening shortness of breath and chronic productive cough. Pulmonary function tests yield the following results:

Total lung capacity (TLC)	3.7 L (65% of predicted)
Forced vital capacity (FVC)	3.1 L (62% of predicted)
Forced expiratory volume in 1 second (FEV_1)	2.8 L (85% of predicted)
Functional residual capacity (FRC)	1.8 L (72% of predicted)
Residual volume (RV)	0.6 L (95% of predicted)

With respect to pulmonary function, which of the following best describes this man's lungs?

A. Normal
B. Exhibiting restrictive airway disease
C. Exhibiting obstructive airway disease
D. Exhibiting a combined restrictive/obstructive airway disease

24. In an attempt to increase his maximum lift on the biceps curl, a professional weight-lifter injects a substance into his elbows. During the lift, a loud sound is heard and it appears that he has ruptured his biceps tendon. Which receptors that monitor the force developed by the muscle was the weight-lifter trying to manipulate?

A. Nuclear bag intrafusal fibers
B. Golgi tendon organs
C. Ruffini corpuscles
D. Pacinian corpuscles
E. Nuclear chain intrafusal fibers

25. A 52-year-old woman complains of anxiety, difficulty sleeping, weight loss, headaches, and muscle tremors. Her blood pressure is 220/110 mm Hg. A computed tomographic scan shows a mass on her left adrenal gland. A diagnosis of malignant hypertension secondary to pheochromocytoma is made. Urinalysis would be expected to show markedly increased levels of which of the following compounds?

A. 5'-hydroxyindoleacetic acid (5'-HIAA)
B. Cortisol
C. Vanillylmandelic acid (VMA)
D. Dehydroepiandrosterone

26. A 43-year-old man complains of abdominal pain after fatty meals and greasy, foul-smelling stools. On examination, sharp pain is elicited by deep palpation at the costal margin in the right upper abdominal quadrant during inspiration (positive Murphy's sign). A right upper quadrant ultrasound study confirms the suspicion of cholecystitis and biliary obstruction. This patient would most likely be expected to be deficient in which of the following compounds?

A. Vitamin C
B. Vitamin K
C. Iron
D. Vitamin B_{12}
E. Intrinsic factor

27. A woman brings her 7-year-old son to the clinic for evaluation of "allergies." She explains that her son frequently experiences trouble breathing. A high-pitched expiratory wheeze is noted on examination, and asthma is suspected. Which of the following statements best explains forced expiration in this patient?

A. As residual volume is approached, the upper airways collapse before the lower airways do.

B. Airway diameter increases during expiration due to a more negative intrapleural pressure.
C. The ratio of forced expiratory volume to forced vital capacity (FEV_1/FVC) is less than 0.8.
D. FEV_1 is increased.

28. A migrant worker with a productive cough, night sweats, and fatigue has a positive tuberculin (PPD) test. If a tuberculosis infection has preferentially affected the apex of the lung, some impairment of gas exchange might be expected. In the healthy patient, the apex of the lung

A. Is at a more favorable position on the compliance curve
B. Displays zone 1 flow
C. Is better ventilated than the base
D. Displays diffusion-limited transfer
E. Displays perfusion-limited flow

29. A 52-year-old man complains of fatigue and shortness of breath. His symptoms have become so severe that he no longer enjoys golf. Cardiac examination reveals a grade 4/6 crescendo-decrescendo systolic ejection murmur best appreciated at the right second intercostal space. Echocardiography confirms the presence of severe aortic valve stenosis and reveals an ejection fraction of 20%. An electrocardiogram (ECG) reveals left ventricular hypertrophy, and his physician tells him that he has left-sided heart failure. Which of the following conditions may be expected in this patient?

A. Right-axis deviation on ECG
B. Peripheral edema
C. Activation of the sympathoadrenal axis
D. Decreased secretion of atrial natriuretic factor
E. Decreased pressure recording from a pulmonary wedge device
F. Increased plasma pH

30. An 8-year-old girl is brought to the clinic by her mother. The mother states that her daughter has always had problems swallowing food, but that recently it seems to be getting worse. She also notes that her daughter frequently vomits at night. Past medical history reveals that the girl has been hospitalized previously for aspiration pneumonia. You suspect achalasia. Which of the following findings would best support your diagnosis?

A. Complete relaxation of the lower esophageal sphincter (LES) with swallowing
B. Decreased resting tone of the LES
C. Increased resting tone of the upper esophageal sphincter (UES)
D. Incomplete relaxation of the LES with swallowing, coupled with increased resting tone of the LES
E. Incomplete relaxation of the LES with swallowing, coupled with increased resting tone of the UES

31. A 28-year-old woman gives birth at 31 weeks to a male infant. The physician notices that the infant is having difficulty breathing and attributes this difficulty to respiratory distress syndrome. Which of the following statements best characterizes this disease?

A. It is caused by the overproduction of surfactant.
B. It decreases the surface tension in the alveoli.
C. It preferentially results in the collapse of smaller alveoli.
D. It causes a decrease in the retractile force of the lung, resulting in a low transmural pressure.
E. It occurs less frequently in premature infants.

32. A 14-year-old girl is concerned because she has not had her first period and she is much shorter than her peers. Her parents ask about potentially starting her on estrogen therapy. Which of the following effects would most likely result from *short-term* treatment with exogenous estrogen in a female patient who has not yet entered puberty?

A. Closure of the epiphyses
B. Ovulation
C. Pronounced nocturnal spikes of follicle-stimulating hormone (FSH)

D. Initiation of a growth spurt
E. Osteoporosis

33. A patient with hyponatremia and hyperkalemia is placed on fluid restriction. After 12 hours of fluid restriction, the urine became increasingly concentrated, until a urine osmolarity of 900 mOsm/L is reached. The hyponatremia continues to worsen. This indicates that the hyponatremia could be attributable to

A. Nephrogenic diabetes insipidus
B. Central diabetes insipidus
C. Syndrome of inappropriate antidiuretic hormone secretion (SIADH)
D. Psychogenic polydipsia
E. Mineralocorticoid deficiency

34. A patient has left-sided heart failure that is being managed with two diuretics to prevent fluid overload. He develops hypokalemia from the diuretic therapy, and an electrocardiogram (ECG) shows characteristic changes, such as the presence of a U wave after the T wave. At a cellular level, what effect of hypokalemia on cardiac muscle cells could provide a rationale for the changes seen in the ECG of a patient with hypokalemia?

A. Hypokalemia hyperpolarizes cells.
B. Conduction velocity is slowed.
C. The potassium current in phase 4 is abolished.
D. The membrane potential moves toward the potassium equilibrium potential.
E. The Nernst equation explains these changes.
F. The membrane potential moves away from the potassium equilibrium potential.

35. A 70-year-old woman with respiratory failure due to pneumonia is intubated and placed on a ventilator with a tidal volume of 700 mL and a respiratory rate of 16 breaths per minute. An arterial blood gas analysis reveals adequate oxygenation, and her ventilatory settings are decreased. Which of the following changes would produce the greatest decrease in this patient's minute ventilation?

A. Increase the respiratory rate to 18 breaths per minute
B. Decrease the respiratory rate to 12 breaths per minute
C. Decrease the tidal volume to 600 mL and decrease the respiratory rate to 14 breaths per minute
D. Decrease the tidal volume to 500 mL
E. Increase the tidal volume to 800 mL

36. A new drug is developed to minimize muscle weakness in neuromuscular disorders such as myasthenia gravis. This drug preferentially opens sodium channels without affecting the permeability of other ions. What effect would this medication have on the resting cell?

A. The membrane potential would move away from the sodium equilibrium potential.
B. The membrane potential would move toward the sodium equilibrium potential.
C. The sodium equilibrium potential would remain unchanged.
D. The sodium equilibrium potential would increase.
E. The cell would hyperpolarize.

37. A 21-year-old woman complains of fatigue, weakness, and recent weight gain. She has the typical moon face, truncal obesity, thin extremities, and abdominal striae of Cushing's syndrome A CT scan of the head reveals an enlarged pituitary gland, and an endocrine workup shows markedly increased levels of plasma cortisol and adrenocorticotropic hormone (ACTH). Which of the following metabolic effects would most likely be observed in this patient?

A. Decreased lipolysis in adipose tissue
B. Increased glycolysis in skeletal muscle
C. Decreased plasma glucose
D. Increased hepatic glycogenesis
E. Decreased plasma protein levels

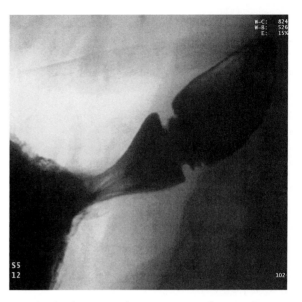

Reproduced with permission from Grainger RG, Allison D, Adam A, Dixon AK: Grainger & Allison's Diagnostic Radiology: A Textbook of Medical Imaging, 4th ed. London, Churchill Livingstone, 2001, Fig. 46-6.

38. A 45-year-old woman presents for evaluation of a long history of "heartburn" which is worse at night. She also complains of occasional dysphagia to solids, particularly when eating meat. A radiograph is obtained (see the accompanying figure) and shows circular strictures about 5 cm above the diaphragmatic opening. The most likely cause of these findings is

A. Hiatal hernia and Schatzki rings
B. Achalasia
C. Barrett's esophagus
D. Epiphrenic diverticulum
E. Pyloric stenosis
F. Crohn's disease

39. An 18-year-old woman presents with high levels of prolactin, estriol, and progesterone and low levels of luteinizing hormone (LH) and follicle-stimulating hormone (FSH). She has missed several periods. This patient is best described as

A. A patient with functional amenorrhea
B. A pregnant patient
C. A patient taking aromatase inhibitors
D. A patient using oral contraception
E. A patient with polycystic ovary syndrome
F. A patient with hyperprolactinemia
G. A patient with resistant ovary syndrome
H. A patient with primary amenorrhea

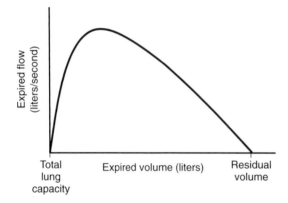

40. A young champion tennis player with asthma requests a pulmonary evaluation before entering a major tournament. The peak expiratory flow rate is assessed both before and after administration of bronchodilator drugs. The volume of gas expelled is plotted during expiration with maximal effort, from the rise to maximal inspir.ed volume to residual volume (see the accompanying figure). Which of the following statements best describes the maximal rate of forced expiratory flow (peak expiratory flow rate) in a healthy lung?

A. It is limited by the rigidity of the thoracic cage.
B. It is a consequence of the length-tension relation for skeletal muscle.
C. It is increased at an optimal intermediate starting lung volume.
D. It is less than in restrictive disorders.
E. It is increased if the initial volume is increased.

41. A 50-year-old man complains of dizziness when he gets out of bed in the morning. To test autonomic reflexes associated with standing rapidly, he is tested on a tilt table. In this test, the patient relaxes comfortably in the horizontal position while immobilized, and the table is then tilted rapidly so that the patient is placed in a vertical position. Before and after the maneuver, blood pressure and electrocardiographic tracings are obtained. Which of the following effects would be expected as part of the baroreceptor reflex when the patient is moved to the vertical position?

A. Increased cardiac output
B. Increased total peripheral resistance
C. Increased preload
D. Increased rate of firing of aortic arch baroreceptors
E. Increased membrane potential of carotid sinus baroreceptors
F. Increase rate of firing of carotid sinus baroreceptors
G. Increased left-axis deviation

42. Which of the following agents could potentially result in the inability to achieve or sustain an erection?

A. Phosphodiesterase inhibitors
B. Nicotinic blockade
C. Sympathetic excitation of the bladder
D. Guanyl cyclase activators
E. α-Adrenergic antagonists

43. A 72-year-old man with a long history of untreated hypertension complains of fatigue and shortness of breath. On examination, jugular venous distention and bibasilar crackles are present. His current blood pressure is 90/50 mm Hg, and echocardiography shows an ejection fraction of 35%. Without treatment, which of the following consequences may occur?

A. Extremely elevated urine production
B. Suppression of the renin-angiotensin system
C. Slight urine production (oliguria)
D. Decreased extracellular fluid volume
E. Decreased plasma levels of atrial natriuretic peptide

44. While on a group expedition in tropical Africa, a 29-year-old woman becomes fatigued and jaundiced. Because of the isolated location, laboratory evaluation of the woman's medical condition depends solely on analysis of urine and stool samples using available testing kits. Based on your knowledge of normal bilirubin metabolism, which of the following findings would be consistent with nonobstructive jaundice caused by a hemolytic anemia?
A. Urine with a positive reaction for conjugated bilirubin
B. Presence of occult blood in the feces
C. Pale stools negative for bilirubin and urobilinogens
D. Urine with a positive reaction for indirect bilirubin
E. Elevated levels of urobilinogens in the urine and feces

45. Antidiuretic hormone (ADH) may occasionally be administered to patients with substantial polyuria caused by central diabetes insipidus. A risk associated with the use of ADH in this context is that acute hyponatremia and volume expansion can occur in a patient receiving intravenous fluids, with consequent brain swelling and death. In this situation, what terminates the physiologic effects of ADH?
A. Increase in plasma volume
B. Decrease in plasma osmolarity
C. Increase in levels of cyclic adenosine monophosphate (cAMP) in collecting duct cells
D. Endocytosis of aquaporin water channels
E. Receptor-mediated endocytosis of ADH from the luminal surface

46. A 55-year-old man diagnosed with hyperthyroidism complains of fevers and insomnia. Physical examination shows tachycardia. He is initially treated with propylthiouracil (PTU) to manage the symptoms of hyperthyroidism prior to surgery. Two weeks later, he develops a sore throat and his fever becomes elevated. Blood cultures reveal a fall in the neutrophil count, so propylthiouracil is discontinued. His physician recommends surgery. The normal preoperative management for a hyperactive thyroid goiter calls for treatment with which of the following agents about 2 weeks prior to surgery?
A. Potassium iodide
B. Allopurinol
C. Thyroxine
D. Corticosteroids
E. Radioactive iodine

47. A 67-year-old woman is evaluated for a 1-week history of worsening fatigue, leg edema, shortness of breath, and a new requirement for use of pillows to sleep at night. Heart failure in this setting is associated with the secretion of high levels of atrial natriuretic factor (ANF). Which of the following is the most likely cause of the increased secretion of ANF in this patient?
A. Improving cardiovascular function
B. Decreased preload
C. Increased preload
D. Increased natriuresis

48. In a normal heart, the period of isovolumic contraction of the left ventricle continues until which of the following pressures is reached?
A. Wedge pressure
B. Positive end-expiratory pressure
C. Aortic pressure
D. Mean arterial pressure
E. Systolic pressure

49. A 10-year-old boy has frequent muscle cramps with exercise and a recent episode of red-tinged urine. Laboratory evaluation reveals elevated creatinine and potassium concentrations. The physician then performs an ischemic forearm exercise test. In this test, an intravenous line is placed in the median vein. The subject is asked to clench and unclench the hand rapidly while the blood supply is occluded, during which a sample of venous blood is taken, and samples are also taken after occlusion is stopped. This test reveals high levels of ammonia and low levels of lactate in the venous blood of the occluded forearm. The cause of the boy's cramping and discolored urine is most likely

A. Hyperkalemic periodic paralysis
B. Type A lactic acidosis
C. Cushing's syndrome
D. Myophosphorylase deficiency
E. Carnitine palmitoyltransferase II deficiency
F. Paroxysmal nocturnal hemoglobinuria
G. Phosphofructokinase deficiency
H. Oxygen debt

50. A 43-year-old woman is diagnosed with a rare inherited form of hypertension known as Liddle's syndrome. In this disorder, hypertension results from a gain-of-function mutation in the amiloride-sensitive sodium channel of the distal nephron. Which of the following findings would be expected in this patient?

A. Elevated plasma renin
B. Hypokalemia
C. Increased sympathetic stimulation of the juxtaglomerular apparatus
D. Decreased plasma cortisol
E. Metabolic acidosis

1. **D** (mitral stenosis) is correct. Although rheumatic heart disease can affect the mitral and aortic valves and cause each of the valvular disorders, it most commonly affects the mitral valve, resulting in stenosis. Mitral stenosis causes a diastolic murmur because of turbulent flow across the stenotic mitral valve during ventricular filling in diastole. Mitral stenosis is most commonly caused by rheumatic fever and typically develops approximately 20 years after the fever. The dyspnea results primarily from blood backing up in the pulmonary veins due to ineffective flow through the stenotic mitral valve. This increases the hydrostatic pressure in the pulmonary capillaries, causing transudation of fluid across the capillaries and pulmonary edema.

A (aortic stenosis) is incorrect. Aortic stenosis causes a systolic murmur because of turbulent flow of blood across the narrowed aortic valve during ejection of blood from the heart.

B (aortic regurgitation) is incorrect. Aortic regurgitation causes a systolic heart murmur and is associated with an increased pulse pressure, neither of which is present in this patient.

C (mitral regurgitation) is incorrect. Mitral regurgitation causes a systolic murmur rather than a diastolic murmur.

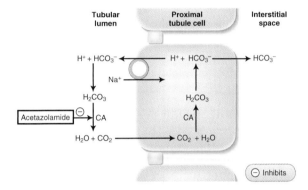

2. **B** (acetazolamide) is correct. Acetazolamide works by inhibiting luminal carbonic anhydrase (CA), an enzyme that promotes the tubular absorption of HCO_3^- by catalyzing the conversion of carbonic acid to water and CO_2 within the proximal tubule (see the accompanying figure). Inhibition of carbonic anhydrase inhibits HCO_3^- reabsorption and results in an alkaline urine, which can worsen an existing metabolic acidosis.

A (bumetanide) is incorrect. Bumetanide is a loop diuretic that works by inhibiting the Na^+-K^+-$2Cl^-$ cotransporter pump located in the loop of Henle. The net result is decreased reabsorption of sodium, potassium, and chloride, leading to diuresis. This drug can possibly cause a metabolic alkalosis from excessive loss of sodium and hydrogen ions, but it cannot cause metabolic acidosis.

C (furosemide) is incorrect. Furosemide, like bumetanide, is a loop diuretic that inhibits the $Na^+-K^+-2Cl^-$ cotransporter. Its use can lead to metabolic alkalosis, but not metabolic acidosis.

D (ethacrynic acid) is incorrect. Ethacrynic acid, like bumetanide, is a loop diuretic that inhibits the $Na^+-K^+-2Cl^-$ cotransporter. Its use can lead to metabolic alkalosis, but not metabolic acidosis.

E (hydrochlorothiazide) is incorrect. Thiazide diuretics increase the excretion of sodium, chloride, and water by inhibiting sodium ion transport at the distal tubules. Acid-base balance usually is not affected. However, the hypochloremia caused by this drug can lead to mild metabolic alkalosis.

3. **C** (atrial natriuretic peptide) is correct. Atrial natriuretic peptide (also referred to as atrial natriuretic factor, or ANF) is released from the atria in response to increased stretching of the atrial wall, which is typically caused by volume overload but also by pressure overload. ANF acts to decrease plasma volume in multiple ways. It acts on the kidneys to increase the glomerular filtration rate (GFR) and decrease sodium reabsorption at the collecting ducts, both of which result in increased elimination of salt and water, thereby lowering plasma volume. Additionally, ANF inhibits secretion of aldosterone by the adrenal cortex. All of the other agents listed increase blood pressure. Renin is secreted by the renal juxtaglomerular cells in response to hypoperfusion of the afferent arteriole. Renin converts the plasma protein angiotensinogen (released from the liver) into angiotensin I. Angiotensin-converting enzyme, found largely in the pulmonary vasculature, then converts angiotensin I to angiotensin II, which has powerful vasoconstrictor effects.

A (arginine vasopressin) is incorrect. Arginine vasopressin is a synonym for antidiuretic hormone (ADH), which stimulates release of aldosterone; this increases renal reabsorption of sodium in the collecting duct and stimulates thirst.

B (angiotensin II) is incorrect. Angiotensin II has multiple target sites, including the kidneys, hypothalamus, adrenal cortex, and vascular smooth muscle cells. Contraction of smooth muscle cells is promoted via binding of angiotensin II directly to receptors found on the cells and by upregulation of sympathetic release of norepinephrine at the neuronal varicosities, both of which increase the cytoplasmic concentration of calcium in the cells.

D (aldosterone) is incorrect. Aldosterone acts on the renal collecting ducts to increase reabsorption of sodium and potassium (water follows passively).

E (antidiuretic hormone) is incorrect. Antidiuretic hormone (ADH) and arginine vasopressin are the same hormone. ADH inhibits diuresis and therefore acts to increase plasma volume and blood pressure.

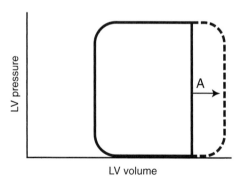

4. **C** (increased preload after brief exercise) is correct. A brief period of exercise increases venous return. This results in an increased amount of ventricular filling, which increases the end-diastolic volume as line A moves to the right. Because the heart rate increases with exercise, there is a greater accumulation of calcium within the muscle (Bowditch treppe), so the contractility of the muscle increases at higher heart rates. Increased contractility lowers the end-systolic volume (see the accompanying figure). The total stroke volume increases with exercise due to the lower end-systolic volume and the increased preload. The increase in both stroke volume and heart rate results in a substantial increase in cardiac output with exercise.

A (less compliant ventricle in hypertension) is incorrect. A stiffer ventricle would result in a shift of the diastolic filling portion of the curve to a higher ventricular pressure and move the systolic ejection to a lower ejection pressure. The end-diastolic volume would shift to the left, opposite to the shift shown in the accompanying figure.

B (increased afterload in hypertension) is incorrect. Afterload is the aortic pressure against which the ventricle contracts. If the afterload is increased, then the systolic ejection phase occurs at a higher pressure and terminates earlier, resulting in a higher end-systolic volume. This reduces the stroke volume without affecting the end-diastolic volume (preload).

D (increased contractility with increased heart rate) is incorrect. Increased contractility at higher heart rates means that systolic ejection is more effective, so the stroke volume increases. This is seen as a shift in the end-systolic volume to the left, correlating with an increased slope in the end-systolic pressure-volume relation (see the accompanying figure). This line is the change in pressure relative to the change in volume (dP/dV) and must not be confused with compliance or the function dP/dT (where T is time).

E (the effect of afterload reduction therapy) is incorrect. Afterload reduction therapy would bring systolic ventricular pressures down, which would increase stroke volume by allowing ventricular ejection to fully occur. This would not affect the end-diastolic volume (preload).

5. **D** (pressure diuresis) is correct. This patient has primary aldosteronism (Conn's syndrome), caused by an aldosterone-secreting tumor of the adrenal cortex. Aldosterone acts on the nephron to increase sodium reabsorption, thereby leading to extracellular volume expansion and hypertension. Because the glomerular filtration rate increases in response to renal perfusion, pressure diuresis by the kidneys limits the severity of the hypertension and hypervolemia that occurs with primary aldosteronism.

A (target tissue insensitivity to aldosterone) is incorrect. Although some receptor down-regulation is expected in response to abnormally high levels of aldosterone, the phenomenon of pressure diuresis appears to play a more important role in limiting the severity of the hypertension that occurs in primary hyperaldosteronism.

B (decreased atrial natriuretic peptide) is incorrect. In hyperaldosteronism, increased levels of atrial natriuretic factor would be expected in response to volume expansion.

C (feedback inhibition of angiotensin-converting enzyme by aldosterone) is incorrect. Aldosterone is not involved in the production of angiotensin II by angiotensin-converting enzyme.

E (increased baroreceptor-mediated sympathetic outflow) is incorrect. Volume expansion in hyperaldosteronism inhibits sympathetic-mediated outflow via the baroreceptor reflex.

6. **B** (celiac sprue) is the correct answer. This clinical picture of chronic diarrhea, weight loss, fatigue, and failure to thrive is typical of a malabsorption syndrome. Celiac sprue is the likely cause for this patient's symptoms in light of the improvement of diarrhea after withdrawal of breads and grains from the diet and the small bowel biopsy findings. The pathology underlying celiac sprue is an immune-mediated reaction against gluten, which is a protein found in grains and wheat. Small bowel biopsy commonly shows atrophy and blunting of the villi. Treatment involves adhering to a diet free of glutens.

A (Whipple's disease) is incorrect. Whipple's disease manifests more commonly in men between the ages 30 and 40 years. Although it does cause diarrhea, weight loss, and symptoms of malabsorption, there typically are additional findings suggestive of this disease. It is caused by a gram-positive actinomycete, *Tropheryma whippelii*. In addition to the gastrointestinal system, it can affect the joints and central nervous system. The key morphologic finding is periodic acid–Schiff (PAS)–positive granules and rod-shaped bacilli by electron microscopy.

C (lactase deficiency) is incorrect. Lactase deficiency can manifest as a malabsorption syndrome. However, this patient seems to have no problems when ingesting milk.

D (pseudomembranous colitis) is incorrect. Pseudomembranous colitis does cause diarrhea but occurs after use of an antibiotic. This patient has not received any antibiotics recently.

E (viral gastroenteritis) is incorrect. This patient's clinical picture is more suggestive of a malabsorptive syndrome than an acute viral syndrome. Viral gastroenteritis typically manifests first with nausea and vomiting, followed by diarrhea. Furthermore, this patient is afebrile, which is not a common presentation of viral gastroenteritis.

7. **B** (adrenocorticotropic hormone–secreting pituitary adenoma) is correct. Any condition that causes an elevation in glucocorticoid levels can produce the symptoms seen in this patient. The dexamethasone suppression test is commonly used to differentiate Cushing's disease (resulting from an ACTH-secreting tumor in the anterior pituitary) from Cushing's syndrome (caused by adrenal hypersecretion of cortisol due to hyperplasia or a tumor), and ectopic ACTH secretion from a nonendocrine neoplasm. If the symptoms are caused by an ACTH-secreting pituitary adenoma, administration of a high dose of dexamethasone will result in decreased plasma ACTH levels, decreased cortisol levels, and decreased urinary secretion of steroids, because the pituitary still retains some responsiveness to feedback inhibition by cortisol.

A (thyroid adenoma) is incorrect. A thyroid adenoma would most commonly manifest as a painless mass. Typically, adenomas are cold nodules and produce only local symptoms such as difficulty swallowing.

C (Ectopic secretion of adrenocorticotropic hormone) is incorrect. Ectopic secretion of ACTH arises most commonly from a small cell carcinoma of the lung, and it can result in Cushing-like features. However, a tumor secreting ectopic ACTH is not controlled via feedback inhibition by cortisol or dexamethasone. Therefore, a high-dose dexamethasone suppression test does not result in decreased levels of ACTH and cortisol or decreased urinary secretion of steroids.

D (adrenal tumor) is incorrect. An adrenal tumor could result in increased levels of cortisol. However, as with ectopic ACTH secretion, high-dose dexamethasone fails to suppress plasma levels of cortisol or urinary secretion of steroids.

E (congenital adrenal hyperplasia) is incorrect. Congenital adrenal hyperplasia causes symptoms much earlier in life and is not associated with hypercortisolism.

8. **B** (prolonging of phase 3) is correct. Phase 3 of the action potential in cardiac myocytes is membrane repolarization due to potassium efflux. By blocking the potassium channels, this drugs extend the duration of repolarization, thereby extending the duration of the action potential.

A (shortening of phase 0) is incorrect. Phase 0 involves fast sodium channels, not potassium channels.

C (shortening of phase 3) is incorrect. Phase 3 of the action potential in cardiac myocytes represents membrane repolarization due to potassium efflux. Blocking of the potassium channels would lengthen this repolarization phase, and thereby lengthen the action potential.

D (prolonging of phase 0). Although potassium channel blockers prolong the duration of the action potential, they do not affect phase 0, which is due to activation of fast sodium channels.

9. **D** (how rapidly the stimulus is applied) is correct. Phasic, or rapidly adapting, receptors are better suited than tonic receptors for encoding the rate of a stimulus. Phasic receptors fire action potentials at a decreasing rate during the application of a stimulus. They are useful for certain stimuli, such as the putting on and taking off of a hat, so that one is aware of it for only a brief moment.

A (strength of stimulus) is incorrect. Tonic receptors, which fire action potentials continuously during stimulus application, are more suited for encoding the strength of a stimulus.

B (duration of stimulus) is incorrect. Tonic receptors, which fire action potentials continuously during stimulus application, are more suited for encoding the duration of a stimulus. Phasic receptors fire action potentials at a decreasing rate as the stimulus

is constantly applied, thus allowing it to be removed from the realm of consciousness.

C (quality of stimulus) is incorrect. Both receptors are equally adept at providing information about the quality of a stimulus.

E (location of stimulus) is incorrect. Both receptors are equally adept at providing information about the location of a stimulus.

10. **A** (activates tyrosine-specific protein kinase autophosphorylation) is correct. This woman is exhibiting common symptoms of diabetes mellitus, most likely type 2. Symptomatic patients typically present with polyuria, polydipsia, polyphagia, and fatigue. Peripheral vascular disease is also a common problem, and patients can present with claudication and nonhealing peripheral ulcers. Diabetes mellitus type 2 pathology results from a derangement in secretion of insulin as well as insulin resistance. Insulin exerts its effects on cells by binding to the α-subunit of the insulin receptor and activating tyrosine-specific protein kinase autophosphorylation, which then increases the number of glucose transporters expressed by the cell.

B (activates adenyl cyclase) is incorrect. Epinephrine and glucagon are examples of hormones that exert their effects by activating adenyl cyclase. Adenyl cyclase converts adenosine triphosphate (ATP) to cyclic adenosine monophosphate (cAMP), which activates protein kinase A.

C (activates phospholipase C) is incorrect. Thyrotropin-releasing hormone and oxytocin are examples of hormones that activate phospholipase C, which then cleaves phosphatidylinositol bisphosphate (PIP_2) to diacylglycerol (DAG) and inositol triphosphate (IP_3). DAG activates protein kinase C, and IP_3 causes calcium to be released from intracellular stores.

D (binds to intracellular receptors which then bind regulatory elements on DNA) is incorrect. Steroids and thyroid hormones are examples of hormones that bind intracellular receptors, which then bind regulatory elements on DNA that either stimulate or inhibit the synthesis of mRNA.

E (activates guanylate cyclase) is incorrect. Atrial natriuretic peptide (ANP) activates guanylate cyclase.

11. **B** (oxytocin by the hypothalamus) is correct. Neuroendocrine secretions are secretions of peptides from specialized neurons into the blood. Examples include the secretion of oxytocin and of antidiuretic hormone (ADH) from hypothalamic neurons, the axons of which project into the posterior pituitary. Endocrine secretions are also secretions of hormones into the blood, but the secretory cells are not neurons. Paracrine secretions are secretions of substances that acts locally on adjacent cells and tissues and do not normally need to be secreted into the blood.

A (cortisol by the adrenal cortex) is incorrect. The adrenal cortex does not fit the criterion of a neuronal tissue: it is not an excitable tissue connected in a network. Secretion by the adrenal cortex is classified as endocrine only.

C (corticotropin-releasing hormone by the neurohypophysis) is incorrect. CRH is not secreted by the neurohypophysis. The secretion of CRH by the hypothalamus, is, however, an example of neuroendocrine secretion.

D (thyroid-stimulating hormone by the anterior pituitary) is incorrect. The anterior pituitary is a true endocrine gland, and secretion of TSH by thyrotrophs is not classified as a neuroendocrine secretion. (The anterior pituitary is an upgrowth of ectoderm from the oral cavity.)

E (insulin by pancreatic β-cells) is incorrect. The endocrine pancreas fulfills some of the criteria of a neuronal tissue: Its cells are electrically connected by gap junctions, it is an excitable tissue, it releases a substance in

response to depolarization, it is capable of synthesizing neurotransmitter amines, and it is connected to the extensive gastrointestinal nervous system. However, it is classified as an endocrine tissue.

12. **E** (an increase in the renal excretion of bicarbonate) is correct. The physiologic changes of the body in response to a higher altitude reflect the decreased partial pressure of oxygen (i.e., a smaller amount of oxygen being delivered to the tissues). The body uses several compensatory mechanisms to increase oxygen delivery to the tissues. The respiratory response is an increase in the ventilatory rate, which produces a respiratory alkalosis as the lungs blow off CO_2. The kidneys attempt to counter this respiratory alkalosis by increasing bicarbonate excretion. The carbonic anhydrase–inhibiting drug acetazolamide further increases renal bicarbonate excretion, creating a mild metabolic acidosis, which can be useful in treating high altitude sickness.

A (a decrease in erythropoietin) is incorrect. Tissue hypoxia, as occurs at higher altitudes, stimulates the release of renal erythropoietic factor (REF) from the kidney. REF then stimulates the formation of erythropoietin in an effort to increase the production of red blood cells. This secondary polycythemia is the body's effort to increase oxygen delivery to the tissues.

B (a decrease in 2,3-DPG) is incorrect. The level of diphosphoglycerate (DPG) increases in response to hypoxia and alkalosis. The increased DPG concentration increases the P_{50} of the hemoglobin (the pressure of oxygen at which hemoglobin is half saturated), which helps to maintain greater tissue O_2 tension than would otherwise be the case.

C (an acute decrease in ventilatory rate) is incorrect. Hypoxia stimulates an increase in acute ventilation in an effort to deliver more oxygen to the tissues.

D (a chronic decrease in ventilatory rate) is incorrect. Hypoxia stimulates an increase in the ventilatory rate. Although the increase in ventilation is more significant in the acute response to higher altitude, the late response still maintains a higher ventilatory rate than at low altitude.

13. C (gonadotropin-releasing hormone) is correct. This boy has Kallmann's syndrome, an X-linked disorder of GnRH release that manifests as a hypogonadotrophic hypogonadism. During fetal development, GnRH is present, but the large pulses that are required to stimulate puberty are absent, probably owing to failure of the neurons to properly complete their passage to the hypothalamus. Maternal GnRH is sufficient to trigger normal development of the male sex. Because the defect is an isolated deficiency of GnRH, normal puberty can be stimulated with GnRH pulses. Normally, pulsatile secretion of GnRH stimulates the release of luteinizing hormone (LH) and FSH from the anterior pituitary. Patients with Kallmann's syndrome may also benefit from exogenous testosterone.

The GnRH neurons migrate from the olfactory placodes to the hypothalamus during normal development. In Kallmann's syndrome, the abnormal development of the olfactory tract and abnormal migration of neurons in this pathway explain the loss of smell (anosmia). Another finding in Kallmann's syndrome is synkinesia, which is defined as symmetric mirror movements, probably related to developmental defects in motor nerve tracts in the brainstem.

A (human chorionic gonadotropin) is incorrect. HCG can be used to try to stimulate the descent of the testes, which are usually not descended in Kallmann's syndrome. Patients with Kallmann's syndrome may produce testosterone in response to HCG, but GnRH does not increase, meaning that fertility will be abnormal. Fertility requires both LH and FSH. Note that Kallmann's syndrome is not an example of constitutional delay of puberty, because these patients have normal height.

B (growth hormone) is incorrect. GH is not deficient in these patients. They do not have normal bone density, and testosterone increases if GnRH pulses are given, which aid in the development of bone structure.

D (clomiphene) is incorrect. Because the disorder is hypothalamic, clomiphene, which stimulates GnRH at the hypothalamus, most likely would not be effective in stimulating GnRH. Clomiphene is used primarily in women with an intact hypothalamus to stimulate GnRH and subsequently LH and ovulation (as an estrogen antagonist, it simulates estrogen deficiency).

E (follicle-stimulating hormone) is incorrect. FSH inhibits GnRH rather than stimulating its release. GnRH is deficient in Kallmann's syndrome, not FSH.

14. D (Kussmaul's respiration) is correct. The patient is a diabetic who is in diabetic ketoacidosis. Kussmaul's respiration is a pattern of rapid, deep breathing seen with severe metabolic acidosis. This type of breathing occurs as the body tries to compensate for a severe metabolic acidosis by increasing the rate at which carbon dioxide is removed from the body.

A (Cheyne-Stokes respiration) is incorrect. Cheyne-Stokes respiration is an abnormal respiratory pattern that occurs as a result of disease, congestive heart failure, and hypoxia. This type of respiration is characterized by a waxing and waning of the tidal volume followed by periods of apnea.

B (Biot's breathing) is incorrect. Biot's breathing is a type of breathing that occurs with brain damage from diseases that increase intracranial pressure. It is characterized by one or more large tidal volumes followed by periods of apnea.

C (apneustic breathing) is incorrect. Sleep apnea is a disorder of respiratory control. It can occur as a result of obstruction, in which inspiration is prevented by a temporary blockage of the airway, or by a central mechanism, in which there is an absence of rhythmic breathing in the respiratory center of the brain.

E (normal respiration) is incorrect. Normal respiratory rates range from 14 to 20 respirations per minute.

15. **C** (expanded plasma volume) is correct. Hypertension due to a known cause (e.g., primary aldosteronism) is referred to as secondary hypertension. Secondary hypertension is most commonly caused by renal artery stenosis, although primary hyperaldosteronism is becoming increasingly recognized. In renal artery stenosis, hypoperfusion of one or both kidneys results in increased secretion of renin. Elevated plasma renin activity leads to volume expansion and increased total peripheral resistance via the actions of angiotensin II and aldosterone. It is for this reason that blood pressure is elevated in this patient.

A (renal hyperperfusion) is incorrect. Renal hypoperfusion is more common in causes of secondary hypertension (e.g., coarctation of aorta, renal artery stenosis).

B (low plasma renin activity) is incorrect. Elevated plasma renin is more common in causes of secondary hypertension (e.g., coarctation of aorta, renal artery stenosis).

D (decreased total peripheral resistance) is incorrect. Elevated levels of renin and angiotensin and volume expansion result in vascular remodeling and increased peripheral arterial resistance.

16. **C** (absence of all ganglion cells in the affected segment of bowel) is correct. This infant is displaying typical symptoms of Hirschsprung's disease, which is caused by the failure of migration during development of precursor ganglion cells to the distal segment of the large bowel. Ganglion cells are missing from the muscle wall (Auerbach's plexus) as well as the submucosa (Meissner's plexus) in the affected area. Barium enema typically reveals a dilated segment of bowel proximal to the aganglionic segment and a segment of narrowed bowel distal to it.

A (absence of Auerbach's plexus only) is incorrect. In Hirschsprung's disease, there is a complete absence of ganglion cells from the both Auerbach's plexus and Meissner's plexus of the affected segment.

B (absence of Meissner's plexus only) is incorrect. In Hirschsprung's disease, there is a complete absence of ganglion cells from the both Auerbach's plexus and Meissner's plexus of the affected segment.

D (failure of involution of the vitelline duct) is incorrect. Failure of involution of the vitelline duct leads to a Meckel diverticulum. Most diverticula remain asymptomatic, although painless rectal bleeding can occur.

E (absence of pathology, because failure to pass meconium is normal for a newborn) is incorrect. Newborns pass meconium during the first 24 hours of life. Abdominal distention and bilious vomiting are not normal findings and should always lead to further evaluation.

17. **B** (transfusion) is correct. Venoconstriction increases the systemic venous pressures, which increases the pressure gradient for venous return to the right atrium, resulting in increased venous return. A transfusion that expands the plasma volume also increases the systemic venous pressure, increasing the peripheral-to-central venous pressure gradient and leading to enhanced venous return.

A (arterial vasoconstriction) is incorrect. Selective arterial vasoconstriction reduces the pressures in systemic veins, because increased resistance causes greater reduction in blood pressure across the constricted arteries, ultimately leading to a decreased peripheral-to-central venous gradient and decreased venous return.

C (hemorrhage) is incorrect. Hemorrhage reduces the plasma volume and thereby reduces systemic venous pressures, which decreases venous return.

D (diuresis) is incorrect. Diuresis causes loss of plasma volume, similar to hemorrhage, and thereby reduces systemic venous pressures and venous return.

18. **D** (ventricular arrhythmia) is correct. The concurrent use of hydrochlorothiazide and digitalis can result in significant hypokalemia, which can predispose patients to ventricular arrhythmias such as torsades de pointes. Potassium supplements should be given to prevent hypokalemia, and potassium levels should be checked frequently.

A (hyperkalemia) is incorrect. Hypokalemia, not hyperkalemia, can result from the concurrent use of digitalis and hydrochlorothiazide.

B (hypouricemia) is incorrect. Hyperuricemia is a possible adverse effect with hydrochlorothiazide. This drug leads to an increase in the serum uric acid levels and can predispose patients with a history of gout to an attack due to the accumulation of crystals in the joints.

C (hypoglycemia) is incorrect. Hyperglycemia is a possible side effect when using hydrochlorothiazide in patients with diabetes mellitus.

E (hypocalcemia) is incorrect. Thiazides can inhibit the secretion of calcium in the renal tubules, thereby possibly leading to hypercalcemia.

19. **C** (increased levels of luteinizing hormone and follicle-stimulating hormone) is correct. Menopause is associated with a diminished production of estrogen and progesterone by the ovaries and decreased responsiveness to LH and FSH. During menopause, LH and FSH levels increase because pulsatile secretion of GnRH is not lost, and the lack of negative feedback exerted by LH and FSH increases the levels of these trophic hormones. The pattern of secretion changes slightly (the level of FSH rise above that of LH), but the pulsatile nature of GnRH secretion is maintained.

A (lack of pulsatile secretion of gonadotropin-releasing hormone) is incorrect. GnRH (also called leuteinizing hormone–releasing hormone, or LHRH), is a difficult hormone to study for technical reasons related to half-life and accessibility in the portal circulation. However, the continued response of LH and FSH to GnRH suggests that GnRH pulsatility continues in the menopause.

B (complete loss of estrogen production) is incorrect. The ovaries become ineffective in producing estrogens in postmenopausal women. The adrenal glands become the source of most postmenopausal estrogen, in the form of androstenedione that is converted peripherally by aromatase to estrone.

D (monthly cycle in which a high ratio of LH to FSH is maintained) is incorrect. The ratio of LH to FSH increases periodically during each menstrual cycle. In postmenopausal women, this pattern is lost, and the secretion of FSH exceeds that of LH.

E (decline in estrogen production only) is incorrect. The synthesis of both estrogen and progesterone declines in the postmenopausal woman.

20. **B** (locus ceruleus) is correct. The locus ceruleus is responsible for most of the norepinephrine released in the brain. Located in the pons, it provides most of the noradrenergic innervation to the forebrain.

A (basal nucleus of Meynert) is incorrect. The basal nucleus of Meynert is a major collection of cholinergic neurons. Stimulation of this structure increases the amount of acetylcholine in the brain.

C (raphe nucleus) is incorrect. Stimulation of the raphe nucleus increases the amount of serotonin in the brain.

D (substantia nigra) is incorrect. The substantia nigra, which normally produces dopamine, is the target structure in this experiment, but the probe was incorrectly placed.

E (caudate nucleus) is incorrect. Stimulation of the caudate nucleus causes release of two types of neurotransmitters, γ-aminobutyric acid (GABA) and acetylcholine.

21. **D** (vitamin B_{12}) is correct. This woman most likely has a vitamin B_{12} (cobalamin) deficiency due to her inadequate diet. Vegetarians are at increased risk for this nutritional deficiency because their diet lacks a good source of this vitamin. Cobalamin is an essential cofactor for DNA replication and erythropoiesis. A deficiency of vitamin B_{12} can result in a macrocytic or megaloblastic anemia, because nuclear maturation lags behind cytoplasmic maturation as a result of impaired DNA synthesis. Neurologic symptoms such as ataxia, paresthesias, and weakness can also result. In severe cases, a deficiency of vitamin B_{12} can also result in damage to the spinal cord, referred to as subacute combined degeneration of the spinal cord.

A (vitamin B_1) is incorrect. Vitamin B_1 (thiamine) deficiency does not result in anemia. Thiamine deficiency typically occurs in underdeveloped countries or in chronic alcoholics. This deficiency can lead to polyneuropathy or Wernicke-Korsakoff syndrome.

B (intrinsic factor) is incorrect. Intrinsic factor is secreted by the parietal cells of the stomach. It is not acquired from the diet.

Intrinsic factor is necessary for the absorption of vitamin B_{12}. Pernicious anemia can lead to a deficiency in intrinsic factor.

C (iron) is incorrect. Iron deficiencies are known for their tendency to produce microcytic rather than macrocytic anemia.

E (pyridoxine) is incorrect. Pyridoxine (vitamin B_6) deficiency is rare but can occur in alcoholics and in patients treated with isoniazid for tuberculosis. Symptoms include seborrheic dermatitis, cheilosis, glossitis, peripheral neuropathy, and, in severe cases, convulsions.

22. **E** (acute cardiogenic pulmonary edema) is correct. Diuretics can resolve acute cardiogenic pulmonary edema because they modify the root problem: increased venous hydrostatic pressure, often as a consequence of reduced ventricular compliance resulting from myocardial ischemia. Diuretics in general are effective in reducing edema only if the fluid accumulation can be reversed by modifying the Starling forces. The most important Starling force modified by diuretics is the capillary hydrostatic pressure. Diuretics remove fluid from the plasma. In order for the edema to resolve, the interstitial fluid must reenter the vasculature, so that it can be removed by the kidneys. Reducing capillary hydrostatic pressure by reducing plasma volume helps return this fluid to the circulating volume and thereby decreases the pulmonary edema.

A (lymphedema) is incorrect. Lymphedema is caused by a block in lymphatic circulation. It cannot be treated by diuretics because the lymphatic fluid is not in communication with the plasma volume.

B (laryngeal edema) is incorrect. Laryngeal edema is a life-threatening swelling of the laryngeal mucosa caused by infections or by acute hypersensitivity reactions. It cannot be treated with diuretics.

C (acute respiratory distress syndrome) is incorrect. A common finding in acute respiratory distress syndrome is an increase in capillary permeability and the formation of an exudate. Because the exudate is rich in protein, the interstitial oncotic pressure rises, which traps fluid in the interstitium. Diuretics are contraindicated, because they reduce the effective circulating volume and are ineffective in removing fluid from the interstitial space.

D (myxedema) is incorrect. Myxedema is the secretion of mucus and proteins in tissues which occurs in hypothyroidism. It results in an increased interstitial oncotic pressure and cannot be cleared by diuretics.

23. B (exhibiting restrictive airway disease) is correct. This patient most likely has a restrictive airway disorder because the FEV_1/FVC ratio (2.8/3.1) is greater than 80% and the various lung volumes (TLC, RV, and FVC) are all reduced.

A (normal) is incorrect. This man most likely has a restrictive lung disease such as asbestosis. His lung volumes are all low, and his FEV_1/FVC ratio is greater than 80%.

C (exhibiting obstructive airway disease) is incorrect. If this man had an obstructive airway disease, elevated lung volumes and an FEV_1/FVC ratio of less than 80% would be expected.

D (exhibiting a combined restrictive/obstructive airway disease) is incorrect. Despite his smoking history, there is no objective evidence on pulmonary function testing for an obstructive airway disease such as chronic obstructive pulmonary disease (COPD).

24. B (Golgi tendon organs) is correct. The Golgi tendon organs are stretched whenever the muscle contracts, and they relay information as to the amount of force generated.

A (nuclear bag intrafusal fibers) is incorrect. When the nuclear bag intrafusal fibers are stretched, the Ia afferents respond by generating a burst of action potentials with a frequency that is proportional to the rate of muscle stretch. Therefore, the nuclear bag intrafusal fibers are useful in monitoring the rate of stretch of the muscle, rather than the force generated.

C (Ruffini corpuscles) is incorrect. Ruffini corpuscles respond to pressure applied to the skin.

D (Pacinian corpuscles) is incorrect. Pacinian corpuscles respond to vibratory stimuli on the skin.

E (nuclear chain intrafusal fibers) is incorrect. Nuclear chain intrafusal fibers stretch as the muscle stretches and then maintains its length. They produce a static discharge that is proportional to actual muscle length. Therefore, the nuclear chain intrafusal fibers are useful in monitoring the lengthening of the muscle, rather than the force generated.

25. C (vanillylmandelic acid) is correct. Pheochromocytoma results in increased plasma levels of the catecholamines epinephrine and norepinephrine. Urinary analysis will show elevated levels of VMA, a breakdown product of catecholamine metabolism. Urinary VMA is a specific test; measurement of metanephrine is most sensitive; and the total catecholamine fraction should be obtained also, because a number of factors interfere with these tests.

Pheochromocytomas occur as a result of abnormal proliferation of chromaffin cells associated with the sympathetic nervous system. The adrenal medulla is the most common site of these growths, probably because the adrenal medulla represents the largest collection of chromaffin cells in the body. These patients present with extreme hypertension that may respond only to powerful antihypertensive drugs such as phenoxybenzamine. Surgical resection of the affected adrenal gland is frequently performed.

A (5′-hydroxyindoleacetic acid) is incorrect. Increased levels of 5′-HIAA are associated with carcinoid syndrome, which classically manifests as vasomotor instability and excessive flushing. This woman does not have the carcinoid syndrome.

B (cortisol) is incorrect. Cortisol levels would not be significantly affected by a tumor of the adrenal medulla. Additionally, steroid hormones are typically metabolized by the liver and excreted in the bile. Because steroids are bound to plasma carrier proteins, the kidneys do not usually filter them.

D (dehydroepiandrosterone) is incorrect. Increased levels of cortisol and dehydroepiandrosterone would be expected in Cushing's syndrome, and increased levels of aldosterone in primary aldosteronism (Conn's syndrome).

26. **B** (vitamin K) is correct. This patient has clinical features suggestive of cholecystitis or inflammation of the gallbladder, which results in gallbladder dysmotility and a decrease in the secretion of bile salts from the gallbladder into the small intestine. Bile salts are needed for the absorption of lipids. Therefore, this patient most likely has decreased digestion of fats, resulting in malabsorption of fats and fat-soluble vitamins, weight loss, and steatorrhea. Of the choices available, only vitamin K is a fat-soluble vitamin.

A (vitamin C) is incorrect. Vitamin C (ascorbic acid) is a water-soluble vitamin, and its absorption is not affected by the presence or absence of bile.

C (iron) is incorrect. Iron absorption in the small intestine would not be affected. Bile

salts are not necessary for the absorption of iron.

D (vitamin B_{12}) is incorrect. Vitamin B_{12} (cobalamin) is absorbed in the ileum after being complexed with intrinsic factor. Absorption would not be severely affected by the absence of bile.

E (intrinsic factor) is incorrect. Intrinsic factor is secreted by gastric parietal cells and stabilizes the intestinal passage of vitamin B_{12}. Its absorption is not dependent on the presence of bile.

27. **C** (the ratio of forced expiratory volume to forced vital capacity is less than 0.8) is correct. Asthma is an obstructive airway disease that is characterized by an FEV_1/FVC of less than 0.8. FVC may decrease only minimally in obstructive diseases. However, the amount of air that can be expired in 1 second (i.e., FEV_1) typically decreases significantly, causing the FEV_1/FVC ratio to decline below 0.8.

A (as residual volume is approached, the upper airways collapse before the lower airways do) is incorrect. In asthmatics, it is the lower airways that collapse initially as residual volume is approached.

B (airway diameter increases during expiration due to a more negative intrapleural pressure) is incorrect. Intrapleural pressure becomes less negative (i.e., more positive) during expiration, resulting in reduced airway diameter.

D (FEV_1 is increased) is incorrect. FEV_1 refers to the maximum amount of air that can be forcefully expired in 1 second after a maximal inspiration. FEV_1 is reduced in all obstructive airway diseases.

28. **E** (displays perfusion-limited flow) is correct. Gas exchange across the pulmonary membrane normally occurs so efficiently that it is said to be perfusion-limited; that is, the amount of oxygen entering the arterial circulation is limited only by the extent of blood flow to the lungs. The lung apices are relatively overventilated compared with the lung bases, because the increased apical intrapleural pressures resulting from the weight of the lung keep the alveoli open. However, blood flow to the apex is significantly reduced in the upright position because of the hydrostatic pressures that must be generated to pump blood to the top of the lungs. Therefore, the ventilation/perfusion (V/Q) ratio is highest at the apex of the lungs, and oxygen exchange is perfusion-limited.

A (is at a more favorable position on the compliance curve) is incorrect. The alveoli at the apex of the lung are more distended and therefore are shifted to the right on the compliance curve.

B (displays zone 1 flow) is incorrect. Normally, zone 1 flow does not occur in the healthy lung because arterial pressure is usually enough to overcome alveolar pressure.

C (is better ventilated than the base) is incorrect. The apex of the lung is not as well ventilated as the base. This is due to the better position of the base on the compliance curve. The base is only poorly ventilated at volumes near the residual volume.

D (displays diffusion-limited transfer) is incorrect. Diffusion limitation primarily develops when a barrier is present or the characteristic of the substance do not favor diffusion (low solubility). The increased oxygen partial pressure in the apex of the lung actually means that the force favoring diffusion is increased at the apex of the lung. The apex is closer to perfusion-limited because the poor perfusion relative to ventilation means that increasing perfusion (which occurs in exercise) increases oxygen transfer substantially.

29. **C** (activation of the sympathoadrenal axis) is the correct choice. This patient has systolic heart failure as a result of severe aortic stenosis. The stenotic aortic valve imposed an increased workload on the left ventricle, causing the left ventricle to hypertrophy and ultimately to fail. The reduced cardiac output results in compensatory activation of the sympathoadrenal axis, which attempts to increase blood pressure through increased vascular volume, arteriolar vasoconstriction, and positive inotropic and chronotropic actions on the heart.

A (right-axis deviation on electrocardiogram) is incorrect. Left ventricular hypertrophy may cause left-axis deviation on the ECG because it requires more time for depolarization of an enlarged left ventricle.

B (peripheral edema) is incorrect. Peripheral edema occurs secondary to right heart failure. Pulmonary edema and respiratory symptoms may occur with left heart failure.

D (decreased secretion of atrial natriuretic factor) is incorrect. Activation of the sympathoadrenal axis with heart failure results in plasma volume expansion in an attempt to increase venous return to the heart to thus to increase cardiac output. The increased atrial stretch results in increased secretion of atrial natriuretic factor (ANF).

E (decreased pressure recording from a pulmonary wedge device) is incorrect. Left-sided heart failure causes congestion of blood in the pulmonary vasculature and would result in an increased pressure recording from a pulmonary wedge device.

F (increased plasma pH) is incorrect. Cardiogenic failure leads to tissue ischemia and an increased dependence on anaerobic metabolism, resulting in acidosis and a decreased plasma pH.

30. **D** (incomplete relaxation of the lower esophageal sphincter with swallowing, coupled with increased resting tone of the lower esophageal sphincter) is correct. This patient is exhibiting symptoms of achalasia. Achalasia is thought to be caused by degenerative changes in the neural innervation to the esophagus. It is characterized by aperistalsis, incomplete relaxation of the LES with swallowing, and increased resting tone of the LES. Symptoms usually arise in childhood to young adulthood. Aspiration pneumonia is a complication of the disorder.

A (complete relaxation of the lower esophageal sphincter with swallowing) is incorrect. This is what occurs in a normal esophagus. With achalasia, there is incomplete relaxation.

B (decreased resting tone of the lower esophageal sphincter) is incorrect. There is increased resting tone of the LES in achalasia.

C (increased resting tone of the upper esophageal sphincter) is incorrect. The UES is not involved in achalasia.

E (incomplete relaxation of the lower esophageal sphincter with swallowing, coupled with increased resting tone of the upper esophageal sphincter) is incorrect. In achalasia, there is incomplete relaxation of the LES with swallowing, coupled with increased resting tone of the LES, not the UES.

31. **C** (it preferentially results in the collapse of smaller alveoli) is correct. Respiratory distress syndrome (RDS) is caused by the underproduction of surfactant, which occurs more commonly in premature infants due to the immaturity of the fetal lungs. It is associated with increased alveolar surface tensions. Recall that surfactant normally decreases alveolar surface tension by minimizing the interaction between alveolar fluid and alveolar air.

According to Laplace's law, alveolar surface tension (T) generates a collapsing pressure (CP) that is inversely proportional to the alveolar radius (R), such that smaller alveoli experience a larger collapsing pressure:

$$CP = 2T/R$$

Therefore, in the absence of surfactant, collapsing pressures in the smaller alveoli are pathologically increased, causing preferential collapse of the small alveoli.

A (it is caused by overproduction of surfactant) is incorrect. Respiratory distress syndrome is caused by the underproduction of surfactant.

B (it decreases the surface tension in the alveoli) is incorrect. Respiratory distress syndrome is caused by a lack of surfactant, which causes an increase in surface tension.

D (it causes a decrease in the retractile force of the lung, resulting in a low transmural pressure) is incorrect. Lack of surfactant causes an increase in the retractile force of the lung, resulting in a high transmural pressure. The increase in surface tension decreases the interstitial pressure, which increases the forces across the pulmonary capillaries and causes pulmonary edema.

E (it occurs less frequently in premature infants) is incorrect. Respiratory distress syndrome occurs more frequently in premature infants due to the immaturity of the fetal lungs.

32. **D** (initiation of a growth spurt) is correct. In addition to its role in the development of female secondary sexual characteristics (e.g., breast maturation, female pattern of fat deposition) and the menstrual cycle in maturing females, estrogen also promotes bone growth. More long-term effects of estrogen include skeletal maturation, increased bone density, and stimulating fusion of the epiphyseal plates in adolescent females.

A (closure of the epiphyses) is incorrect. Although estrogen is responsible for the closure of the epiphyses, this is not a short-term effect of exogenous prepubertal estrogen therapy; it occurs only with chronic therapy.

B (ovulation) is incorrect. Fertility requires a periodic cycling of the gonadotropic hormones, including luteinizing hormone (LH), which usually begins after puberty. Although short-term estrogen is critical for ovulation to occur, chronic estrogen therapy suppresses fertility.

C (pronounced nocturnal spikes of follicle-stimulating hormone) is incorrect. Nocturnal spikes of FSH are not characteristic of puberty, nor are they a result of exogenous estrogens. Although FSH levels do fluctuate with levels of gonadotropin-releasing hormone (GnRH), the amplitude of the LH pulsations is much more noticeable.

E (osteoporosis) is incorrect. Estrogens have positive effects on bone mass and inhibit resorption. They do not cause osteoporosis.

33. **E** (mineralocorticoid deficiency) is correct. The primary mineralocorticoid secreted from the adrenals is aldosterone. Aldosterone functions to preserve intravascular volume, and it does this in part by stimulating reabsorption of sodium (and therefore water) by the kidneys. It also stimulates renal excretion of potassium and hydrogen ion. A deficiency in mineralocorticoids can therefore result in hypotension, hyponatremia, hyperkalemia, and a metabolic acidosis. Fluid restriction is inappropriate for these patients, and the plasma volume should be expanded with isotonic saline (not hypotonic saline).

A (nephrogenic diabetes insipidus) is incorrect. Nephrogenic diabetes insipidus would not be expected to result in an initially high urinary sodium level, nor would the urine osmolarity increase after fluid restriction, because the kidneys are not able to respond to ADH.

B (central diabetes insipidus) is incorrect. Central diabetes insipidus is excluded because the kidneys in this case had a normal

response to fluid restriction (i.e., they were able to form concentrated urine).

C (syndrome of inappropriate antidiuretic hormone secretion) is incorrect. SIADH should be treated by fluid restriction, because water is retained excessively in SIADH when ADH levels are inappropriately high. The resulting hyponatremia may or may not be corrected by fluid restriction, and diuretics may be necessary to remove water in conjunction with hypertonic saline administration, or demeclocycline may be used. In this case, the presence of hyperkalemia before treatment suggests that the disorder is not SIADH, as does the finding that the urine only becomes more concentrated after fluid restriction.

D (psychogenic polydipsia) is incorrect. Although psychogenic polydipsia should result in hyponatremia in response to fluid restriction, this hyponatremia should normalize. The fact that it does not normalize suggests some disorder of sodium reabsorption.

34. **F** (the membrane potential moves away from the potassium equilibrium potential) is correct. Hypokalemia is associated with a more excitable membrane. The basic ECG changes with hyperkalemia and hypokalemia are rational, despite the chaotic constellation of changes. Normally, the permeability of cells to potassium is 20 times that of sodium. This is why the normal membrane potential is closer to the potassium equilibrium potential (approximately −90 mV) than to that predicted for sodium (approximately +65 mV). In hyperkalemia the potassium permeability increases, whereas in hypokalemia the membrane permeability to potassium decreases. This is important, because atrial pacemakers in the resting state are less permeable to potassium (i.e., they have a higher membrane potential, farther from the potassium equilibrium potential).

Therefore, in hypokalemia, the permeability of the membrane to potassium decreases, resulting in a move of the resting membrane potential away from the potassium equilibrium potential. For this reason, the membrane becomes more excitable (despite the more negative potassium equilibrium potential). In hyperkalemia, the permeability of the membrane to potassium is increased, and the resting membrane potential moves toward that predicted by potassium. The net effect is stabilization, not excitation, and this prominently affects the atrial cells with their less negative potential.

A (hypokalemia hyperpolarizes cells) is incorrect. With hypokalemia, the ECG changes are more consistent with those of more excitable cells, which repolarize more slowly (e.g., shortened repolarization T vector, longer QT interval).

B (conduction velocity is slowed) is incorrect. Slower conduction velocity would be expected if the QRS interval widened and the PR interval was prolonged. Neither of these changes occurs in hypokalemia. Lengthening of the QT interval suggests prolonged ventricular depolarization.

C (the potassium current in phase 4 is increased) is incorrect. The disappearance of the depolarizing P wave in hyperkalemia is consistent with increased potassium efflux in phase 4 of the cardiac action potential. In hypokalemia, however, the permeability to potassium decreases. This suggests that the potassium currents that have a generally hyperpolarizing effect would be less effective. The repolarization vector (T wave) would be less strong, and the QT interval, reflecting action potential duration, would be prolonged because the phase 3 potassium efflux is less effective. This effect of hypokalemia equivalent to the effects that Vaughan Williams class III antiarrhythmics (e.g., amiodarone, bretylium) have on the action potential: potassium channel blockade prolongs QT intervals.

D (the membrane potential moves toward potassium equilibrium potential) is incorrect. In hypokalemia, the permeability to potassium decreases. This explains why the membrane becomes more excitable with hypokalemia.

E (the Nernst equation explains these changes) is incorrect. The ECG changes observed with variation in potassium levels are opposite to the rationale predicted by the Nernst equation. According to the Nernst equation, the equilibrium potential for potassium (the point at which the electrical potential matches the given separation of ionic charge due to concentration) is as follows:

$$E_{ion} = -61 \log\left(\frac{[K^+]_{in}}{[K^+]_{out}}\right)$$

where $[K^+]_{in}$ is the potassium ion concentration inside the cell and $[K^+]_{out}$ is the concentration outside the cell. In hypokalemia, the denominator ($[K^+]_{out}$) gets smaller, so the equilibrium potential becomes more negative. In contrast, the membrane potential becomes less negative in hyperkalemia. Therefore, the Nernst equation predicts a more hyperpolarized membrane with hypokalemia. In fact, the T waves shrink or disappear (shortened repolarization vector), and the QT interval gets longer (suggesting that phase 3 potassium-mediated repolarization is not as effective), changes generally consistent with more excitable cardiac membranes.

35. **D** (decrease the tidal volume to 500 mL) is correct. Minute ventilation can be calculated as the product of tidal volume and respiratory rate. On the initial ventilatory settings, the patient's minute ventilation was 11.2 L/minute (16 breaths/min × 700 mL/breath). Decreasing the tidal volume to 500 mL per breath would reduce her minute ventilation to 8 L/minute.

A (increase the respiratory rate to 18 breaths per minute) is incorrect. This modification would increase the minute ventilation to 12,600 mL/minute.

B (decrease the respiratory rate to 12 breaths per minute) is incorrect. This modification would decrease the minute ventilation to 8,400 mL/minute.

C (decrease the tidal volume to 600 mL and decrease the respiratory rate to 14 breaths per minute) is incorrect. This modification would decrease the minute ventilation to 8,400 mL/minute.

E (increase the tidal volume to 800 mL) is incorrect. This modification would increase the minute ventilation to 12,800 mL/minute.

36. **B** (the membrane potential would move towards the sodium equilibrium potential) is correct. In a resting skeletal muscle cell, because of the actions of the sodium-potassium-adenosine triphosphatase (Na^+,K^+-ATPase) pump, the cell maintains a high extracellular sodium concentration coupled to a high intracellular potassium concentration. Opening of sodium channels in a resting cell causes the influx of sodium ions and moves the membrane potential toward the sodium equilibrium potential. The influx of sodium ions also causes the cell to depolarize.

A (the membrane potential would move away from the sodium equilibrium potential) is incorrect. Opening of the sodium channels causes the membrane potential to move toward the sodium equilibrium potential.

C (the sodium equilibrium potential would remain unchanged) is incorrect. The gradient caused by the sodium-potassium-adenosine triphosphatase (Na^+,K^+-ATPase) pump results in an influx of sodium ions once the sodium channels are opened.

D (the sodium equilibrium potential would increase) is incorrect. The sodium equilibrium potential decreases once the channels are opened.

E (the cell would hyperpolarize) is incorrect. The influx of sodium ions, as occurs during conduction of an action potential, causes depolarization of the cell.

37. **D** (increased hepatic glycogenesis) is correct. Cortisol has a myriad of metabolic effects on the body, most of which are catabolic. However, its effects on the liver are generally anabolic in nature, resulting in increased production of plasma proteins, increased storage of glycogen (glycogenesis) in the liver, stimulation of glucogenesis, and potentiation of the actions of Epi and glucagon.

A (decreased lipolysis in adipose tissue) is incorrect. Cortisol stimulates lipolysis in adipose tissue, thereby increasing plasma levels of glycerol and fatty acids and providing gluconeogenic substrates to the liver. It also inhibits glucose uptake by adipose tissue.

B (increased glycolysis in skeletal muscle) is incorrect. Cortisol increases plasma glucose in a variety of ways, including inhibition of both glycolysis and glucose uptake by all tissues (including skeletal muscle) and stimulation of hepatic gluconeogenesis. It also forces tissues to combust fatty acids for energy, rather than glucose, by mobilizing fatty acids from adipose tissue.

C (decreased plasma glucose) is incorrect. Hypercortisolism leads to elevated glucose levels (e.g., adrenal diabetes).

E (decreased plasma protein levels) is incorrect. Cortisol has anabolic effects on the liver, thereby increasing hepatic production of plasma proteins.

38. **A** (hiatal hernia and Schatzki rings) is correct. A hiatal hernia is most likely when Schatzki rings are seen above the diaphragmatic opening, as in this patient. Schatzki rings are webs of the lower esophagus that are always located just above the gastroesophageal boundary; their cause is unknown. They are more common in women older than 40 years of age, and they may produce dysphagia due to narrowing of the lumen. This condition does not improve with nitrates but may improve with hot water or liquids. Pain is rare. Herniation of the stomach through the diaphragm is the most likely cause of the reflux in this patient.

B (achalasia) is incorrect. Achalasia results in inability of the lower esophageal sphincter to relax. The ring seen here is not caused by achalasia, because it is located far above the diaphragm. In achalasia the sphincter relaxes if exposed to nitrates, whereas this may not be the case with an esophageal web. Achalasia also does not usually result in heartburn.

C (Barrett's esophagus) is incorrect. Barrett's esophagus describes the histopathologic changes that occur in the esophagus in response to prolonged gastric reflux. Barrett's esophagus is characterized by a replacement of the normal esophageal squamous epithelium with a columnar epithelium.

D (epiphrenic diverticulum) is incorrect. This patient does not have diverticula in the esophagus. A diverticulum is an outpouching of the esophagus, not an inpouching as might be imagined with the shape of the Schatzki rings.

E (pyloric stenosis) is incorrect. Pyloric stenosis is a narrowing of the pylorus, which is the muscular band surrounding the junction between the duodenum and the stomach, not the esophagus and the stomach. It is associated with regurgitation and projectile vomiting (especially in male infants), not dysphagia and heartburn.

F (Crohn's disease) is incorrect. Crohn's disease is an inflammatory bowel disease characterized by granulomatous, full-thickness, ulcerative, noncontinuous lesions that rarely affect the esophagus. Because the inflammation results in thickening of the mucosa, the lumen may be narrow, and this could result in a stricture that produces dysphagia in the esophagus. The lower esophageal sphincter would still be competent, however. Additionally, this option does not explain the symptom of heartburn in this patient.

39. **B** (a pregnant patient) is correct. In a pregnant patient, high levels of hormones produced by the placenta result in suppression of LH and FSH, which are not required for estrogen and progesterone synthesis during pregnancy. Human chorionic gonadotropin (hCG) maintains the synthesis of the placental hormones during pregnancy, in cooperation with substrates derived from the fetal adrenal gland. Because of this alternative source, estriol is the major source of estrogen in pregnancy. Note that the most common cause of amenorrhea in teenage girls is pregnancy, which should always be ruled out before any provocative hormone stimulation tests are performed.

A (a patient with functional amenorrhea) is incorrect. In a patient with functional amenorrhea, ovulation and ovarian function are impaired due to disruption in the pulses of gonadotropin-releasing hormone (GnRH), which results in low levels of LH and FSH and consequent low levels of ovarian hormones as well. Other hormonal disturbances may characterize this disorder, but the elevations in progesterone and estrogens in this patient suggest that functional amenorrhea is not a likely cause.

C (a patient taking aromatase inhibitors) is incorrect. A patient taking aromatase inhibitors would have low levels of estrogen, because these drugs interfere with estrogen synthesis. LH and FSH would be elevated as a compensatory response.

D (a patient using oral contraception) is incorrect. Although oral contraceptives increase the levels of estrogen and progesterone, prolactin secretion does not increase in response to these drugs. Prolactin increases during pregnancy.

E (polycystic ovary syndrome) is incorrect. Polycystic ovary syndrome is characterized by ovarian dysfunction leading to increased levels of LH and androgens. Estrogen is secreted, but peaks do not occur; therefore, ovulation usually is impaired, and progesterone is absent. Hirsutism, cysts, insulin resistance, acanthosis nigricans, increased prolactin, growth hormone excess, and an increased risk of endometrial cancer may also characterize this syndrome.

F (a patient with hyperprolactinemia) is incorrect. If a patient had elevated prolactin as a primary event, gonadotropin-releasing hormone (GnRH) would be suppressed, leading to lack of LH and FSH secretion, with consequent amenorrhea and low levels of both estrogen and progesterone. Hyperprolactinemia is commonly caused by a pituitary tumor or by the use of dopamine antagonists. Although prolactin is elevated in pregnancy, it is antagonized by progesterone, so lactation does not occur during pregnancy. The fall in progesterone after birth removes this inhibition.

G (a patient with resistant ovary syndrome) is incorrect. Resistant ovary syndrome may be caused by autoimmune processes that shut down ovarian function, resulting in amenorrhea, usually as part of a constellation of autoimmune findings (known as type I polyglandular insufficiency) in which primary amenorrhea may occur. Because the disorder is confined to the ovary, low or absent ovarian hormones would be expected, with higher levels of LH and FSH. This is essentially premature menopause, and it can occur in teenage girls. Additional disturbances associated with this rare autosomal recessive disorder include hypoparathyroidism, diabetes mellitus, pernicious anemia, hypothyroidism, adrenal insufficiency, and chronic hepatitis.

H (a patient with primary amenorrhea) is incorrect. In endocrinology, the terms "primary" and "secondary" often are used to describe the cause of a disorder. For example, primary hyperparathyroidism describes an increase in secretion of parathyroid hormone, which is a primary event unregulated by the normal feedback control system and is usually caused by a tumor. This is not the case in the nomenclature of amenorrhea. "Primary amenorrhea" is defined as the lack of normal menarche by age 16 years, and "secondary amenorrhea" is defined as a lack of menses for longer than 6 months in a woman with previously regular cycles. The cause of either type of amenorrhea can lie in the ovary itself or in the hormonal control systems; therefore, the term "primary amenorrhea" does not indicate isolated ovarian failure independent of control systems.

40. **E** (it is increased if the initial volume is increased) is correct. The expiratory flow rate curve is the mechanical equivalent in the lung of the ventricular function curve (Starling curve) in the heart or the length-tension curve in skeletal muscle. Essentially, it states that, over the course of a forced expiration, the rate of expiratory gas flow rises and then falls. In a healthy lung, the maximal flow rate increases with effort until a certain volume is reached. After that point, the rate of flow declines linearly with lung volume, independent of effort. If the initial lung volume were increased, the highest rate of flow obtained would also increase, but the rate would then fall similarly from that point. Although the phrase "effort independent" is often used to describe this curve, it should be clear that, if the initial force of expiration is greater, the flow rate is more rapid at the beginning of expiration, when lung volume is greater. This is essentially what happens at the beginning of a cough, when the glottis is occluded and abdominal muscles are compressed. The built-up force is rapidly expelled in the cough, with the fastest expiratory flow rate coming at the beginning.

The effort-independent portion of the expiratory flow comes after the maximal flow rate is exceeded and dynamic compression begins. Effort independence means that there is a fixed relation between maximal flow and lung volume that cannot be exceeded at a given lung volume by increasing the effort. Because expiratory rates are higher for higher volumes, increasing the volume is the only way to increase the expiratory flow rate. In this sense, the lung is mechanically similar to the heart: it pumps out what is given to it. In the heart, cardiac output (liters/minute) is increased if end-diastolic volume is increased. However, in the heart, the cardiac output for a given preload is not fixed, because physiologic adaptations can shift the Starling curve by increasing contractility. In the lung, the position of the expiratory flow rate curve cannot be physiologically altered. Exercise does not shift the curve itself; it only alters the highest expiratory flow rate by increasing the inhaled volume. However, pharmacologic intervention can alter the expiratory flow curve; for example, in asthmatics, the use of bronchodilators improves expiratory flow for any given volume and shifts the curve to the right.

A simple, handheld, noncostly plastic device is often used to record the expiratory flow rate, in place of measurement of the ratio of forced 1-second expiratory volume to forced vital capacity (FEV_1/FVC). Although it cannot distinguish obstructive from restrictive disorders, this device is helpful for triage of patients into "normal" and "abnormal" groups.

A (it is limited by the rigidity of the thoracic cage) is incorrect. The thoracic cage helps to keep the lungs inflated, so it might be thought that the lungs would deflate faster were the ribs not in place. However, the thorax and the cartilage in the airways actually help the forced expiratory flow by preventing airway collapse as air is forced out by the increase in intrapleural pressure resulting from abdominal contraction.

B (it is a consequence of the length-tension relation for skeletal muscle) is incorrect. The length-tension relationship for skeletal muscle states that the maximal force developed in a skeletal muscle contraction depends on the initial length of the muscle before contraction. Less than maximal force is developed if muscles are initially too short or too long. Expiration is normally a passive process, but in forced expiration the abdominal and internal intercostal muscles are used. The greater the inhalation, the greater the distention of the abdomen, and the more the initial position of the abdominals is altered. Up to a point, this expansion increases the maximal force developed in these muscles, yet even expirations from a small starting lung volume are well within the range of maximal force development for abdominal muscle. Therefore, the expiratory flow rate cannot be explained by the initial length of the abdominal muscles.

C (it is increased at an optimal intermediate starting lung volume) is incorrect. This curve is obtained for a single forced expiration and shows the absolute expired volume. It does not relate starting volume to maximum flow rate. Although the shape of the curve looks similar to the length-tension relationship in muscle, the curve is not equivalent.

D (it is less than in restrictive disorders) is incorrect. The maximal expiratory flow rate in restrictive disorders is limited because the expired volume is usually small. Even though any given restrictive flow rate is greater when normalized for the small lung volume (due to increased recoil), the maximal flow rate is less in absolute terms.

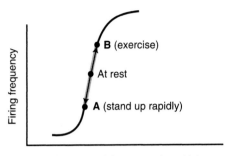

Mean arterial pressure (mm Hg)

41. **B** (increased total peripheral resistance) is correct. The main outcome of the baroreceptor reflex is an increase in the total peripheral resistance, which is mediated by sympathetic innervation. The fall in blood pressure is detected by the carotid sinus baroreceptor (the aortic arch is insensitive to a fall in pressure) as a reduction in stretch, which reduces its membrane potential. The tonic inhibitory rate of firing of the baroreceptor is thus reduced, which leads to disinhibition of the sympathetic vasoconstrictor center in the medulla, as well as inhibition of the vagal response. The net effect is vasoconstriction, venoconstriction, increased cardiac contractility, increased atrioventricular (AV) node conduction velocity, increased sinoatrial (SA) node firing rate, and, ultimately, increased heart rate, pulse pressure, and stroke volume, with maintained cardiac output. Once blood pressure rises, the response is turned off rapidly by the baroreceptors (see the accompanying figure). To turn the response off, both the carotid sinus and the aortic arch detect increased stretch; the rate of firing increases, and this sends inhibitory signals to the sympathetic output and stimulatory signals to the vagal center. The vagal response is quicker than the adrenergic response, and the vagal response also interferes with sympathetic release in the heart; in this way, the cutoff in the feedback loop occurs faster than the positive stimulus (which prevents a runaway effect).

A (increased cardiac output) is incorrect. The cardiac output is the product of heart rate and stroke volume. When the patient is tilted, preload decreases due to venous pooling. In response, either the stroke volume must increase, through an increase in contractility and venous return, or the heart rate must increase. Both events do happen, but the result is maintenance of the cardiac output rather than an increase, because the response is turned off by the baroreceptors.

C (increased preload) is incorrect. The preload is immediately reduced by the tilt table test, due to a reduction in end-diastolic volume caused by reduced venous return.

D (increased rate of firing of aortic arch baroreceptors) is incorrect. The aortic arch baroreceptors are less sensitive to a reduction in pressure than the carotid sinus baroreceptors. Also, the rate of firing would be expected to decrease in response to a decrease in pressure.

E (increased membrane potential of carotid sinus baroreceptors) is incorrect. The membrane potential of the carotid sinus baroreceptors decreases in response to decreased stretch, leading to a decreased rate of firing of action potentials.

F (increased rate of firing of carotid sinus baroreceptors) is incorrect. The rate of firing of baroreceptors is normally tonically inhibitory to the pressor center, so a decrease in pressure results in a decrease in firing. This explains why hypertension can result from denervation of the carotid sinus or periods of syncope from hypersensitivity.

G (increased left-axis deviation) is incorrect. The axis of the heart can shift when a patient moves from the supine position to the standing position. However, this move causes deviation of the mean electrical axis to the right.

42. **B** (nicotinic blockade) is correct. Nicotinic blockade results in blockade of the sympathetic and parasympathetic ganglia, all of which utilize acetylcholine as their neurotransmitter. This can result in hypotension and impotence due to the failure of vasodilation to occur and the loss of driving pressure to maintain the erection. It also results in loss of sympathetically mediated ejaculation.

> **A** (phosphodiesterase inhibitors) is incorrect. The effect of phosphodiesterase inhibitors such as sildenafil is to increase cyclic guanosine monophosphate (cGMP), which stimulates vasodilation and erection.
>
> **C** (sympathetic excitation of the bladder) is incorrect. In contrast to the process of ejaculation, voiding of the bladder is under parasympathetic control. Sympathetic discharge to the bladder simply contracts the bladder neck and prevents sperm from entering the bladder during ejaculation (retrograde ejaculation).
>
> **D** (guanyl cyclase inhibitors) is incorrect. Activation of guanyl cyclase leads to vasodilation, which aids erection.
>
> **E** (α-adrenergic antagonists) is incorrect. α-Adrenergic antagonists are sometimes used to aid erection because they cause vasodilation.

43. **C** (slight urine production [oliguria]) is correct). Congestive heart failure (CHF) is characterized by hypotension and inadequate perfusion of the tissues (i.e., cardiac insufficiency), resulting in a reduced glomerular filtration rate (GFR) and slight urine production. Compensatory responses to maintain an adequate perfusion pressure include activation of the renin-angiotensin-aldosterone system, with a resultant increase in sodium retention and plasma volume (this explains the edema seen in patients with CHF). Increased plasma volume places a further demand on the heart, which increases the rate at which it fails, further stimulating the renin-angiotensin system. Thus, a vicious cycle is propagated. Treatment of CHF includes administration of diuretics (e.g., furosemide), which can dramatically increase the production of urine, thereby reducing extracellular fluid volume and reducing the workload of the failing heart. Cardiac glycosides such as digoxin can also be given to patients with CHF. Cardiac glycosides have a positive inotropic effect on the heart, and at the same time they increase the amount of time spent in diastole, which allows for more optimal perfusion of the ischemic heart.

> **A** (extremely elevated urine production) is incorrect. Cardiac insufficiency leads to reduced renal perfusion and a decreased glomerular filtration rate, resulting in oliguria.
>
> **B** (suppression of the renin-angiotensin system) is incorrect. Compensatory responses to maintain an adequate perfusion pressure in congestive heart failure (CHF) include activation of the renin-angiotensin-aldosterone system, with a resultant increase in sodium retention and plasma volume (this explains the edema seen in patients with CHF). Increased plasma volume places a further demand on the heart, which increases the rate at which it fails, further stimulating the renin-angiotensin system. Thus, a vicious cycle is propagated.
>
> **D** (decreased extracellular fluid volume) is incorrect. In congestive heart failure, compensatory endocrine responses result in volume expansion.
>
> **E** (Decreased plasma levels of atrial natriuretic peptide) is incorrect. In congestive heart failure, volume expansion results in increased secretion of atrial natriuretic peptide (factor) from the right atrium, as a response to increased venous return.

44. **E** (elevated levels of urobilinogens in the urine and feces) is correct. Remember that the breakdown of red blood cells leads to an increase in the amount of unconjugated bilirubin in the bloodstream. The liver processes the unconjugated bilirubin to produce conjugated bilirubin, which is soluble and secreted in bile. Gut bacteria then deconjugate most of the conjugated bilirubin and degrade it into colorless urobilinogens, which are secreted in the feces. Therefore, hemolytic anemia leads to an increase of bilirubin in the bloodstream and, ultimately, to increased levels of urobilinogens in the feces. (Urobilinogens are also elevated in the urine, because some are absorbed from the colon via the enterohepatic circulation).

A (urine with a positive reaction for conjugated bilirubin) is incorrect. Conjugated bilirubin in the urine would occur with an obstructive jaundice in which there is an increase of conjugated bilirubin in the bloodstream. The excess conjugated bilirubin can be excreted in the urine because it is water soluble.

B (presence of occult blood in the feces) is incorrect. Occult blood in the feces could occur as a result of loss of blood somewhere along the gastrointestinal tract, but this is not typically seen in nonobstructive jaundice.

C (pale stools negative for bilirubin and urobilinogens) is incorrect. Absence of bilirubin and urobilinogen in the stool implies the presence of an obstruction.

D (urine with a positive reaction for indirect bilirubin) is incorrect. Indirect (unconjugated) bilirubin is insoluble and cannot be excreted in the urine.

45. **D** (endocytosis of aquaporin water channels) is correct. Ultimately, the effects of exogenous ADH (Desmopressin) are mediated by endocytosis of the aquaporin water channels. This is caused by the reduced level of cAMP, which declines as soon as ADH is no longer stimulating the V2 receptors in the basolateral membrane (i.e., when ADH is cleared from the circulation by hepatic and renal metabolism and excretion). If a patient with central diabetes insipidus is receiving intravenous fluids and Desmopressin simultaneously (e.g., after cranial surgery), the result could be acute hyponatremia; therefore, close monitoring is required. This is usually a concern only in hospital settings where intravenous hydration is possible. In the outpatient setting, Desmopressin is most commonly used to manage nocturia. In this case, the evening dose should be titrated by determining the time course of resumption of polyuria the next day. If the evening dose is too high, the polyuria will resume too late the next day, and if the dose is too low, the nocturia will resume in the night or early the next day.

A (increase in plasma volume) is incorrect. High-volume states send a tonic inhibitory signal to the paraventricular nuclei by way of the baroreceptors, inhibiting ADH release. This effect is secondary to that of osmolarity. However, in central diabetes insipidus, this central control mechanism is lost, as is secretion of ADH.

B (decrease in plasma osmolarity) is incorrect. The effect of a decrease in plasma osmolarity is mediated by the hypothalamic osmoreceptors, which terminate ADH release. In a normal individual, this is the most important factor controlling ADH release; however, if central diabetes insipidus is present, both this control mechanism and ADH release are extinguished.

C (increase in levels of cyclic adenosine monophosphate in collecting duct cells) is incorrect. The effect of ADH at the V2 receptor is mediated by an increase in cAMP in response to activation of adenyl cyclase. An increased insertion of aquaporin channels occurs with the increase in cAMP, and a reduction in cAMP is required for cellular termination of the ADH effect.

E (receptor-mediated endocytosis of ADH from the luminal surface) is incorrect. ADH acts at the basolateral surface of the collecting duct, not the luminal surface. Receptor-mediated endocytosis is probably not an important means of removing ADH from the circulation, although one hypothesis maintains that ADH is internalized in clathrin-coated pits on the basolateral surface, and that the presence of ADH in these vesicles inhibits the breakdown of apically recycled aquaporin 2 and promotes recycling to the membrane, thereby prolonging the effect of aquaporins.

46. **A** (potassium iodide) is correct. Supraphysiologic levels of iodide make the thyroid gland substantially less vascular before surgery, which reduces bleeding risks. The transient decline in thyroid hormone levels that occurs with the administration of iodide is known as the Wolff-Chaikoff effect; it is caused by inhibition of iodide binding to thyroglobulin. The high levels of exogenous iodide inhibit iodide transport into the thyroid, resulting in depletion of iodide within the gland. The fever associated with hyperthyroidism can mask fever as a sign of life-threatening agranulocytosis. Agranulocytosis is a decline in the count of neutrophils (among other blood cells) that can occur as an idiosyncratic reaction to the drug PTU.

B (allopurinol) is incorrect. Allopurinol is used to treat gout.

C (thyroxine) is incorrect. Thyroxine (T_4) is usually indicated after surgery, because hypothyroidism is a common outcome of radioactive ablation and surgical excision of the thyroid, particularly after a total thyroidectomy. It takes about four half-lives for a drug to be eliminated, and T_4 has a prolonged half-life of about 8 days, so thyroid

hormone replacement typically is not started until 1 month after surgery.

D (corticosteroids) is incorrect. The use of corticosteroids before surgery would impair wound healing after surgery and would not affect the vascularity of the gland. Although corticosteroids inhibit the conversion of thyroxine (T_4) to triiodothyronine (T_3), they are typically used only in the treatment of thyroid storm.

E (radioactive iodine) is incorrect. Radioablation is another option for managing hyperthyroidism, but it is not used as preoperative preparation. Furthermore, radioactive iodine competes with iodide for uptake in the gland, so a patient being given iodide before surgery cannot be immediately switched to radioablation therapy. (This competition is also the reason that iodine tablets are advised in the event of a nuclear disaster.)

47. **C** (increased preload) is correct. ANF is secreted primarily in response to atrial stretch. Congestive heart failure is a syndrome in which the heart is unable to supply an output that sufficiently meets the metabolic demands of the body. The decreased cardiac output results in a number of compensatory adaptive mechanisms, including stimulation of the renin-angiotensin-aldosterone system and release of antidiuretic hormone (ADH, vasopressin) in order to increase circulatory volume and thereby maintain perfusion. Normally, increased preload stretches atrial myocytes and stimulates increased secretion of ANF; the resulting increased renal loss of sodium and water reduces plasma volume and, consequently, venous return and preload. However, in advanced heart failure this adaptive mechanism is unable to eliminate enough excess fluid; as heart failure worsens, increased vascular congestion and increased preload lead to pulmonary edema and peripheral edema.

A (improving cardiovascular function) is incorrect. It is actually deterioration of cardiovascular function that leads to the greater preload and subsequent increased secretion of ANF. This occurs because reduced cardiac output causes fluid retention by the kidneys, and the increased fluid retention increases preload.

B (decreased preload) is incorrect. Decreasing preload reduces atrial stretch and would be expected to reduce secretion of ANF.

D (increased natriuresis) is incorrect. Although increased secretion of ANF causes increased natriuresis, the opposite is not the case.

D (mean arterial pressure) is incorrect. The mean arterial pressure is an average of the systolic and diastolic pressures and is the diastolic plus one-third the systolic pressure. Because the aortic valve opens once the aortic pressure is exceeded, this occurs at about the diastolic pressure. Therefore, the period of isovolumic contraction occurs at a lower pressure than the mean arterial pressure.

E (systolic pressure) is incorrect. The systolic pressure is the maximum pressure obtained during systole. It occurs midway through the ejection phase. The ejection phase is nonisotonic and nonisometric; the pressure-volume profile changes due to the dynamic interaction between ventricular muscle and the aorta.

48. **C** (aortic pressure) is correct. In a typical heart, the left ventricle must work against an afterload of approximately 80 mm Hg in the aorta. Once this pressure is exceeded, blood begins to move and contraction is no longer isovolumic (isometric). At this point, enough pressure has been generated to open the aortic valve, and the ejection phase of the cardiac cycle begins. In the ejection phase, the potential energy generated during isometric contraction is used to eject blood. Although this is typically referred to as the isotonic phase, it is not completely isotonic. This is because the pressure in the ventricles rises nonlinearly and reaches a maximum approximately two-thirds of the way through ejection, after which the resistance of the arterial walls in the aorta comes into play.

A (wedge pressure) is incorrect. The wedge pressure is a good estimate of the left atrial pressure (i.e., left ventricular filling pressure). It is obtained by inserting a catheter into the pulmonary artery. Closure of the mitral valve occurs when the ventricular pressure exceeds wedge pressure.

B (positive end-expiratory pressure) is incorrect. The positive end-expiratory pressure occurs only when a patient is artificially ventilated.

49. **D** (myophosphorylase deficiency) is correct. This is an inherited metabolic disease, also known as McArdle's disease or glycogen storage disease V. Myophosphorylase is the enzyme that liberates glucose from glycogen. Muscle is an important storage site for glycogen, and the enzyme serves to provide fuel for glycolysis. In myophosphorylase deficiency, fast-twitch muscle (type II) fibers, which depend on anaerobic metabolism for energy, cannot produce enough glucose once extracellular glucose stores are depleted. The result is cramping. This causes necrotic destruction of muscle, leading to rhabdomyolysis and myoglobinuria as well as hyperkalemia. A high-carbohydrate diet may be helpful in preventing the symptoms.

In contrast, the slow-twitch muscle (type I) fibers, which can use both fats and carbohydrates for energy, function normally. This property of the type I slow fibers is responsible for the "second wind," which develops as muscles switch back to their resting fatty acid substrate after plasma glucose is depleted.

The ischemic forearm occlusion test is helpful in distinguishing myophosphorylase deficiency from other disorders. The rise in lactate that would be predicted in normal ischemic anaerobic muscle does not occur, indicating that the disorder is either glycogen storage disease V or a defect in glycolysis (e.g., phosphofructokinase [PFK] deficiency). The clinical history is helpful in distinguishing these conditions, as is the absence of hemolytic anemia in glycogen storage disease V.

A (hyperkalemic periodic paralysis) is incorrect. Hyperkalemic periodic paralysis is an autosomal dominant disorder that results in high levels of potassium, which depolarizes cells, causing contraction of muscle that can result in cramping. The key distinguishing feature is that the contractions are interspersed with periods of paralysis in which the muscle is refractory. The ischemic forearm test would reveal normal increases in lactate.

B (type A lactic acidosis) is incorrect. Type A lactic acidosis is caused by hypoxia, whereas other types are metabolic in nature. Hypoxia is unlikely in this case, because lactate accumulation is not present. (The "second wind" effect is not attributable to an increase in tissue oxygenation, but rather to the switch in metabolic substrates from glucose to fatty acids.)

C (Cushing's syndrome) is incorrect. Cushing's syndrome is caused by an excess of cortisol. Cortisol stimulates breakdown of type I aerobic oxidative red muscle fibers, the opposite pattern to that seen here. A patient with Cushing's syndrome would have a normal lactate response to exercise.

E (carnitine palmitoyltransferase II deficiency) is incorrect. Carnitine palmitoyltransferase II is an enzyme required for fatty acids to enter the inner mitochondrial matrix. A deficiency results in an inability of muscle to oxidize fatty acids. The clinical picture also includes muscle damage and myoglobinuria. Because fatty acid oxidation is impaired, the disorder either results in cramping after the activity (when muscles switch substrates from glucose to fatty acids) or manifests as an increase in

muscle stiffness or tenderness in resting muscle. Because glycolysis is normal, the ischemic forearm test results in increased lactate levels.

F (paroxysmal nocturnal hemoglobinuria) is incorrect. Paroxysmal nocturnal hemoglobinuria is an acquired disorder of bone marrow that results in hemolytic anemia. It is diagnosed by a positive Ham's test. A positive result is hemolysis of 10% to 80% of red blood cells in an acid (pH 6.5) medium.

G (phosphofructokinase deficiency) is incorrect. Phosphofructokinase is the rate-limiting enzyme in glycolysis. Deficiency results in severe cramping (more severe than in McArdle's disease), because the actual process of glycolysis is impaired rather than just the supply of substrates. Because erythrocytes depend on glycolysis, this disorder is characterized by a hemolytic anemia. The disorder is aggravated by high-carbohydrate diets, and the initial presentation is often in early childhood. Because glycolysis does not occur, lactate levels do not rise in the forearm test.

H (oxygen debt) is incorrect. The oxygen debt hypothesis states that the lactate built up during anaerobic exercise results in an oxygen debt, which must be repaid by oxidative reconversion of the lactate to glycogen. This is because lactate does not accumulate normally, so any oxygen consumption during the recovery period cannot be attributed to lactate reconversion.

50. **B** (hypokalemia) is correct. The gain-of-function mutation responsible for Liddle's syndrome causes excess reabsorption of sodium ions in the distal nephron. Because potassium ions are exchanged for sodium ions, increased reabsorption of sodium ions results in increased secretion of potassium and hydrogen ions, resulting in hypokalemic metabolic alkalosis. Because reabsorption of sodium ions at the nephron is the main determinant of extracellular fluid volume, overactivity of the amiloride-sensitive transepithelial sodium channel results in hypertension. Increased blood pressure inhibits activity of the sympathoadrenal axis, and increased delivery of sodium to the macula densa inhibits secretion of renin. Therefore, patients with Liddle's syndrome present with low-renin hypertension and hypokalemic metabolic alkalosis.

A (elevated plasma renin) is incorrect. Patients with Liddle's syndrome typically present with low-renin hypertension and hypokalemic

metabolic alkalosis. Hypernatremia caused by increased renal reabsorption of sodium inhibits secretion of renin by the juxtaglomerular apparatus.

C (increased sympathetic stimulation of the juxtaglomerular apparatus) is incorrect. Compensatory responses to hypertension include decreased sympathetic outflow.

D (decreased plasma cortisol) is incorrect. Plasma cortisol levels are elevated in Liddle's syndrome.

E (metabolic acidosis) is incorrect. Hypokalemic metabolic alkalosis occurs in Liddle's syndrome.

Index

Note: Page numbers followed by f indicate figures; those followed by t indicate tables.